Physiology and Behaviour
of Animal Suffering

The Universities Federation for Animal Welfare

UFAW, founded 1926, is an internationally recognised, independent, scientific and educational animal welfare charity concerned with promoting high standards of welfare for farm, companion, laboratory and captive wild animals, and for those animals with which we interact in the wild. It works to improve animals' lives by:

- Promoting and supporting developments in the science and technology that underpin advances in animal welfare;

- Promoting education in animal care and welfare;

- Providing information, organising meetings, and publishing books, videos, articles, technical reports and the journal *Animal Welfare*;

- Providing expert advice to government departments and other bodies and helping to draft and amend laws and guidelines;

- Enlisting the energies of animal keepers, scientists, veterinarians, lawyers and others who care about animals.

"Improvements in the care of animals are not now likely to come of their own accord, merely by wishing them: there must be research ... and it is in sponsoring research of this kind, and making its results widely known, that UFAW performs one of its most valuable services."

Sir Peter Medawar CBE FRS, 8th May 1957
Nobel Laureate (1960), Chairman of the UFAW Scientific Advisory Committee (1951–1962)

For further information about UFAW and about how you can help to promote and support its work, please contact us at the address below.

Universities Federation for Animal Welfare
The Old School, Brewhouse Hill, Wheathampstead, Herts AL4 8AN, UK
Tel: 01582 831818 Fax: 01582 831414 Website: www.ufaw.org.uk

Physiology and Behaviour of Animal Suffering

Neville G. Gregory
Royal Veterinary College
and
Biotechnology and Biological Sciences Research Council

Blackwell
Science

© 2004 Universities Federation for Animal Welfare (UFAW)

Series editors:
James K. Kirkwood, Robert C. Hubrecht and Elizabeth A. Roberts

Blackwell Science, a Blackwell Publishing company
Editorial offices:
Blackwell Science Ltd, 9600 Garsington Road, Oxford OX4 2DQ, UK
 Tel: +44 (0) 1865 776868
Blackwell Publishing Professional, 2121 State Avenue, Ames, Iowa 50014-8300, USA
 Tel: +1 515 292 0140
Blackwell Science Asia Pty Ltd, 550 Swanston Street, Carlton, Victoria 3053, Australia
 Tel: +61 (0)3 8359 1011

First published 2004

ISBN 978-0-632-06468-7

A catalogue record for this title is available from the British Library

Gregory, Neville G.
 Physiology and behaviour of animal suffering / Neville G. Gregory.
  p. cm. – (UFAW animal welfare series)
 Includes bibliographical references and index.
 ISBN 978-0-632-06468-7
 1. Pain in animals. 2. Pain–Physiological aspects. 3. Perception in animals. 4. Animal behavior. 5. Veterinary physiology. I. Title. II. Series.

SF910.P34G74 2004
636.089′60472–dc22

2004006542

For further information on Blackwell Publishing, visit our website:
www.blackwellpublishing.com

Contents

Colour plate sections falls after page 148

Foreword

The human population of the world exceeds six billion and is still growing rapidly. We live in a closed system with finite resources. Whether we like it or not, our interests are frequently in conflict with those of other species. We use animals for food, for companionship, and in research, and we compete with many free-living animals for habitat and food. Side-effects of many of our activities present threats not just to individual animals but to species viability. We cannot avoid having to manage this situation and, frequently and unavoidably, this involves having to weigh the interests of individuals of one species against the interests of individuals of another.

During the last century (and coincident with the period over which much of the human population growth has occurred), remarkable advances in comparative neuroanatomy, physiology and behavioural sciences have provided strong evidence that the capacity for subjective experience of unpleasant (and pleasant) feelings is not limited to humans only. In contrast to the view, commonly-held among influential thinkers prior to this scientific enlightenment, it is now generally accepted that subjective experience, and thus the capacity to suffer, are widespread in the animal kingdom (at least in the vertebrate branch). This knowledge has brought with it a particular responsibility, when pursuing human interests or environmental management for the preservation of biodiversity, to avoid or minimise the risks of causing harm to individuals of other species.

Growing awareness of this responsibility has led, around the world, to a striking proliferation of codes and legislation aimed at protecting and improving animal welfare. In practice, pursuit of these aims depends frequently upon making valid assessments of welfare status. Concern for an animal's welfare is concern about its subjective quality of life – on how it feels. This cannot be measured but can only be inferred from observations of its physical state and behaviour in the light of our own experiences of what it is like to have feelings and of what these are like under various circumstances. Subjectivity cannot be avoided in this process – in the step from what is observed to what is inferred. But, the greater our knowledge of the neurological and other machinery that generates feeling, and of how and when it operates, the safer and surer our inferences are likely to be.

This is a very valuable and timely book in this context. It provides a wide-ranging and informative overview of the physiological and behavioural responses to many diseases, injuries and other stresses, and of the mechanisms that underlie the associated subjective experiences. Improvements in animal welfare do not come about merely by wishing them (to quote Sir Peter Medawar), but depend upon a proper understanding of the causes of suffering and of the ways in which these can be prevented or alleviated. In this book, Neville Gregory makes a major contribution to promoting understanding of animal suffering and thus, both to tackling many forms of it and also to properly taking suffering into account in cost/benefit judgments when pursuit of human or environmental interests put other animals at risk.

James K Kirkwood
June 2004

Preface

Suffering is a state of mind that is difficult to grasp from a conceptual and scientific standpoint. It is not a single entity and it cannot be directly assessed or measured. Instead it is a collective term that indicates unpleasant states of mind.

Suffering can be inferred from observation, enquiry and reasoned analysis. That analysis uses conventional reductionist appraisal of a particular situation. From a knowledge of the accepted causes of suffering, and the responses that usually accompany suffering, we can judge whether or not suffering is likely to be present for that situation.

This book brings together some of the knowledge that should help people arrive at informed judgements using the approach indicated above. It describes the effects and responses during various deprivations and insults in animals, along with the perceptions that occur in some comparable situations in humans. The scientific knowledge is, however, incomplete, and so our judgements will be limited by some uncertainties.

We are not always in a good position to appreciate what goes on in an animal's mind, and so our judgements on suffering will also lack rigorous proof. Dismissing the presence or existence of suffering on the grounds of absence of proof is sometimes used as an obtuse way of dismissing a concern about suffering. However, absence of proof is not proof of absence. Instead, logical constructs that argue for the presence of suffering in a particular situation, call for equally logical constructs if those concerns are to be dismissed or discounted.

This book does not provide the reader with moral judgements or views. The aim is to help the reader in his or her thinking, rather than telling him or her what to think. It intentionally avoids giving opinions about the acceptability of causes of animal suffering. Instead it provides a technical base that can be incorporated into ethical thinking.

Nevertheless, some of the descriptions of the work on injuries and insults that went towards compiling this book were harrowing to read, and in the author's view it would be unacceptable ever to repeat some of those experiments. A few of those descriptions have been included along with the pathophysiology because they are helpful to understanding suffering, and should help in treating similar cases that may occur in practice in the future.

The ideas on how this book should be written were developed from discussions with Professor David Mellor of Massey University, and I am grateful to David for his constructive thoughts.

N.G. Gregory

Introduction

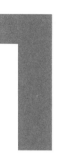

1.1 What Is Suffering?

Suffering is an unpleasant state of mind that disrupts the quality of life. It is the mental state associated with unpleasant experiences such as pain, malaise, distress, injury and emotional numbness (e.g. extreme boredom). It can develop from a wide range of causes. For example, it occurs when there is misery during exposure to cold, with the sense of fatigue and depression during cancer and when there is unremitting pain from chronic headache. Some of the general mental states that contribute to suffering in humans are given in Table 1.1.

1.2 Why Worry about Animal Suffering?

The main reason for being concerned about human and animal suffering is a sense of respect and fairness towards others. Many people feel that needless suffering is unfair, and should be controlled or avoided. Society should not be responsible for needlessly ruining other peoples' or animals' lives. This is a moral outlook, and it inevitably varies between individuals. Some people care. Others do not.

1.3 When Can We Stop Worrying about Animal Suffering?

One of the dilemmas of worrying about suffering is in knowing when to stop being concerned. Do you stop worrying at a human, a mouse or an earthworm? Buddhists strive to minimise all death and suffering, and in some sects it is inappropriate to kill even an earthworm, because it might be a reincarnation of a human. Others take the view that there is no need to be concerned about suffering

Table 1.1 Examples of emotional and mental states that can lead to suffering when they become severe or protracted.

Negative emotional and mental states		
fear	anxiety	sadness
irritation	phobia	bitterness
starvation	boredom	anguish
sickness	depression	mental illness
frustration	pain	paranoia
fatigue	distress	despair
thirst	nausea	torment
	loneliness	longing

in 'lower' life forms because they do not have the capacity to suffer (Rose, 2002). Where can we draw the line and say that suffering no longer exists?

The forms of suffering listed in the third column in Table 1.1 have a higher degree of complexity than those on the left. Intuitively, one might expect the features on the right to be unique to humans or a limited number of mammals, whilst those on the left occur in a larger number of species. This seemingly obvious statement introduces the first dilemma: when trying to decide whether a particular species has the **capacity to suffer**, one has to make clear which form of suffering is being considered.

One approach which might pre-empt that complication, and help simplify decision making, is to consider which species seem to be able to think for themselves. Ability to learn might be considered a sign that a species has some **cognitive capacity**, and cognition is presumably a prerequisite for suffering. Scientifically, a more convenient starting point would be to assume the inverse. Let us take the position that animals that show limited **ability to learn** probably have limited cognitive capacity. We may be concerned with conserving them as individuals and as a species, but we are let off the hook from worrying about whether they can suffer.

Agar (1925) approached this question by testing whether water fleas (*Daphnia carinata*), water mites (Hydrachnidae) and freshwater crayfish (*Parachaeraps bicarinatus*) could learn to avoid an aversive stimulus (Figures 1.1 & 1.2). Each type of animal was placed in the centre leg of a Y-maze and subjected to an unpleasant stimulus, which was either CO_2 in the water or decreasing water depth, to encourage them to swim into one of the side limbs. In one of the side limbs they always experienced an electric shock and in the other there was no shock. By repeating this test many times, their ability to learn, remember and execute a correct decision was evaluated. The *Daphnia* and Hydrachnids failed to learn and adapt, even though they showed a violent reaction to the electric shock. The young crayfish, on the other hand, quickly mastered the situation and avoided the wrong limb. It was more proficient at learning and remembering.

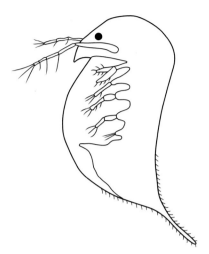

Figure 1.1 Water flea *(Daphnia)*.

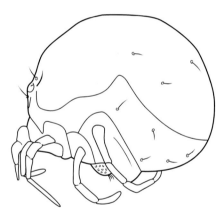

Figure 1.2 *Hydrachna* sp. (Hydrachnidae).

Crayfish also seem to be clever at learning whether a threatening stimulus is a real threat. When a wild-caught crayfish is first handled it is defensive and, if it has cognitive capacity, the impression is that it is apprehensive. It raises its claws in a defensive manner when approached. It wheels round to keep facing the approaching hand and, when seized, it fights to escape. We could interpret this as apprehension and fear. After some days, these fear reactions completely disappear. The animal ceases to threaten the approaching hand with its claws, and remains quiet when picked up. One interpretation is that it learns that the experience was not so bad, or, maybe it adopts a form of learned helplessness. Alternatively, was it a form of subconscious adaptation?

Another tantalising but perplexing finding is the impact of stress on the single-cell organism *Euglena*. They show a more rapid flight response away from a bright light if they have previously been exposed to a pressure shock wave (Murray, 1971). The pressure-shocked *Euglena* were sensitised to the next unpleasant stimulus, which happened to be the light. If this sensitisation to stress was subconscious, then can stress-induced sensitisation be subconscious in other members of the animal kingdom? If so, what are those behavioural situations?

The conclusion from many other studies on protozoa and on coelenterates is that it is not clear whether or not members of these phyla can learn (Jensen, 1964). They can show learning-like behaviour, but the problem is in distinguishing between learning, acclimatisation, habituation, facilitation and adaptive responses. The importance of these distinctions becomes clearer by considering the following example of an acquired response in the sensitive plant (*Mimosa pudica*), which has no cognitive capacity.

Each leaf of this plant is divided into 10 to 20 leaflets, which fold together in pairs when the plant is touched or mechanically shaken. The folding reaction following shaking is immediate. The plant also folds its leaflets at night, but this is a much slower response. A key feature is that the rapid folding response can be conditioned, using darkness as a conditioned stimulus before shaking which is the unconditioned stimulus. The plant folded its leaflets more rapidly to darkness once it had been trained to 'expect' a vigorous shaking as soon as the lights went out. This finding gives the impression that this plant can anticipate a good shaking, but because this occurred in a plant we cannot conclude that it was a cognitive 'anticipatory response'. Instead, it must have been a functional adjustment (Armus, 1970). The same applies to many studies which have examined simple life forms in the animal kingdom. For the purposes of understanding the ability to suffer, we need to distinguish between true cognitive learning and non-cognitive adaptation.

Some simple animals show very interesting learning or adaptive capacities. The earthworm *Lumbricus terrestris*, for example, can learn to distinguish between the limbs of a T-maze to gain access to moist earth or moss, rather than a sandpaper floor and an electric shock. Earthworms were slower at acquiring this skill in the morning compared with the evening (Arbit, 1957). An even more 'primitive' life-form, the planarian worm *Cura foremanii*, 'learnt' to move faster to intercept a photodiode beam in order to extinguish a bright light for 15 minutes (Best, 1964). This was an operant conditioning response, which in other species would usually be assumed to be a form of intelligence. But was it a subconscious response?

There is no doubt that habituation and some forms of learning in animals can be subconscious. Locusts, grasshoppers and wetas can be trained to switch off a noise source set at an irritating vibration frequency. Perhaps this was subconscious learning, as decapitated locusts and grasshoppers also learnt to turn off the sound. Decapitated wetas were not so adept, but this was because head removal was too traumatic for this particular insect.

Subconscious learning also seems to exist in the mammalian foetus. The level of oxygenation *in utero* is thought to be insufficient to support conscious activity in the foetal lamb brain (Mellor & Gregory, 2003). However, a number of studies have shown that the foetus is capable of learning. For example, in experiments by Hepper (1991), the rat foetus was found to be capable of associative learning, and recall of that learning persisted into infancy. Other studies have shown that aversive conditioning can be induced in the rat foetus.

Both conscious and subconscious learning have a molecular basis. In the case of long-term potentiation (LTP), which is a form of associative learning, there are chemical changes which involve activation of N-methyl-D-aspartate (NMDA) receptors (Skuse, 2000). These receptors control calcium entry into neurones, which in turn sets off a chemical cascade that ends with the phosphorylation of a protein called cyclic AMP-responsive element-binding protein (CREB). CREB is a transcription factor which regulates genes that enable the maintenance of LTP at the cellular level. In mice, CREB is involved in fear conditioning, spatial learning and social learning. It also serves a function in invertebrates. For example, it is important in forming long-term memory in the fruit fly (*Drosophila melanogaster*) and soil nematode *Caenorhabditis elegans* (Figure 1.3). It is quite plausible that proteins such as CREB form a common link between conscious and subconscious memory processes.

None of these findings tells us when to stop worrying, but they do tease our curiosity and they help us form impressions. Let's take a different approach. Can we stop worrying about suffering in a species if it is unable to experience **pain?** This begs the question, which life-forms can experience and suffer pain? An animal can feel pain at a conscious level if it meets the following criteria:

- it possesses receptors sensitive to noxious stimuli;
- its brain has structures analogous to the human cerebral cortex;
- nervous pathways link the receptors to the higher brain;
- painkillers modify the response to noxious stimuli;
- the animal responds to noxious stimuli by consistently avoiding them;
- the animal can learn to associate neutral events with noxious stimuli;
- it chooses a pain killer when given access to one, when pain is otherwise unavoidable.

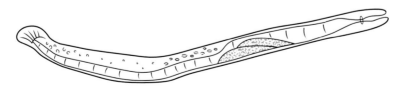

Figure 1.3 Soil nematode *(Caenorhabditis elegans)*.

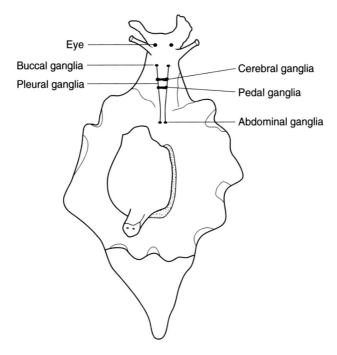

Figure 1.4 Sea hare *(Aplysia californica)*.

There are few species which have been evaluated for all these criteria, and so, for the time being, we have to accept an incomplete picture and form impressions instead of making conclusions.

One school of thought considers that some invertebrates are able to experience pain. This is supported by particularly convincing work done by Kavaliers *et al.* (1983) in the land snail. When placed on a hot plate at 40°C, the snail lifted the anterior portion of its foot. Morphine increased the time taken to respond, whereas naloxone reduced it, and abolished the effect of morphine. In other species, the mollusc *Aplysia californica* withdraws its tail when the skin is pinched (Figure 1.4). This animal can express sensitisation which is equivalent to hyperalgesia, and it is being used as a model for neuropathic pain (Woolf & Walters, 1991). The nematode *Caenorhabditis elegans* has a primitive nervous system with only 302 neurones, one of which is the so-called ASH neurone which is functionally analogous to vertebrate mechano-nociceptive neurones that mediate pain (Kaplan & Horvitz, 1993). This species is used in experimental models of hyperalgesia (Wittenburg & Baumeister, 1999). Lastly, the leech *Hirudo medicinalis* has polymodal neurones which respond to temperatures over 38°C, and to noxious chemicals such as acetic acid and capsaicin (Figure 1.5). Together, these findings help to focus our question, but more studies along the lines of Kavaliers *et al.* (1983) are needed in other

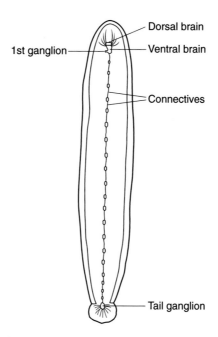

Figure 1.5 Leech *(Hirudo medicinalis)*.

invertebrates before we know where in the evolutionary tree the capacity for pain emerged.

People will inevitably vary in their judgement as to when suffering should be managed. In addition, decisions will depend on the feasibility of treating or preventing the suffering, the alternatives that may be available and whether they also present hazards of suffering, the cost of controlling the suffering and whether the individual actually cares. Not everyone wants to get involved with situations where there is animal suffering. However, society in general can have responsibilities to guard against suffering, even though it may be a select group of people who are the guardians. That responsibility applies particularly to animals that depend on or are strongly influenced by human activities.

1.4 Recognising Suffering in Animals

Many scientific disciplines use experimental **animals as models** for human disease or dysfunction. This book takes the opposite approach. It takes the human as a model for animals in understanding pain, unpleasant sensations and suffering. This is a logical approach because experience in humans is the only context in which we learn what pain and suffering are like. The weaknesses in doing this are much the same as using animals as models for the human. We do not always know how relevant the model is to the target species. This does not mean that the model can be dismissed because of uncertainty. Instead, it means that the human model should be used wisely, in a considered way, and its main value is in highlighting potential forms of suffering.

Recognising suffering is of obvious importance if we really care about animal suffering. How do we recognise when an animal has a specific type of suffering, such as a headache? Presumably it would look ill or depressed, but we have no way of knowing whether this is due to a general sense of sickness, a headache or simply a bad mood. One approach to understanding the signs associated with specific forms of suffering is to see what they are like when induced pharmacologically. This has been done in studying the signs associated with **nausea**.

Apomorphine causes nausea and vomiting in humans, and it is an emetic in a wide range of species. Normally, birds do not vomit. They can regurgitate crop contents when feeding young, but it would be unusual for a bird to bring up the contents of its proventriculus. In the pigeon, instead of inducing emesis, apomorphine causes the bird to peck rapidly at the floor and other objects, without eating anything. This behaviour comes on very rapidly and is so compulsive that in some cases the beak has been injured. After this pecking phase the bird is subdued and seemingly depressed. It is thought that the pecking phase is analogous to the chewing phase that is seen in other species before they vomit.

Learning from practical experience is another way of recognising the signs of sickness and understanding what the animal might be feeling. Veterinary practitioners are in a particularly strong position to do this because their job brings them into contact with animal suffering every day. The detailed descriptions they provide can be very helpful. Take the following account of the signs associated with **sinusitis** that occurred when dirty dehorning equipment had been used in a herd of cattle:

- the animals rested their muzzles on a stationary object, such as a water trough;
- they head pressed or extended their head and neck with their nose held parallel to the ground and their eyes partially or fully closed;
- palpation over the sinus elicited signs of pain in some animals.

Anecdotes such as this form the basis for diagnosis and understanding the behaviours associated with particular types of suffering.

1.5 Can Animals Go Mad?

In the past, psychological research into **neuroses** using animals was scorned by psychiatrists because it was assumed that insanity only occurs in humans. It was thought that animals cannot go mad, even though the signs of rabies in dogs were fully appreciated. In 1921, a significant experiment was conducted on a dog, which helped to change that outlook (Abramson & Seligman, 1977). This dog was a good-natured animal and easy to handle. It was trained to be led to a room where it received its food. In that room a circle of light was shone onto a screen in front of the dog, and this was followed by food. Once the dog had developed a salivation response when the light was turned on, the shape of the projected light was altered the following day. If the light was elliptical instead of a circle, there was no food, but when it was a circle, the dog was always given its food. The dog learnt over a period of days to anticipate food on this basis. However, its discrimination broke down as the ellipse got closer in shape to a circle. At a 9:8 ratio of the axes, the dog became confused, and there was a dramatic change in its behaviour. The once-quiet dog became highly aroused. It began to squeal and tried to destroy the experimental equipment. It refused to enter the feeding room, and barked violently when feeding time approached. This dog did not go mad, but it developed neurotic responses out of frustration. Since that experiment there have been many other experimental and clinical reports on neurotic behaviour in domesticated animals, and the general view is that some animals can and do become neurotic, which in extreme cases is the equivalent of madness.

Some animals seem to be able to **hallucinate**. This has been observed in cats, and the behaviours were similar to those seen in other cats given the psychogenic drug LSD, and included:

- staring;
- limb flicking;
- abortive grooming;
- looking around the floor, ceiling or walls, tracking invisible objects with their eyes and sometimes hissing, batting or pouncing at them.

1.6 What Constitutes Animal Suffering?

One of the shortcomings in using the human as a model for studying animal suffering is that humans do not share all the same senses as animals. These deficiencies limit the inferences we can make from self-experimentation and observation. We do not have:

- an electrosensory lateral line;
- a vomeronasal organ;
- ability to detect infrared radiation;
- magnetoreceptors;
- specific pheromones.

In addition, the frequency range of our hearing is limited in comparison with insects and some other animals. Our proficiency at chemoreception is inferior to that of many aquatic animals. We do not know what life is like for cavefish (*Astyanax hubbsi*) or mole rats (*Spalex ehrenbergi*) which are naturally blind, or for whales which have limited ability to smell, taste, feel with their skin and see. Other senses are more important to these animals, and the implications are difficult to appreciate fully.

One of the most exciting advances in neuroscience is **neuroimaging**. This technique is allowing us to recognise which cortical regions of the human brain are activated when we have particular feelings. We are now beginning to understand where in the cortex the different forms of suffering are integrated. For example, we now recognise that thirst perception involves the posterior cingulate cortex, and that several forms of pain are registered in the anterior cingulate cortex and insula. When the cortical sites associated with suffering have been fully mapped, we may be in a position to identify the corresponding cortical and telencephalon sites in animals. This in turn could lead to the experimental diagnosis of suffering based on the activation or inhibition of particular brain regions.

1.7 Conclusions

The main points made in this chapter are as follows:

- Deciding when to care about suffering has moral as well as practical considerations. Morals may be influenced by personal outlook, but society in general has a responsibility to care about animal suffering.
- The forms of suffering that can be experienced by 'lower' life forms are narrower than those experienced by 'higher' life forms, and so it is helpful to specify the form of suffering when discussing capacity for suffering.
- Cognition is a prerequisite for mental suffering. In some cases, inability to learn can be an indication of limited cognitive capacity. However, learning can be a subconscious activity and so, in 'lower' life forms, an ability to learn does not necessarily demonstrate cognitive capacity or capacity to suffer.
- Pain is an important perception that can lead to suffering. Scientifically, there are seven criteria that have to be met before there is adequate proof that a species can experience pain. On its own, one of the most convincing criteria is the self-selection of a pain killer during chronic or otherwise unavoidable pain. Few species have been tested in this paradigm.
- Experience in the human provides a useful model for recognising insults and situations where suffering could occur in 'higher' animals.
- Some pharmaceuticals can provoke specific types of discomfort or distress. In the future they may be helpful in allowing us to recognise the behavioural signs associated with specific types of suffering in 'higher' animals.
- 'Higher' animals can display neurotic behaviour patterns which are analogous to some forms of mental disorder in humans.

- Some species have sensory modalities which humans do not possess. This makes it difficult for us to appreciate the importance of loss of those sensory modalities in terms of potential suffering.
- In the future, we may get greater insight into different species' repertoire for suffering through comparative neuroimaging of cortical homologues in the brain.

Stress

2

Stress is a physiological disturbance that is imposed by a stressor, such as a threatening or harmful situation. It is associated with suffering when there is mental distress. It occurs following physical trauma, during disease and in emotional conflicts. When the stress is severe, homeostatic processes are put under abnormal pressure, behaviour becomes disorganised and there can be pathological effects. Stress is usually classified according to the stressor, which can be either the stimulus that provokes the stress response or the context in which the stress occurs. The physiological responses are not necessarily the same for all stressors, but some common features are highlighted in this chapter.

2.1 Stress Physiology

The **physiological stress pathways** in the brain are channelled along two main routes:

(1) corticotrophin releasing hormone activation of the hypothalamic–pituitary–adrenal (HPA) axis;
(2) activation of the sympathetic nervous system (SNS).

Corticotrophin releasing hormone (CRH) is synthesised at a number of sites in the brain including the hypothalamus, amygdala, *stria terminalis*, prefrontal cortex and cells surrounding the *locus coeruleus* (LC) (Figures 2.1 & 2.2). CRH from the hypothalamus stimulates the secretion of adrenocorticotrophic hormone (ACTH) from the anterior pituitary, which in turn stimulates the secretion of glucocorticoids from the adrenal cortex.

When CRH is administered centrally into the brain of a laboratory animal, it has anxiogenic effects and can enhance behavioural signs of **fear**, panic or depression. These and the other main roles of CRH are listed below. Some of these effects are mediated by the amygdala, and the prefrontal and cingulate cortical areas in

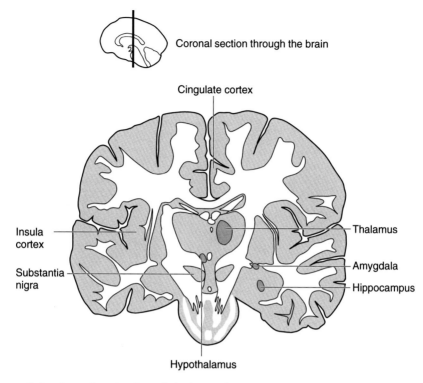

Coronal section through the brain

Cingulate cortex

Insula cortex

Thalamus

Substantia nigra

Amygdala

Hippocampus

Hypothalamus

Figure 2.1 Coronal section through the human brain.

the brain (Steckler & Holsboer, 1999), and in humans, an overactive CRH pathway has been implicated in stress-related anxiety, depression disorders, and anhedonia. Central administration of ACTH can also produce some anxiety-like behaviours in rats. These include excessive grooming, increased submissive behaviour, and protracted avoidance responses (see below).

Stress effects that are produced by central administration of CRH in the rat are:
- increase in heart rate and blood pressure;
- defecation;
- suppression of exploratory behaviour;
- induction of grooming behaviour;
- increased activity;
- reduced feeding;
- disruption of reproductive behaviour;
- exaggerated acoustic startle response;

continued

- enhanced fright-induced freezing and fighting behaviour;
- enhanced fear conditioning.

The functions of CRH are:
- activation of the HPA axis through the release of ACTH from the pituitary;
- stimulation of the release of β-endorphin from the pituitary;
- enhancing central activation of the autonomic nervous system;
- stimulation of noradrenaline release centrally;
- activation of the gastrointestinal system;
- mediation of aversive behavioural responses;
- production of anxiogenic-like effects.

One of the main **roles of the HPA** axis is in combating disease. Cytokines produced in response to disease organisms stimulate ACTH release from the pituitary, partly through activating CRH release. ACTH passes to the adrenal cortex by the bloodstream where it stimulates the release of glucocorticoids. The glucocorticoids check the development of inflammation, preventing it from getting out of control, and promote the supply of substrates required during repair and recovery. They

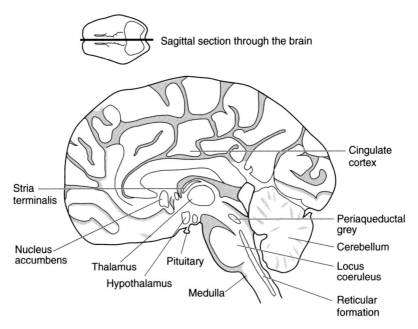

Figure 2.2 Sagittal section through the human brain.

- promote skeletal muscle and liver proteolysis and gluconeogenesis;
- exert anti-inflammatory effects and suppress immune responses;
- reduce pain through their anti-inflammatory effects.

The HPA axis is also activated by trauma, psychological stress and pain. Measuring hormones associated with the HPA axis has been useful in comparing the impact on an animal of different husbandry stressors. These measurements have been used in evaluating the stress of:

- antler removal;
- branding;
- castration;
- confinement;
- disbudding;
- force-feeding;
- laparotomy;
- restraint;
- shearing;
- social dominance;
- social isolation;
- tail docking.

This has been helpful in determining the least stressful ways of performing some of these procedures.

In general terms, psychological stressors which activate the HPA axis include:

- learned helplessness, in which animals anticipate an inescapable unpleasant experience;
- fear;
- anticipation of food;
- starvation.

In situations where there is chronic psychological stress, there is a risk of down-regulation within the HPA axis. In people this has been known to occur in cases of repeated assault and can result in post-traumatic stress disorder. Interpretation of HPA hormonal measurements becomes more complex in these situations.

Corticosteroids can pass through the blood–brain barrier, and if the brain is exposed to excessive amounts of these hormones the viability of neurones declines. Neurones in the CA1 region of the hippocampus are often affected, and as this region is involved with learning and memory, these faculties deteriorate. In addition, chronic exposure to high levels of corticosteroids in young animals results in an overall reduction in numbers of brain cells in the cerebrum and cerebellum, through the suppression of nerve growth factor.

Activity of the **autonomic nervous system** is controlled through interconnecting nuclei in the brain, which are collectively known as the central autonomic network. This network supplies signals to both vagal and sympathetic neurones which mediate autonomic functions. The main regions in the forebrain that contribute to the central autonomic network are the:

- hypothalamus (paraventricular hypothalamic nucleus, lateral hypothalamus, posterior periventricular area, zona incerta);
- basal forebrain (central nucleus of the amygdala, bed nucleus of the stria terminalis);
- cerebral cortex (insula and medial frontal cortices).

The paraventricular nucleus of the hypothalamus is involved in regulation of the cardiovascular system and adrenal nerve activity. Activation of this nucleus leads to an increase in blood pressure. The lateral hypothalamus is involved in feeding, insulin release, reductions in blood pressure, heart rate and coronary blood flow. The zona incerta subserves thirst, plus some aspects of arousal and locomotion. The central amygdala is involved in fear and affective stress-related states. The insula receives substantial inputs from the viscera, and it projects to many of the subcortical autonomic regions. Stimulation of this cortical region produces a rise in blood pressure, and parts of this region are involved in pain recognition. The medial prefrontal cortex is involved in limbic functions. The effects of many of these forebrain structures is facilitated and modulated through the *locus coeruleus* (LC).

The *locus coeruleus* synthesises and stores noradrenaline. When the animal is resting, asleep or absorbed in self-focussed behaviour, the LC is almost inactive. When the LC is activated in non-stressful situations, it helps the animal maintain vigilance. Typically, the animal's attention is directed at a particular stimulus, or it might start scanning the environment (Valentino *et al.*, 1998). These are characteristic fear-related responses. When stress fully activates the LC through exposure with CRH, there are more dramatic responses, including anxiety behaviours, conditioned fears, despair responses, defensive withdrawal, potentiation of the acoustic startle response, defecation and suppression of immune function independently of HPA activation. Some of these behaviours involve pathways in the amygdala, and chronic stressors have been shown to increase CRH synthesis in the amygdala. Neurones in the LC project to the dorsal horn of the spinal cord where they have an inhibitory effect on afferent pain pathways and a facilitatory effect on motor neurones. This form of spinal analgesia is mediated at the spinal level by α_2 adrenergic receptors. When noradrenaline stores in the LC are exhausted through over-activation, stress-induced depression sets in.

In general terms, the **sympathetic nervous system** (SNS) prepares the individual metabolically for the muscular effort involved in defence or flight. Responses to sympathetic nervous stimulation include:

- mobilisation of glycogen from the liver;
- mobilisation of free fatty acids from adipose tissue;
- dilation of the pupils;
- increased heart rate and contractility;
- vasoconstriction in body regions not directly involved in fight or flight mechanisms;
- reduced upper intestinal secretions and motility.

The sympathetic nervous pathways and hormones from the adrenal medulla serve similar functions, but they tend to act reciprocally. For example, when sympathetic nervous activity is suppressed during fasting, adrenomedullary responses take over. In addition, during some stress responses, activity in the sympathetic nervous pathways is biphasic, there being an initial suppression followed by activation. Adrenomedullary secretion occurs during the initial phase. The complementary patterns of the two systems can also be seen in the division of functions between the two systems. For example, cold stress activates the sympathetic nervous system, whereas stress associated with competitive mental concentration is more adrenomedullary.

The CRH–HPA axis and the LC–SNS pathway do not operate independently of each other. Activation of one system tends to activate the other as well. In fact, CRH activates the LC besides stimulating ACTH release.

During recovery from stress, the balance between parasympathetic and sympathetic nervous function shifts towards the **parasympathetic nervous system**. With the resumption of parasympathetic activity, gut and other visceral functions return to normal. The parasympathetic nervous system aids digestion by stimulating saliva secretion in the mouth, acid, pepsinogen, mucus and gastrin secretion in the stomach and lipase, trypsinogen, chymotrypsin, enterokinase, cholecystokinin and vasoactive intestinal peptide secretion in the small intestine. It also enhances gut motility and coordinates these movements with sphincter action. In these ways, the parasympathetic nervous system promotes functions associated with growth and restoration of tissue reserves and function. The sympathetic nervous system has the opposite effects.

2.2 Stress-related Disorders

Excessive stress can have pathophysiological effects. In the cardiovascular system these include:

- tachycardia and arryhthmias;
- hypertension;
- increased tendency for blood clot formation;
- vasodepressive syncope;

- cardiac ischaemia through coronary vasoconstriction;
- arteriosclerosis.

These effects can cause three life-threatening conditions:

(1) a rise in heart rate which is followed by rebound suppression that is well below the normal resting rate;
(2) arrhythmias;
(3) myocardial necrosis.

Myocardial necrosis from insufficient perfusion of the heart is the more common life-threatening effect. It has been observed in a wide range of species and situations, including wild arctic ground squirrels that were held in captivity for two weeks and in wild rats that were made to listen to a tape recording of a cat–rat fight. Occasionally, farm animals die from cardiac arrest when they are restrained and myocardial ischaemia plus dysrhythmias have been implicated. There are laboratory animal models for susceptibility to myocardial necrosis. A strain of rat has been bred that is prone to developing myocardial lesions when injected with the β-adrenergic agonist isoprenaline (Starec *et al.*, 1994). This strain is also leaner, less aggressive and more anxious when subjected to an open field test in comparison with an isoprenaline-resistant strain. It is more likely to freeze when threatened. Paradoxically, it is less susceptible to stress-induced gastric ulcers, and it shows less severe arthritis in response to a standardised infectious challenge.

Hypertensive disease is unusual in free-living animals, but hypertensive episodes are common during stress. There are laboratory animal models for spontaneous hereditary **hypertension**. Cardiac irregularities are also common stress responses in people and animals who are not affected by cardiac disease. For example, arrhythmias and suppression of the S-T segment of the electrocardiograph (ECG) have been noted during public speaking, driving and during tests or audits in normal people with no heart problems. Nevertheless, it has been difficult to use some of the subtle changes in the electrocardiogram as stress indicators in animals (Gregory & Wotton, 1981).

Heart rate and blood pressure are more commonly used as stress indicators. They are not unequivocal indicators of stress and suffering, and they have to be used selectively in respect to the stressful context. A remarkable study which implied that heart rate can be 'willed' to rise or fall to obtain a reward was performed by Miller and Di Cara (1967). Part of this effect was mediated through control of vagus nerve activity, and changes in heart rate in this instance were not stress-related.

Psychological stress can impair **reproduction**. In males it can inhibit spermatozoa production through glucocorticoid-induced suppression of testicular sensitivity to luteinizing hormone (LH). A cockerel that is dominated by another cock may become impotent in this way, and the testes atrophy resulting in psychological castration. In females, stress can cause reduced LH and follicle stimulating hormone (FSH) secretion and inhibition of ovarian responsiveness to LH. This is the mechanism that probably operates in baboons (*Papio cynocephalus anubis*), where the dominant female physically harasses subordinates into anovulation. In other situations, acute stress can cause anoestrous animals to ovulate. This has been observed for example in ewes experiencing transport stress on their way to slaughter (Lang, 1964). It was also the basis for using the central nervous system (CNS) stimulant yohimbine to bring anoestrous cows into oestrus.

Fear-induced stress can inhibit **milk let down**. For example, fear inhibits the release of oxytocin, which would normally induce contraction of the myoepithelial cells surrounding the acini in the mammary gland, from the posterior pituitary.

Exposure to high levels of glucocorticoids early in life can lead to behavioural abnormalities later in life. For example, rats show retarded maturation of swimming behaviour, and this may be due to deficits in cerebellar neurone development. In addition, animals subjected to corticosterone treatment early in life are more reactive emotionally when they mature. They seem to be less adept at responding to changes in their lifestyle or daily routines. One sign of this in laboratory rats is increased water intake which is thought to indicate anxiety. They also show less exploratory behaviour and more frequent defecation (Kalin, 1989).

Stress responsiveness may have an **hereditary** component. When rainbow trout (*Oncorhynchus mykiss*) were subjected to confinement stress, some developed a high plasma cortisol response whilst others were low responders. The heritability of the size of the cortisol response was 0.4–0.6. The high responders were more likely to show flight behaviour instead of freezing when confronted by an unfamiliar smaller intruder, and the low responders showed less stress-induced suppression of appetite (Øverli *et al.*, 2002).

2.3 Restraint Stress

Restraint is probably the single most common stressor that is applied directly by humans to animals. It is particularly stressful for animals that are unfamiliar with the handler or the handling method, but training from an early age helps to reduce the effects of restraint stress (Levine, 1957).

Restraining methods which can be stressful include:

- yoking;
- roping;
- hobbling;
- confinement in a chair (laboratory primates), tube (rodents) or slings (dogs);
- securing with a head or neck halter;
- holding upside down by the legs;

- restraint during religious and conventional slaughter;
- leghold trapping;
- snares;
- rodent glue boards;
- birdlime traps used for birds and rodents;
- muzzling;
- electroimmobilisation.

Severe restraint provokes large increases in plasma adrenaline and noradrenaline, and this can bring on a heart attack (Chiueh & Kopin, 1978). In particular, the heart becomes more sensitive to stimuli that can provoke ventricular fibrillation (Lown *et al.*, 1973). Restraint by muscle paralysis using succinylcholine in stress-sensitive pigs has been sufficiently stressful to kill them from catecholamine-induced myocardial ischaemia, and this response has been prevented by prior amygdalectomy (Johansson *et al.*, 1981). This type of pig has an unduly responsive sympathetic nervous system, as well as skeletal muscle that is prone to excessive production of lactate and heat when the animal is stressed (Gregory & Lister, 1981). It has been known for a stress-sensitive pig to die suddenly when a pig in a neighbouring pen was restrained in order to give it an injection.

Stress can lead to an increase in body temperature, especially when there is greater physical activity. One exception occurs in the rabbit, which can develop hypothermia when restrained. This is known as **emotional hypothermia** and is due to increased heat dissipation (Grant, 1950). It is not necessarily accompanied by shivering and so it is not always easy to recognise.

Pigs and birds are sometimes **restrained upside down**, but they should not be held in this position for long periods. This position causes a fluid shift to the head, increased central venous pressure, and alterations in renal function including increased diuresis and natriuresis (Bouzeghrane *et al.*, 1996). If held in the head-down position for long periods, plasma renin is increased, aldosterone is reduced and hypovolaemia is likely to develop. Part of this effect may be due to decreased physical activity (hypokinesia).

Electroimmobilisation is sometimes used for restraining cattle, and a shearing system has been developed which uses electroimmobilisation in sheep. The advantage of this shearing system is that it is easier for the shearer. Research has shown that electroimmobilisation is stressful for sheep. For example, it is more aversive than physical restraint (Rushen, 1987). In these and all other studies carried out to date, the electroimmobilisation current was continuous. This prevented the animal from breathing properly. A new electroimmobilisation-shearing system uses an interrupted current that allows the animal to breathe, but it is not known whether it is more or less stressful than conventional shearing systems.

Restraint can be difficult under free-range conditions where there are no handling yards or equipment. For example, providing assistance to a beef cow with dystocia is sometimes impossible, and instead the attitude is that evolutionary pressure should be allowed to take its course, and animals prone to dystocia be left to survive or die by their own means.

2.4 Stress-induced Analgesia

Stress can inhibit the transmission of pain signals in the spinal cord and brain. This serves as a useful protective mechanism against becoming overwhelmed by pain during a dangerous situation.

The following stressors have been shown to provoke stress-induced analgesia (SIA):

- uncontrollable footshock;
- anticipation of footshock;
- centrifugal rotation;
- inescapable swimming in cold water;
- heat pain;
- injection of intraperitoneal saline;
- restraint;
- social isolation;
- body pinching;
- brief exposure to the scent of a predator.

These stressors do not need to be severe in order to provoke SIA. Not all of them are opioid mediated, but those that are usually involve the dorsolateral funiculus of the spinal cord.

2.5 Stress-induced Seizures and Fits

In some situations, mental distress can precipitate a seizure or fit. Physical seizures are not a direct cause of suffering, as in most types of seizure the subject is unconscious. However, the physical activity of the fit, coupled with absence of breathing can leave the subject feeling exhausted when consciousness returns, and there is a risk of inflicting self-damage during the convulsions. Stress-induced seizures are not common. One example is the case of a servant who witnessed his officer being killed during World War I. This provoked a fit in the servant, and he had recurrent fits thereafter. In sheep, lambs can develop seizures when docked and castrated, but here again this is not a common reaction. Dogs have been known to develop hysterical epilepsy following the death of an owner, and fear-provoked group seizures have been reported in a pack of dogs.

Anxiety and Fear

3

3.1 Introduction

This chapter discusses fear and its associated disorders.

In humans fear and anxiety can be associated with terror, irritability, a desire to hide, run away or cry, and, in some cases, a sense of faintness or falling. There is often a sense of unreality as well as desperation, and a tendency towards aggression or lashing out. Prolonged fear and anxiety result in depression, tiredness without being able to sleep, restlessness, anorexia and avoidance of novel or tension-producing situations.

In animals, the situations that can produce fear and distress include:

- capture, especially in an unfamiliar environment;
- exposure to unfamiliar noises, objects and odours;
- sudden movement which appears threatening;
- separation from familiar companions;
- exposure to strangers in the home environment;
- aggressive or threatening encounters;
- alarm vocalisations or displays;
- exposure to predators or predator-related cues;
- exposure to a situation that was previously unpleasant.

In extreme cases, fear can lead to abnormal behaviours, of which there are two main types. The animal may show restlessness and **hyperexcitability** or it may start with timidity that develops into **depression**. In humans, the categories used to describe **fear-** or **anxiety-related disorders** are quite complicated, and the different types of disorder are partly distinguished by behavioural signs and by the drugs which correct them. Different drugs are effective in reversing different anxiety-based symptoms. For example, panic disorders and obsessive compulsive disorders

(OCDs) usually respond to tricyclic antidepressants or selective serotonin re-uptake inhibitors, whereas generalised anxiety disorders often respond to the anxiolytic benzodiazepines. Phobias are usually best treated with monoamine oxidase inhibitors, or selective serotonin re-uptake inhibitors, and subjects with post-traumatic stress disorders can experience some relief with monoamine oxidase inhibitors or tricyclic antidepressants. Anxiety, fears, phobias and OCDs are neurochemically related, and can be treated with selective serotonin re-uptake inhibitors. Although **pharmacodiagnosis** of these states is not an exact science, it is useful as a practical tool and it is finding clinical application in treating behavioural problems in dogs.

In the past, a common alternative to managing anxiety-related disorders in companion animals has been to destroy the animal. Even now, about 80% of the urban dogs that are surrendered to pounds and animal shelters are submitted because of a behaviour problem (Seksel & Lindeman, 2001). Anxiety-related disorders are probably the single most common category in those dogs, and they take one or more of the following forms:

- generalised anxiety;
- separation anxiety;
- fears;
- obsessive compulsive disorders;
- phobias;
- aggression.

3.2 Anxiety

In humans, anxiety is a distress or uneasiness of mind caused by dread or uncertainty. It is less focussed than a fear, which is usually caused by an identifiable worry. Anxiety-like behaviour is fear-like behaviour, but it may occur in the absence of external triggers. It can develop into behavioural regression.

Separation anxiety is the earliest form of anxiety experienced by humans. In infants the feelings range from a heightened sense of awareness to a deep fear of impending disaster. In young animals it is usually accompanied by increased responsiveness, vocalisation, restlessness, and autonomic stress responses.

In older dogs, the main signs of separation anxiety are excessive vocalisation, inappropriate elimination, salivation, escaping and destructive behaviour. The dog becomes distressed when the owner prepares to leave, and on the owner's return there is excessive enthusiasm. The dog may even hold onto the owner with its mouth to prevent departure. Other signs of this type of anxiety can include pacing, panting, anorexia and depression. Destructive behaviour is often directed towards entry and exit points, such as doors or windows, and objects that are frequently handled or worn by the owner.

Anxiety disorders that do not have a genetic basis, but instead develop from experience, are known as **acquired anxiety disorders**. A characteristic sign of the start of an acquired anxiety disorder is a complete reversal of emotional patterns. This was noticed in soldiers that developed anxiety disorders during World War II. The quiet retiring individual became garrulous and vivacious, whereas good-humoured sociable men became morose and sullen (Anon., 1943). In both personality types, the change in behaviour preceded either a sudden outburst of weeping, which had no apparent cause, or sudden aggression.

In civilian life, anxiety is common in people with breathing disorders such as obstruction of the airways, and they are particularly fearful of taking a shower, shaving, going to the toilet, eating alone, going into lifts or being away from home without an inhaler or a companion (Yellowlees *et al.*, 1987). Anxiety is itself conducive to hyperventilation, and this may help to reduce panic-provoking increases in p_aCO_2.

An example of a clinical case of an acquired **anxiety disorder** in cats occurred in a group that had been rescued from a boarding cattery that was flooded. On the sixth day after the rescue most of them went off their food and abnormal behaviour developed first in a young tortoiseshell. She began chasing imaginary beings which seemed to appear to her like flying objects. She tried to grab them in mid-air and cowered down presumably as they zoomed towards her. Then one after another six more cats took up the chase. Three of them acted as if they were wading through water, picking their feet high and shaking them. After four days, the cats resumed eating and they gradually returned to normal behaviour patterns. Another anecdotal example, also involving a flood, was the case of a dog that belonged to Pavlov's laboratory in Leningrad. It was trapped in a room that gradually filled with water during a violent and noisy storm. None of the animals drowned, but when the dog's responses were tested with a simulated flooding, it jumped onto a table, dashed around yelping, and looked anxiously at its feet.

Anxiety during pregnancy can influence behaviour in the subsequent offspring. Rats that develop anxiety during pregnancy produce offspring that are more emotional in early life. The offspring show more pronounced freezing responses when threatened and are more likely to defecate. In addition, cross-fostering studies have shown that pups which have been nursed by anxious females are likely to be more emotional. Both effects can be reduced by handling either the mother during pregnancy or the pups during infancy. The offspring and the anxious mothers have higher corticosterone responses to stress (Vallée *et al.*, 1997). Similar effects have been observed in other species.

Early postnatal experience can also play a role in anxiety-like behaviours. When the mothers of macaque monkey infants were subjected to variable, unpredictable foraging conditions, the infants grew into adults that were considerably more timid, less social, more subordinate socially and more reactive emotionally to the CNS stimulant yohimbine, in comparison with offspring from mothers that received constant foraging conditions. They also had higher concentrations of CRH in their cerebrospinal fluid as adults.

3.3 Experimental Models

There are about 30 animal behaviour tests that have been used to test anxiety. The models include:

- motivational conflict tests;
- mother–infant separation;
- pharmacological challenges;
- symptomatic cases.

Most of the models are based on acquired anticipatory anxiety, as distinct from unsignalled anxiety where there is no clear cause for the fear.

Motivational conflict models are thought to be similar to generalised anxiety in humans. An example is the test where a rat is trained to press a lever to obtain a feed reward. After the initial training period, the feed reward is coupled with an electric shock, and so every time the rat presses the lever it obtains a feed pellet at the expense of also getting a shock. This creates an approach–avoidance motivational conflict. The model is used for screening potential anxiolytic drugs, as is a comparable test where an electric shock is delivered through the drinker. When motivational conflict has been used to induce an anxiety disorder in dogs, they have shown compulsive patterns of escape or hiding, exaggerated avoidance responses to stimuli, frequent startle reactions and apparent automatism (Harris, 1989). An example of a naturally-occurring conflict situation that can be linked to anxiety is *neophobia* (fear of novel things or experiences).

The X-maze (or elevated maze) test is probably the most commonly used test of anxiety in rats and mice. The animal is placed in an X-shaped maze which is elevated from the floor. Two opposite arms of the maze are open sided, and the other two have side and end walls. Rats show an aversion either to the openness of the arms or their elevation or a combination of both. The aversion is enhanced by anxiogenic drugs and reduced by anxiolytics (Handley & McBlane, 1993).

Beta-carboline-3-carboxylic acid is used for studying drug-induced anxiety. It blocks benzodiazepine receptors, and in rhesus monkeys elicits extreme agitation, distress vocalisation, defecation and freezing responses (Skolnick *et al.*, 1984).

Inducing frustration has been another way of creating anxiety experimentally in rats. Frustration can be assessed with non-reward tests, or the defensive burying test. Both types of frustration can be reversed by anxiolytics. In the defensive burying test, rats are confined with a threatening object. Sometimes they try to bury the object. This response is suppressed by anxiolytic drugs, and so it is thought to be a sign of anxiety.

3.4 Fear

Four types of fear are commonly recognised in animals:

(1)   innate fears – e.g. isolation, fear of the dark, snakes, spiders;
(2)   novelty – e.g. strange objects, sudden movements;
(3)   fears learned by experience – e.g. anticipated pain;
(4)   fear provoked by signs of fear in others.

It is thought that most species have **innate fears,** but we do not have a good understanding of all the innate fears that exist in animals. A common innate fear is aversion to heights, which can be tested experimentally with a visual cliff apparatus. When the animal is placed on a pedestal or finds itself at the edge of an apparent precipice, it will back away from the edge if fearful, or descend if unconcerned. For example, newly-hatched chicks showed no fear of a drop of 25 cm, they had some hesitancy with 40 cm, but never attempted to descend a drop of 98 cm. These findings have some value in designing automated chick-handling systems in hatcheries. An innate fear that has been discovered recently is the fear of the sound of fire in frogs (Grafe *et al.*, 2002).

Things which are very frightening for one species may be only mildly so for another. Species variation may be linked to differences in dependence on the different faculties. The water turtle seems to show no fear of heights. Rats are myopic and their fear of heights has to be acquired. The presence or smell of a predator, however, provokes immediate innate fear in rats, and does not require a learning process: laboratory rats spent much of their time hiding when exposed to a cat's collar, even though they had never been exposed to a cat before (Dielenberg & McGregor, 1999). They also showed increased anxiety in the X-maze test after exposure to the collar. When rodents are confronted by a snake for the first time, they show a variety of responses including kicking sand at the snake, tail flagging, foot-drumming or freezing. Innate fears in primates include fear of dead bodies, mutilated bodies, strangers, a head detached from its body, and an anaesthetised primate. Ostriches seem to have an innate fear of dogs and are prone to stampeding and fence charging, but they can be trained out of this reaction by early familiarisation.

Fearfulness has a hereditary component. This has been demonstrated for humans, rats and some bird species. In children the **heritability of fear** is 0.29 and, in the case of fear of the unknown and fear of injury, it is 0.46 (Stevenson *et al.*, 1992). In rats fearfulness in a given individual resembles more closely its genetic parent than its foster mother. When rats have been genetically selected for or against fearfulness, using the defecation response in an open field test, the fearful genetic line (known as Maudsley reactive) developed more pronounced stress behaviours. They groomed themselves more when placed in a novel environment, showed less exploratory behaviour, were readily distracted from feeding by a threatening stimulus, and made more vigorous attempts to escape from stressful situations. As pups they produced greater levels of ultrasonic vocalisation when removed from their mothers.

The **signs of fear** can be obvious once one is familiar with the species. In some situations fear can provoke hostility. For example, in cats there is erection of the hair, arching of the back, bristling of the whiskers and spitting. These occur even in kittens before the eyes have opened. There can also be salivation, sweating from the paws and panting. Tremors can occur in humans when there has been a severe emotional strain or terror. There is rigidity of the part that is showing tremor, and once the muscle contraction controlling that rigidity is overcome, the tremor usually subsides. When fish are alarmed by the presence of a predator they hide, freeze, shoal, flee to the surface, jump out of the water or conceal themselves by disturbing mud on the water bed and making the water turbid, but these signs are not necessarily evidence of fear.

Behavioural fearfulness is sometimes over-exaggerated. Oversubmissive dogs raise a paw, lie down, roll over and raise a hind leg. In adolescent dogs this may be followed by urination. Excessively nervous or fearful dogs overexpress these behaviours, and if they occur in front of a stranger they may be followed by fear biting (Fox, 1962). This form of paw raising is not to be confused with a displacement behaviour or psychogenic lameness, where the behaviour is part of a reward–sympathy schedule that has developed with the owner. There is also the case of an army horse that began limping whenever the troops started to pack-up camp. This could have been a conditioned response, or possibly a reluctance to work, or a learnt fear from previous combat (Schmidt, 1968). Clearly, recognising fear simply from behaviour patterns is not always as straightforward as might at first be thought.

Some **psychosomatic disorders** can be produced or made worse by chronic fear. This has been noted in cases of gastrointestinal disorders, alopecia, hypertension and asthma. The psychosomatic gastrointestinal disorders include anorexia, nervous vomiting, oesophageal and gastric spasms, peptic ulcers, incontinence, chronic diarrhoea, spastic colon and chronic constipation. Dogs have been known to develop fear-associated salivation and vomiting during repeat visits to a veterinary clinic, and many species void when stressed. Some cats also evacuate their anal glands when stressed by fear.

Fear and other intense emotions can cause some people to faint. This is due to activity in limbic structures in the brain in response to emotions, which results in vasovagal syncope. As with other forms of reduced perfusion of the brain, the impending loss of consciousness is associated with blurred vision, cold sweating, nausea and abdominal discomfort. The subject turns pale, blood pressure falls and heart rate is greatly suppressed.

Methods that are commonly used for **quantifying fear** experimentally in a frightening context include:

- freezing or reduced exploratory behaviour;
- amount of defecation;
- failure to feed whilst in a strange environment;
- time to emerge from safe hiding.

Some methods used by animal owners to manage their animals' fears are controversial. In the short term they may cause distress whilst aiming at reducing suffering in the longer term. One example is the succinylcholine method used for breaking-in horses and for treating over-reactive or vicious horses. The animal is immobilised using an injection of succinylcholine, and, whilst paralysed but conscious, it is subjected to gentle handling which allows it to become familiar with relatively innocuous procedures. This is used to reduce unwarranted fear.

3.5 Fright

Fright occurs when an animal encounters a perceived danger without being prepared for it. A sudden fright usually elicits a **startle response**. In humans the response is usually a jolt. Normally, when a rat experiences a sudden loud noise, it jumps off the ground. Similarly a chicken leaps in the air whilst flapping its wings. These responses are increased in anxiety states created by conditioned fear. The rat becomes more jumpy, and the chicken more flighty. In fish, the startle response propels it away from the immediate danger.

Following the startle response there are two types of behavioural response to a fright: **active avoidance** or **passive avoidance**. Animals that run away when frightened, or stand and fight, have sympathoadrenomedullary activation, whereas those with a passive response freeze or hide, and often show a sudden and marked fear-bradycardia (Smith *et al.*, 1981). Fear-bradycardia is brought about by vagus nerve activation, and it is associated with reduced ventilation depth and oxygen consumption.

Sudden fright can precipitate a cardiac arrest, especially during exercise or when there is a pre-existing cardiac disorder (Meisel *et al.*, 1991): the emotional component induces myocardial ischaemia through catecholamine-induced vasoconstriction.

3.6 Phobias

A phobia is a type of fear that is out of proportion to the reality of the situation. It leads to avoidance of the feared situation and, in general, phobias are less easily extinguished than fears.

An example of a phobia case is the story of Alpha, a female chimpanzee. She was born and raised in captivity. When she was about 15 years old, at one of her night feedings, she refused her food. She did not seem to be ill, and she was clearly hungry the next day, even though there was food lying untouched in her cage. She avoided the food, making a wide circle around it when moving about the cage. Four months later, when the avoidance of food was less marked, she showed a sudden and marked avoidance of the attendant who had been feeding her. This lasted seven days. On the eighth day there was fear of food but not of the attendant. Over time there were further alternating bouts of fear of food and the attendant. The cause of the phobias was not reported.

When hens are kept loose-housed indoors it is common to find a number of victimised birds. These are poorly-feathered, underweight or emaciated birds which can be found hiding in corners or under nest-boxes. They appear to be highly fearful of other birds to the extent that they spend most of their time in partial isolation, usually crouching in a timid manner with the head lowered or retracted and the back facing the other birds. Generally they avoid contact with flockmates, but when they move amongst other birds to reach a feeder or drinker they often scurry with the head down, and this seems to incite pecking and mobbing. The fear that these birds develop can be severe enough to result in emaciation, dehydration and death, and in these cases it can be regarded as a phobia. It is not clear what causes the phobia, nor whether it is reactive or endogenous. Phobias can also develop in pet animals. For example, dogs can develop noise phobias, especially to loud bangs.

3.7 Panic

A panic attack in humans is defined as sudden fear accompanied by a feeling of terror and an intense urge to escape. It is accompanied by at least four of the following symptoms:

- dyspnoea (difficult breathing);
- chest pain or discomfort;
- choking or smothering sensations;
- shortness of breath;
- tachycardia;
- sweating;
- trembling or shaking;
- nausea;
- dizziness;
- numbness or tingling sensations.

There are often thoughts of going crazy, losing control or dying, and there seems to be no obvious cause for the attack.

People suffering from recurrent panic attacks find it more difficult to interact socially because of the threat of an attack. Claustrophobia may occur when there is a fear of confinement or suffocation and agoraphobia when there is fear of open spaces. If those fears escalate, a panic attack may set in. The majority of people with a panic disorder have breathing-related problems, and they are very sensitive to asphyxia-related cues. A panic episode can be induced pharmacologically either with certain end products of metabolism such as intravenously injected lactate or carbon dioxide inhalation, or with CNS stimulants such as yohimbine. There are some strong similarities between panic attacks and asthma attacks, but the latter have a stronger respiratory component.

Collective panic in a herd or flock often starts with a signal from an individual animal. It is not uncommon in horses, cattle and hens and results in so-called 'hysteria' if there is wild flight which is impossible to stop. In cattle it has been known to be provoked by seemingly trivial causes, such as insects. In hens it can lead to smothering if the birds pile up at one end of a shed, or into nest-boxes and under feeders. The best solution is to put the shed immediately into darkness if there is controlled lighting. Hysteria has been accompanied by birds pulling at their own feathers when the excitement stopped.

Hysterical vomiting tends to be a perpetuation of vomiting caused by a pathological condition, such as poisoning. It was common amongst World War I soldiers who vomited in response to gas poisoning, and subsequently vomited as a habitual or conditioned response to emotional upsets. It can be accompanied by epigastric pain, which is relieved by being sick.

3.8 The Role of the Amygdala

The amygdala in the brain is important in mediating anxiety, fear, rage and associated protective behaviours. There is increased activation of the amygdala during anxiety-provoking events (Davidson *et al.*, 2000). It is involved with learned fear, as distinct from fear associated with new experiences. It serves as a centre where neural pathways involved in learned threats converge. It has projections to the periaqueductal grey, which is a centre that mediates stress and fear-induced analgesia. Along with the anterior paralimbic regions of the right side of the brain, the amygdala also plays a key role in activating panic, phobias and anxiety. During a panic attack, the *insula, claustrum* and *putamen* are also activated. The limbic system in the temporal lobe is responsible for initiating fear-related defensive responses through the amygdala and brainstem centres.

Stimulation of the amygdala can amplify the expression of anxiety states. For example, the amygdala helps to exaggerate the acoustic startle response. It also plays a role in mediating the freezing response to a conditioned fear. It is involved in fear-provoked aggression and escape behaviour in recently-captured wild animals, and it mediates pain-induced aggression that is directed at conspecifics.

3.9 Losing One's Mother

In young animals, the threat of isolation from a parent can be a very frightening experience. Once the animal or infant realises that the mother has gone there is an outburst of vocalising as it tries to draw the mother back. In some species of monkeys this is a 'whoo' call. If this does not work, there may be periods of protest along with crying and, after a time, despair and depression set in. Infant rats display an equally dramatic response, especially when separation is at 15 days of age, which coincides with eye-opening but precedes normal weaning. The activity level in the separated offspring can be tenfold greater than normal, and there is a true separation fear that is not connected with suckling deprivation or hunger.

Some species have more than one type of separation call. Puppy dogs have two types of call. One of them occurs soon after birth and can be provoked simply by cooling its body. The other can be detected from the second week of life and occurs when there has been separation from the mother it has bonded with. Many altricial rodent pups produce an involuntary ultrasound vocalisation when they start to cool, and this emission can also be provoked by stimulants that have anxiogenic effects. Guinea pigs are somewhat different. They are precocial at birth, and instead of producing an ultrasound call they emit a whistle, which serves as a call to establish contact rather than a call for rescue.

In modern farming there are three groups in which the newborn has virtually no contact with its parent: dairy calves, chicks and Karakul lambs. Allowing a calf and cow to bond for one to two days and then separating them is more distressing for both partners than to separate them immediately at birth. Chicks show filial imprinting in the absence of their mother. The chick approaches any conspicuous object and snuggles up to it, frequently emitting 'twitters'. If there are no siblings, the object could be inanimate, and if the object is removed the chicks become restless and emit shrill calls (Bolhuis, 1991). Once bonding with a surrogate mother or sibling has taken place, the chicks actively avoid novel objects.

Emotional Numbness
and Deprivation

4

This chapter is concerned with features associated with emotional numbness that can contribute to suffering, and it discusses:

- anhedonia;
- depression;
- barren environments;
- social isolation;
- sensory deprivation;
- dissociative disorders;
- stereotypies;
- learned helplessness;
- post-traumatic stress disorder;
- sleep deprivation.

4.1 Anhedonia

Anhedonia is an inability to experience pleasure. In humans it is the main symptom of endogenous depression. Depressed mood can be inferred from behaviour in animals, but there are three experimental models that are more specific for anhedonia.

One of those models is failure to self-stimulate the lateral hypothalamus to achieve a pleasurable reward. Rats which had electrodes implanted in this region of the brain can be trained to activate the electrodes in response to a cue provided by a light. The light indicated the opportunity for a pleasurable experience from **self-stimulation**. When the trained rats were injected with the cytokine interleukin-2 (IL-2), they stimulated themselves less, and this was thought to be analogous to the anhedonia that occurs during some forms of sickness and disease (Anisman *et al.*, 1998). The physiological basis underlying these effects is a disturbance of dopamine release.

The other models of anhedonia are based on suppression of sexual behaviour or appetite for sweet things. In rats, chronic mild stress suppresses the drive to work for palatable sucrose solutions, and the suppression is reversed by antidepressants (Bertrand *et al.*, 1997). Administration of lipopolysaccharide results in anhedonia for sex as well as sugar.

Inescapable electric shocks applied to the foot produce a depression-like syndrome in rats which is known as learned helplessness. This appears to be an anhedonic type of depression, as these rats show reduced self-stimulation. Administration of the antidepressant desmethylimipramine reversed the suppression of self-stimulation rewarding behaviour (Koob, 1989).

4.2 Depression

In humans the common signs associated with depression are appetite disturbance, change in weight, sleep disturbance, psychomotor agitation or retardation, decreased energy, feelings of worthlessness or guilt, difficulty in concentration and thoughts of death. There is an inability to obtain pleasure from activities that previously brought enjoyment (anhedonia). Mood is sad, hopeless and discouraged, and there may also be irritability. Depression can also take the form of a boredom or emptiness, or a sense of longing for a nonexistent object or experience. Depression is often accompanied by a loss of self-esteem and a sense of failure, or there may be remorse, or a sense of 'inner badness', which can lead to self directed aggression. Clearly there are many aspects to depression. We know little about these individual facets in depressed animals. For example, we would be hard-pressed to decide whether a chronically-confined depressed dog was feeling predominantly bored, helpless, hopeless or lonely.

One of the experimental models for depression is based on the sugar glider (*Petaurus breviceps*). These animals usually adapt well to captivity and confinement. They form stable social groups, comprising one dominant male and up to eight females plus subordinate males. The dominant male plus the females control access to the nest-box, and the dominant male shows more social sniffing, scent marking and usually wins any fights. If, however, a dominant male is removed from its group and placed in an unfamiliar stable social group, it becomes submissive and expresses behaviours which have been used as an experimental model for depression (Jones *et al.*, 1995). In its new environment it rarely fights, it becomes isolated socially, does not explore the environment, becomes apprehensive, eats less and its plasma testosterone concentration falls while cortisol level rises. It is as if the sudden **social inferiority** results in a depression through loss of self-esteem. In humans this would be diagnosed as an affective disorder with mild depression.

This example is a case where depression develops from a particular denigrating social experience. At the other extreme, elevation in social status in primates has been used as a model for **mania**. Other experimental models of depression have included:

- separation models – e.g. separation of dog from a person with whom it has bonded;
- mother–infant separation – e.g. anaclitic depression in primates;
- behavioural despair tests – e.g. tail suspension test in rats;
- learned helplessness – e.g. unavoidable electric shock in rats;
- drug models – e.g. the reserpine model.

Behavioural despair tests have similarities to tests inducing learned helplessness, except that they do not inevitably involve a painful or traumatic stimulus. They have been widely used by the pharmaceutical industry for screening potential antidepressant drugs. For example, when rats are forced to swim with no opportunity for escape, they eventually give up and just maintain sufficient activity to keep their heads out of water (McKinney, 1992). On subsequent immersion, they give up sooner. If the rats are pre-treated with an antidepressant, they swim for longer and are less likely to give up. This is used as an anti-despair test, but clearly it could be complicated by differences in physical fitness.

4.3 Social Isolation in the Newborn

Rearing young animals in isolation affects their subsequent behaviour. In general they show stronger fear and emotional responses to change or novel stimuli. They have poorer exploratory drive and are more prone to stress responses such as defecation when confronted by a new object or environment. Dogs show more self-directed behaviour, such as whirling and tail chasing when excited. They can be more fearful and this has been reversed with the sedative chlorpromazine. They also show more undirected behaviour when confronted by a threat, whereas dogs reared in a socially enriched environment are more effective at avoiding the threat.

In rats, isolation-rearing from two days of age produces a hyperactive animal which shows anxiety when confronted by the X-maze test. This effect is probably mediated by dopaminergic pathways in the brain, and in particular by the nucleus accumbens. There may also be down-regulation of serotonin function.

In the case of monkeys, the length of the isolation-rearing period is critical. They can withstand at least three months of total isolation from birth without affecting their ability to socialise properly with other monkeys. If they are orphaned, and the isolation period lasts for six or more months, their ability to learn how to socialise and play with other monkeys is compromised (Harlow, 1965). They show self-directed behaviours such as self-clasping, rocking and oral stereotypies; they can be aggressive and are usually sexually incompetent. This form of depression can be corrected to some extent by gradually exposing them to young socially-competent monkeys. Monkeys which could still see their mothers during the period of separation were worse affected than those that were totally removed from their mothers.

Motherless monkeys also make poor mothers. When reared in the absence of a mother, these monkeys fail to show strong bonding with their own offspring, and their mothering ability does not improve as they become more experienced at raising young. Their offspring show a preference for adult females over peers, which was the opposite to the situation with normally reared infants (Sackett et al., 1967).

4.4 Sensory Deprivation in Early Life

Sensory deprivation (loss of a sensory faculty) has quite different effects to social isolation. When animals have been **born blind**, or when kittens have had their eyelids sutured closed at birth, they quickly adapt to the deprivation. They become adept at orienting themselves and avoiding obstacles by using auditory cues and by learning how to manoeuvre safely. However, when the sutures are removed to permit vision, their orientation is totally disrupted. They move about recklessly bumping into objects and they may crawl instead of walk. Similar responses have been noted in cataract patients once they had their cataracts removed and in animals that have been reared from birth in a dark environment. Part of the reason is that the subject finds itself in a new, highly-arousing situation and it seems to become emotionally over-reactive. In addition, it takes time to learn how to use visual cues. Long-term light deprivation is even more disruptive because it causes atrophy of the retina and optic nerve.

The effects of other forms of sensory loss include the following:

- Early auditory deprivation leads to reduced ability to learn from auditory cues once the animal is able to hear properly.
- Anosmia in newborn animals impairs their ability to locate and grasp a teat.
- Early restriction of physical movement leads to reduced use of the limbs or body part that was constrained (Riesen & Zilbert, 1975).
- Preventing young animals from expressing play behaviour caused them to move and explore their environment more.

4.5 Sensory Deprivation in Later Life

If a traumatic experience leaves a mammal unable to smell, hear, vocalise or see, it will usually be able to survive but it may be more prone to accidents and further injury. A few examples highlight some interesting complexities in other phyla. If an octopus (*Octopus vulgaris*) becomes blind, it can maintain good equilibrium and balance whilst walking and swimming. The animal can cope with the debility and survive. Loss of statocyst function, however, is much more serious. The statocysts are important in interpreting the position of the animal's head in relation to gravity and angular acceleration, and if these organs are damaged, the animal loses its orientation when forced to swim. It can only compensate by feeling with its arms, and this limits satisfactory movement considerably (Boycott, 1960).

It is difficult for us to put ourselves in the position of animals, such as the octopus, that depend on senses we do not possess. Similarly, fish have a pressure-sensitive lateral line which allows them to sense water depth, and we do not have the same capacity. Fish also have sensory hairs that project into the mucus layer that covers their body surface, and these help sense eddies and allows them to swim in the dark. In terms of suffering, this means that fish are not so severely compromised if they are visually blind. They can get by satisfactorily with their other senses. **Blindness** in a bird, on the other hand, would be catastrophic. Some fish can also sense electric fields, using electroreceptors in their ampullary organs. This allows them to detect the presence of other fish from their electric charge. Some terrestrial burrowing species are highly sensitive to ground vibration. Mice make good use of their whiskers, and the part of the sensory cortex in the brain which represents vibrissal pad sensations becomes functional at a very early stage of development.

Humans have little reliance on smell in their daily routine. This makes it difficult for us to appreciate the potential impact of being **unable to smell**. Rats subjected to olfactory bulbectomy show some unexpected behaviour changes. They seem to be more irritable, hyperactive and they have elevated levels of plasma corticosteroids. They also show reduced passive-avoidance learning. All these changes are reversed by antidepressant drugs (Willner, 1984).

4.6 Social Isolation and Barren Environments

There is a tendency to think that animals are happiest when they are active and showing their innate behaviours. This is not always the case. Sometimes people are quite content to sit at home doing nothing, just relaxing. The same is probably true for animals like the koala (*Phascolarctos cinereus*), which spends 19 hours in the day resting in a tree, seemingly doing nothing.

Nevertheless, other captive or confined animals find the environment they live in unrewarding. Animals, like humans, strive for benefits from their activities, and uniform environments provide limited new benefits. For some animals, the lifestyle in a **barren environment** may not cause suffering but it is unrewarding.

In many situations it is difficult to consider the effects of a barren environment independently of the effects of social isolation. The two often occur together. A pen- or cage-mate provides company and helps to compensate for an otherwise unenriched environment. However, there are situations in zoos where animals are kept in social isolation in an otherwise moderately enriched environment. There are also a few instances, such as dry sow stalls, where the environment is barren but there is a degree of social contact. Chronic social isolation and confinement in an unrewarding environment can lead to pathological behaviour such as stereotypies.

The effects of social isolation depend on the species. Mustelids and felids often have a solitary lifestyle for part of their lives, and it may not be a great imposition. In fact, keeping some of those animals in colonies can be more stressful than keeping them separate. Keeping animals that normally live in family, herd or flock groups in social isolation, on the other hand, can have pathological behavioural effects. For these animals social contact provides security, it is a rewarding experience, and social isolation is a deprivation which leads to suffering. Socially-deprived animals are easily upset by small changes or disturbances.

4.7 Stereotypies and Neurotic Behaviours

Frustration can lead either to displacement activities, such as irrelevant behaviour, or to redirected activities, including aggression. Pacing and preening can be displacement activities during frustration in hens, and in unconfined dogs it is often body-scratching. Jungle fowl kept in visual isolation from other birds have been known to mutilate themselves trying to fight their own tails, and cockerels deprived of sexual experience from hatching do not mate readily. In extreme situations, **stereotypies** and obsessive compulsive disorders (OCDs) can develop from a frustration behaviour, but they can also arise from depression or conflict caused by an inappropriate environment or management.

OCDs and stereotypies are persistent, recurrent and sometimes unwanted thoughts and actions. The actions can be linked to types of automatism or repetitive comfort behaviours. Examples of OCDs in humans are the mother who is plagued by urges to strangle her baby in its sleep, or the person who has a fixation about hand-washing. OCDs are sometimes diagnosed in companion animals. An example of an OCD in dogs is acral lick dermatitis. This is a repetitive licking of the foot or leg, associated with confinement, boredom or separation anxiety. A common OCD in farmed red deer is fence-pacing, which often causes erosion at fencelines (Figure 4.1). As a stereotypy or OCD develops it is expressed outside

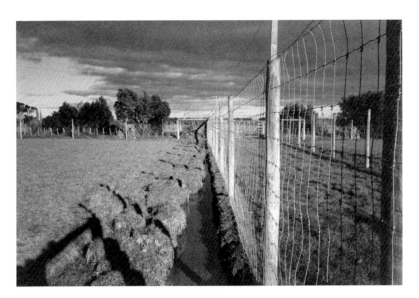

Figure 4.1 Gully worn during fence-pacing by red deer.

the context that originally induced it. This can make it difficult to identify the underlying cause of the abnormal behaviour, which is unfortunate, as the best form of treatment is to remove the cause of the conflict.

Some causes of stereotypies are:

- absence of social partners;
- absence of appropriate objects to chew on;
- absence of opportunity to express prey-catching behaviour.

These deprivations cause the release of **redirected behaviour** towards less useful or suitable activities, including neurotic behaviours and vacuum activities. The behaviours that are taken up are classified according to the normal behaviour from which they appear to be derived (Luescher *et al.*, 1991). For example, dogs show grooming stereotypies and cats can develop running and jumping stereotypies. Stereotypic barking is seen most often in dogs that are tied up or confined outside for long periods.

In hens, confinement-induced stereotypies and displacement behaviours include head-shaking or head-tic, playing with the feed, preening and wing or leg stretching. **Vacuum behaviours** may develop where a bird seems to pretend to make a nest without any nest material or dust-bathes without any dust. The imposition produced by a deprivation can be assessed from **rebound behaviour**. When the deprivation is lifted (e.g. by providing straw for nest building or dry earth for dust-bathing) the animal immediately performs excessive amounts of the thwarted behaviour. There is a rebound into overindulgence. This response indicates that the behaviour provides satisfaction for the animal, and it is often called a comfort behaviour. Some authorities consider that displacement behaviours also act as comfort behaviours.

Stereotypies are common in confined **zoo animals** and include fence-pacing, pathway-pacing, head-weaving and body-rocking. The causes of stereotypic pacing are thought to include:

- lack of space;
- absence of natural surroundings, such as cover;
- imminent feeding time;
- inability to escape or roam;
- threat from a pen or cage mate;
- inability to join a group of animals it can see.

The pacing often stops when the animal is given more space. Sometimes zoo animals take to compulsive licking, gnawing or scratching, and these can develop into self-mutilation. Causes of these behaviours include insufficient exercise, unsatisfied drive to hunt prey and sexual frustration.

The behaviour styles adopted in a stereotypy have species-specific characteristics (Mason, 1993). For example, in amphetamine-induced stereotypies, humans have repetitive thoughts, and may wash their hands repeatedly, groom and search, whereas monkeys make repetitive hand and head movements, cats look from side to side, dogs run back and forth and birds peck. Amphetamine induces stereotypies by activating **dopaminergic systems**, and disturbances in dopamine turnover are also responsible for other stereotypies as well as some of the symptoms associated with schizophrenia. Dopaminergic neurones are activated by endogenous opioids that are released in the brain during the expression of the stereotypic behaviour. The opioid surge brings mental relief, and the induction of opioid release through performing the stereotypy becomes addictive. In this way, stereotypic behaviours are anxiety-reducing.

In young animals, early social isolation has caused stereotypic behaviours in chimpanzees. Intensively-reared veal calves sometimes develop tongue-playing and coat-licking stereotypies, and tongue-playing has been reduced by providing roughage. Stereotypies are common in stabled horses. In a study of 1035 thoroughbred horses in Italy it was found that over 7% were affected by either wind-sucking, head-weaving or stall-walking (Vecchiotti & Galanti, 1986).

Neurotic behaviours are defined as abnormal behaviours that are not an obvious extension of normal behaviour. They are often exaggerated defensive behaviours or alarm responses and include unpredictable aggression towards humans. Sometimes the aggression is self-directed. Self-destructive chewing of the tail occurs in some breeds of dog, especially the German Shepherd and Bull Terrier.

In laboratory rats there is a neurotic disorder known as **activity-stress ulcers**. It occurs when young rats are fed only once a day for one hour. Some of them become hyperactive, and the condition is probably an endogenous opiate-driven compulsion as it can be reduced by naloxone, but it may arise in the first place from frustration.

4.8 Learned Helplessness

Hopelessness and helplessness are two core features of severe human depression. The depressed individual seems to adopt a helpless outlook because of the apparent dissociation between any response and outcome, based on previous experience. Actions seem futile.

Various models based on learned helplessness have been used in the context of clinical depression. The most common model has involved delivering a small number of inescapable electric shocks to the foot of a rat in combination with either a particular environmental situation or some other cue. When learned helplessness has set in, subsequent exposure to the environment or the cue, without the electric shock, produces the same passive response or absence of an escape response. The rats fail to re-learn that their behavioural responses can be used to terminate or avoid the threat. They also show escape deficits when challenged by other situations. They have more passive defensive styles and behaviours, and these responses are not necessarily stimulus specific. They lose weight from a reduced appetite and they groom and play less. Their depressed-like behaviour can be corrected by antidepressant drugs, but less so by anxiolytics. This form of depression is associated with increased release of noradrenaline from nerve endings in the forebrain that originate in the locus coeruleus, and decreased release of **serotonin** in the forebrain. Learned helplessness has been reversed by selective serotonin reuptake inhibitors and by serotonin receptor agonists. Serotonin receptors in the dorsal hippocampus may play a role in preventing learned helplessness along with increased release of monoamines in the prefrontal cortex.

Experimental learned helplessness has also been seen in a range of invertebrates including crayfish (*Procambarus clarkii*), slugs (*Limax maximus*) and cockroaches (*Periplaneta americana*).

4.9 Post-traumatic Stress Disorder

Post-traumatic stress disorder (PTSD) is a dissociative disorder that occurs in people who have witnessed, experienced or been confronted with serious injury or stress to themselves or others. Typically, it occurs in war veterans, rape victims and victims of natural disasters or motor accidents. They experience flashbacks to the traumatic episode and react to cues that symbolise or resemble the episode. It is a non-benign adaptation to trauma. They may suffer from insomnia, irritability, difficulty in concentrating, hypervigilance and an exaggerated startle response, and in severe cases have difficulty in adapting socially. It only occurs in a percentage of those exposed to trauma.

So far there have been no unequivocal reports of PTSD in animals in a clinical context. However, there are laboratory-animal models that share some features with human PTSD. Studies on earthquake victims have shown that situational reminders of the catastrophe, such as living amongst the debris and at the scenes where deaths were witnessed, can be important in reinforcing the development of PTSD.

A comparable effect has been demonstrated in laboratory mice. When mice were given repeated exposures to a reminder of a situation where they had had a prior electric shock, they became hyperactive and developed progressive increases in their acoustic startle response. There was also increased fighting amongst the male mice during the reminder situation, and on some occasions there was catastrophic cohort violence (Pynoos et al., 1997). In this model, and in the clinical state in people, repetitive jogging of the memory seems to precipitate this stress disorder. The **hippocampus** in the brain plays an integral physiological part, linking recall and the developing disorder.

The hippocampus is important in memory storage and retrieval, and in clinical contexts it is involved in amnesia, generalised anxiety, panic disorders and dissociative states. It receives inputs from the *entorhinal cortex* which in turn is supplied with signals from the association cortices. The functions of the hippocampus are integrated with higher centre activity through the amygdaloid nuclei, and this enhances or modulates in other ways the emotional components of memory.

PTSD is associated with degeneration of the hippocampus in humans. When a stress is severe and recurring, the circulating corticosterone levels can be chronically elevated. During overexposure to corticosteroids, there is glutamate-mediated dendritic atrophy within the CA3 region of the hippocampus. This stress effect has also been observed with restraint stress in rats, and psychosocial stress in tree shrews (McEwen & Magarinos, 1997). In humans suffering from PTSD, the atrophy can lead to reductions in hippocampal volume by up to 26%. As PTSD progresses, there is down-regulation of the hypothalamic–pituitary–adrenal (HPA) axis. Plasma and urine cortisol levels are reduced, but CRH levels in the cerebrospinal fluid are elevated. There appears to be hypersensitivity to the negative feedback effects of cortisol, and ACTH secretory responses to CRH are reduced.

Finally, it is worth recalling the story of a horse that experienced an aerial bombardment during World War II. After the exposure it became very nervous, but after a rest period, it seemed to recover. However, it had a serious relapse when it returned to the site where it experienced the blasts. This could have been due to the exercise involved in moving it, or to a relapse from a reminder of its previous experience. Perhaps it was a clinical animal case of PTSD.

4.10 Sleep Disorders

The most common sleep disorders that cause or are caused by suffering are sleep deprivation, disturbed sleep, insomnia and nightmares. Cattle, sheep and pigs may experience sleep deprivation when transported long distances. In humans, **sleep deprivation** can lead to irritability, illusions, visual hallucinations, paranoid thinking, slow thinking, memory loss, a sense of depersonalisation, numbness and dissociative states. Irritability can be expressed as open hostility, especially when aroused from a drowsing state. Interrupting a person's sleep can be more disturbing than reduced sleep time. For example, waking a person up every ten minutes produced extreme daytime sleepiness and restlessness, even though the subject had a normal total sleep time (Gillin *et al.*, 2000). This type of sleep disturbance occurs in people suffering from painful arthritis, sleep apnoea or a bad cough.

Sleep problems need to be assessed from a knowledge of the species' normal sleep requirement and the age of the animal. For example, the sloth often sleeps as much as 20 hours per day. At the other extreme, the shrew may not sleep at all. In general, predators tend to sleep more deeply than prey species. Not all species show rapid eye movement sleep, and some aquatic species, such as the dolphin, exhibit unihemispheric sleep – while one hemisphere is sleeping the other is awake.

There are two neurochemical processes during sleep which have an important influence on mood. Most mammals have two major phases of sleep: rapid eye movement (REM) sleep; and non-rapid eye movement (NREM) sleep (Figure 4.2). REM sleep is associated with dreaming and starts once noradrenergic neurones in the *locus coeruleus* of the brain have ceased being active. It is also associated with reduced activity in serotonergic neurones in the *raphe nucleus*, and with lower heart rate, cerebral glucose metabolism, brain temperature and respiratory rate (Jacobs *et al.*, 1990). Drugs that block serotonin synthesis are conducive to sleeping, and drugs that increase the availability of noradrenaline reduce REM sleep and elevate the mood by improving wakefulness and reducing depression. It is thought that sleep helps to restore noradrenaline and serotonin synthesis and storage to normal levels, and failure of these processes during sleep deprivation helps explain the subsequent dullness in mood and increased irritability.

When laboratory rats had been deprived of sleep, their plasma corticosterone concentrations were elevated, and if they were fasted as well, they were more prone to developing gastric ulcers (Murison *et al.*, 1982). During sleep deprivation, a somnogenic substance accumulates in cerebrospinal fluid, which on transfer to a normal animal causes the recipient to sleep more (Takahashi *et al.*, 1997). Prolonged sleep deprivation can result in death, and in rats this takes about three weeks in the case of total sleep deprivation and five weeks for selective REM sleep deprivation. Death is probably due to metabolic exhaustion, concomitant with falling body temperature and increasing food intake. Failure to sleep occurs if young rat pups are removed from their mother too early (Hofer, 1975).

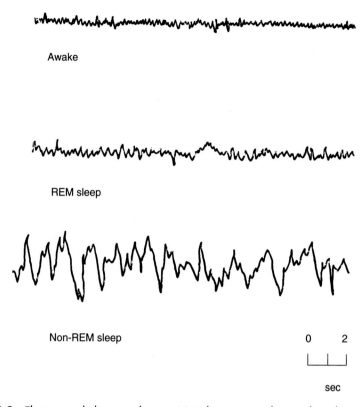

Figure 4.2 Electroencephalograms showing REM sleep, NREM sleep and awake patterns.

Cattle and sheep normally sleep for about four hours at night and drowse for a further six hours. During REM sleep their ears twitch, the eyes move and the eyelids blink. During **rumination**, the EEG shows high amplitude/low frequency activity which merges into an REM sleep episode with the head held low (Bell & Itabisashi, 1973). Feeding sheep or dairy cows a complete pelleted ration, which does not allow rumination because of insufficient long fibre, leads to sleep deprivation. The signs are lethargy, refusal to move, apparent exhaustion, poor exercise tolerance, and, in the case of sheep, proneness to panting (Morag, 1967). Providing additional roughage corrects this, and the animals become alert and responsive and lose their lethargy.

Narcolepsy is a disorder where there is an uncontrolled desire to sleep. Narcoleptic-like conditions have been reported in cats and dogs, and in some cases there were cataplectic attacks as well (Mitler *et al.*, 1974). Damage to the upper part of the brainstem, or pressure on the brainstem from a tumour, can cause excessive sleep.

Nightmares are frightening dreams which occur during REM sleep, and are remembered on awakening. They differ from night terrors, where the subject wakes from a deep sleep in a frightened state and in a sweat without any recall of dreaming. It is not known whether animals experience nightmares, but it is suspected that dogs can have disturbing dreams.

4.11 Weaning

Normally, when a young animal becomes disturbed or frightened it runs to its mother and starts sucking. Nursing is a comfort behaviour, and it provides a sense of security from the touch, smell and sounds normally produced by the dam. Separating the dam and young at weaning time disrupts the young animals' security, removes a source of fluid and feed, and often involves introduction to a new environment. There may also be the stress of mixing the weaned offspring with animals from other litters or groups. Both the young animal and the dam can become frantic whilst attempting to find each other, and sometimes this leads to injuries, particularly with fencelines or pen walls.

The psychological stress of weaning can cause immune suppression and diarrhoea, which, in pigs, can be reduced with psychotropic drugs (Pluske & Williams, 1996). It can also increase the weaned animals' susceptibility to gastrointestinal ulcers (Apter & Householder, 1996). One way of reducing this stress is to wait until the mother–young bond has weakened.

In horses, the mother–young bond begins to weaken as early as two or three months of age, and weaning at two months is not uncommon, although abrupt weaning at four to six months would be the norm. Weaning at two months is sometimes advocated if the mare has an undesirable temperament and the owner wishes to reduce the chance of the foal acquiring the mare's habits. It has been suggested that weaning foals in pairs is less stressful than singly, and this has been confirmed by studies where the plasma cortisol response to ACTH was examined. However, if the foals take to fighting each other, they will need to be separated.

When animals are weaned too early they can develop bizarre behaviours. Kittens nuzzle and knead soft fabrics, and piglets root repetitively at the floor and chew or suck on objects, including the tails of littermates. In rats, early weaning can be fatal. Laboratory rats are often weaned at three to four weeks of age, and they will survive weaning at 15 days of age. However, if separation occurred two days earlier, over 80% of the weaned rats died within eight days. The rats that died had been eating solid feed. This mortality can be prevented by housing the pups with a non-lactating female, indicating that it is not due to deprivation of milk. However, if the surrogate mother was separated from the pups by a wire screen, mortality was high (Plaut et al., 1974). Evidently, physical contact, nest maintenance or warmth were important for the pups' survival. Weaning puppies at three instead of 15 weeks of age results in a dog that has poor exploratory responses,

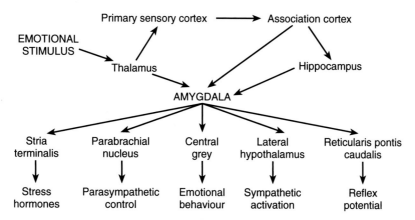

Figure 4.3 Role of the amygdala in brain processing of emotions.

both to humans and towards a companion. These responses are improved if the dogs are given chlorpromazine (Fuller & Clark, 1966).

4.12 Physiology of Emotions

Emotions and instinctive behaviours are coordinated by the **limbic system** in the brain. This system includes the cingulate cortex, hippocampus, amygdala and stria terminalis. These regions are particularly well represented in terms of their size in mammalian species that developed early in evolutionary history. The limbic system is involved with mediating autonomic nervous system responses and integrating them with emotional responses. The central nucleus within the amygdala is the single most important centre within the brain for the expression of emotional responses associated with aversive stimuli. It is the output centre for the part of the brain where emotional responses are coordinated. However, the amygdala is not necessarily the centre where emotions are perceived.

Emotion-provoking signals reach the **amygdala** by two routes: direct projections from the thalamus; and indirectly via cortical structures (Figure 4.3). The direct pathways transmit information to the amygdala, usually through only one synapse, and therefore they are fast. They do not usually represent complex stimuli. In contrast, the cortical–amygdala pathways are slower and they incorporate complexity. They can include signals which suppress the activity of the amygdala, in which case they control emotional responses. Examples of separate output pathways from the central nucleus of the amygdala are pathways to the:

- central grey for conditioned activities such as freezing;
- lateral hypothalamus for raising blood pressure;
- *stria terminalis* for neuroendocrine responses.

Aggression, Overcrowding and Discomfort

This chapter examines the causes and consequences of aggressive competition and cannibalism, and it briefly considers some of the problems associated with confinement and discomfort.

5.1 Aggression

5.1.1 Physiology of aggression

Aggression has been produced experimentally by stimulating the **hypothalamus** with small electrical currents. The attack is directed at animate objects, and in the cat involves stalking, chasing and biting, but the prey is not eaten (Flynn, 1967). The biting reaction depends on sensory input from around the mouth. If this region is deafferented, the cat rubs its muzzle back and forth against the prey instead of biting it. These and other findings originally led scientists to infer that the hypothalamus is an important centre for the control of aggression and predation, but that view has now been modified. Hypothalamic stimulation increases the expression of other motivated behaviours, and this region of the brain is now regarded as a channel that amplifies and initiates a broad range of emotional behavioural expression. The particular behavioural response depends on the situation the animal is in when the stimulation is applied.

Instead, it is the **amygdala** that plays a major role in aggression especially when it involves memory. Electrical stimulation of the dorsomedial part of the amygdala elicits growling and hissing behaviours in cats (Fernandez de Molina & Hunsperger, 1962). The amygdala activates the hypothalamus and central grey matter of the midbrain which in turn initiate threatening and aggressive defence responses when the animal is presented with the appropriate context. Removal of the amygdala seems to disrupt the ability of environmental stimuli to influence aggression. Associative memory is particularly affected, but recognition memory can also be impaired if the hippocampus is damaged along with the amygdala (Murray, 1991).

Serotonin (5-HT,5-hydroxytryptamine) plays an important role in aggression and predation. Aggression has been reduced in humans and chickens when they drank or ate increased amounts of the serotonin precursor tryptophan, and, in primates, aggressive behaviour is linked to lower cerebrospinal fluid concentrations of the serotonin metabolite 5-hydroxyindoleacetic acid (5-HIAA).

Muricide (mouse killing behaviour) can be induced in rats by bilateral lesioning of their olfactory bulbs. This reaction is reversed by lesioning of the medial amygdala or by antidepressant drugs. The attack is often directed at the back of the neck of the mouse.

5.1.2 Situations leading to aggression
Aggression and offensive behaviour occur in the following contexts:

- predation;
- cannibalism and infanticide;
- protecting young;
- protection of territory or social structure;
- establishing a new social or mating hierarchy;
- frustration and hysteria;
- competition for feed, lying area or other facilities;
- pain;
- fear.

It leads to suffering through the injuries that occur during the fight, and the aggression can itself be a sign of suffering when it is due to pain, fear or frustration. When animals fight they often attack sensitive regions of the body, and facial injuries are a common form of trauma during fights for dominance.

5.1.3 Predation
Predators attack and kill their prey in one of three ways:

(1) stalking;
(2) gathering;
(3) harrying.

Harrying is arguably the least humane method.

When a wild pig harries a lamb, it usually runs at the flock, splitting off 20 to 30 ewes and lambs, which it chases before taking a lamb that falls behind. Typically, at the time of lambing, this is successful in 24% of chases (Pavlov & Hone, 1982). Coyotes have a much higher success rate. The coyote selects either the biggest lamb, or the weakest and slowest, and it may kill up to 16 sheep during a single attack, many of which are uneaten (Nass, 1977). It usually attacks a ewe at the throat and a lamb at either the head or throat. This is probably a relatively quick and efficient kill, whereas kills by domestic dogs have a messy appearance, as they are apt to bite the sheep anywhere.

Foxes generally attack lambs from below, often grasping the skin at the sternum, but they have been known to latch onto the thigh, tail, lower jaw and even the tongue (Dennis, 1969). Golden eagles take smaller lambs, with the talons entering anywhere along the back or sides, but it is unusual for them to break any bone larger than a rib (Tigner & Larson, 1977). In Australia, ravens have been known to attack live lambs when there was little carrion about. However, they usually excavate holes in dead or downer animals at natural orifices such as the eyes, mouth, anus, vulva and umbilicus. Roadside goats are at high risk of dog attacks especially at night. The erratic running behaviour of the tethered goat tends to excite the dog to chase it.

In Australia and New Zealand, muzzles are used on dogs, especially yard dogs at abattoirs, to reduce **bite injuries** in sheep. Muzzles are generally recognised as a humane option, but they can cause skin irritation in the dog. Sometimes a veterinarian is asked to remove the canine teeth from working dogs that are inveterate sheep biters, but there is growing resistance to this practice. Electronic collars can be hired from municipal councils for training-out sheep biting amongst working dogs. This is accepted as a more humane method than giving the dog a beating, and is often preferred to destroying the dog. At one time, chain bits, secured through the mouth under the tongue to the dog's collar, were used and they prevented the dog from closing its jaws sufficiently when biting a sheep. Muzzles are generally more comfortable.

Predation in fish farms by birds is a common nuisance. Besides the loss of whole fish, it is a cause of injury in fish that escape. Characteristic scars are produced on both sides of the fish by cormorants (Barlow & Bock, 1984).

Some species are **obligate hunters** and they hunt for the chase, besides food. Holding wild predators in captivity, and depriving them of the opportunity to hunt, may constitute a deprivation.

5.1.4 Cannibalism and infanticide

Cannibalism or infanticide are quite common in chickens, turkeys, pigs, hyenas, ferrets, hamsters, mice, gerbils and a number of gastropods. On pig farms, a sow sometimes develops the habit of eating her own piglets, and, less commonly, mares savage their foals, for no obvious reason.

Cannibalism between adults is a serious problem in layer hens. It can be linked to social disruption, bright lighting, onset of sexual maturity, overcrowding or close confinement, large group size, any factor which has caused healthy birds to go off their feed and the presence of sick, victimised or dead birds. It often erupts unexpectedly. For example, introducing a new batch of feed can cause the birds to stop eating, even though there is nothing obviously wrong with the feed. It is merely different from the previous batch. If the hens go off their feed, they tend to be drawn by unusual features such as a white feather within brown plumage, or by a visible scar on the skin, or by an exposed or everted vent. Exploratory hunger-pecking leads to bleeding which leads to cannibalism. In this situation it is particularly important to recognise the early signs before cannibalism spreads through the flock. A good way of counteracting the early signs is to scatter feed on the floor for several days, until they get used to the new ration.

The home environment can influence cannibalism. For example, providing a family of tree shrews with two nest-boxes helps control pup eating. Presumably the second nest-box gives the mother a break from the pups. Cannibalism also develops from severe hunger. This is the case with broiler breeder hens that are kept on a limited feed allowance to promote fertility and avoid prolapses. Mass cannibalism occurs during mouse plagues, once the source of feed for the mice has been exhausted.

The **speed of the kill** is all-important in determining the length of suffering. In pigs, the usual method of cannibalism is to bite the piglets through the head. Piglets that have been rescued from this situation had depressed fractures of the cranium, and teeth marks on the jaws or neck. It should have been a relatively humane death provided the sow or gilt completed the process promptly. Female Golden hamsters attack their victims with a slight spring followed by a series of bites, usually directed at the head. This is similar to the fighting behaviour seen between adults, and it can be provoked by a pup attempting to suckle a non-lactating female (Richards, 1966). Gerbils, however, do not attack the pups. Instead they eat them in a normal manner. The pup is picked up in the mouth and carried to a corner, held in the forepaws, and eaten much as if it was a piece of food. The interval between first approach and the first bite was usually 15–25 seconds.

In mice, death by infanticide is very quick, and it is the male which attacks the pups. This has been related to testosterone production. Castration of male mice reduces pup-killing, and giving virgin female mice testosterone induces pup killing (Berryman, 1986). Wild mice are more prone to infanticide than laboratory strains when kept in confinement, and environmental noise can provoke infanticide (Busnel & Molin, 1978).

5.1.5 Protecting young
In rodents, maternal aggression towards unwelcome intruders develops after suckling has occurred. Suckling acts as an important endocrine stimulus for defensive maternal aggression. However, it is not directly attributable to prolactin release. In monkeys, maternal aggression is suppressed if the mother was socially deprived when it was young (Meier, 1965).

5.1.6 Protecting territory
When an animal defends its territory, there are three separate phases:

(1)   detection of the intruder;
(2)   chasing or tracking;
(3)   attack.

The mouse relies on sound for detecting and pursuing an intruder, and vision for the attack phase. In rats, defence of a territory is promoted by testosterone in dominant males and by low progesterone status in the females.

Some species engage in **territory battles**. Wild chimpanzees (*Pan troglodytes*) make gang attacks on solitary animals, and, less frequently, they attack an entire neighbouring group as a gang. The naked mole-rat (*Heterocephalus glaber*) also has intergroup warfare, but since the battles occur in underground burrows they take the form of consecutive duels at a battlefront.

5.1.7 Hierarchy
The chicken pecking order helps establish access to limited or preferred resources including feed, water and nest sites. Where resources are unlimited there is little need for reinforcing the pecking order with fighting. However, if a critical resource is limited fighting may erupt. Sometimes this seems haphazard and unpredictable, but the experienced stockperson should be able to recognise the early signs and manage imminent problems.

Bullying can be a problem when heifers and gilts are first introduced into the main breeding herd. The young females usually stay at the edge of the herd and they may have less opportunity to feed. It is best to introduce them as a group rather than individually.

5.1.8 Frustration
Aggression can develop from frustration. It is produced experimentally by preventing an animal from obtaining food when it expects to be fed. For example, pigeons have been trained to operate a switch when a light comes on, and successful pecking at the switch gives them a feed reward. If feed is not delivered even though the bird responds correctly, it is prone to attacking a nearby bird or a look-alike stuffed bird. In chickens, temporary feed deprivation also leads to aggression against subordinates, which are pecked more by middle-ranking hens than by dominant hens (Duncan & Wood-Gush, 1971). Humans also develop rage from frustration when a drinks dispenser or slot machine takes their money without providing the goods, but the aggression is more likely to be directed at the machine than a passer-by.

There are many other situations where aggression is directed at subordinates in response to frustration. Depriving birds of the opportunity to dust-bathe can lead to increased feather-pecking. The bird on the receiving end is not necessarily the source of frustration.

5.1.9 Fear and pain

Aggression can occur from retaliation when an animal is fearful, and it can be a spontaneous response to sudden pain. Cats are prone to defence aggression, and handling unfamiliar cats is an acquired skill, requiring tolerance, gentleness and forward thinking. Forcible restraint provokes considerable resistance.

Aggression is also a constant hazard when handling foxes at fur farms. The foxes are aggressive against the handlers, and are best moved in boxes. When the pelt is being graded or the animal slaughtered, a special type of callipers, similar to a cat-grabber, which grasps the animal at the back of the head, is used.

5.1.10 Genetic and familial aggressiveness

Aggressiveness has a genetic and a familial basis. Young monkeys which experience a hostile mother during the first months of life are more likely to become aggressive adults. Practical experience has also shown that there are docile and aggressive strains of domesticated animals. This applies to breeds of dog, pig, chicken and duck.

The neuroendocrine basis for the differences has not been established, but there is growing evidence which implicates serotonin. Mice with the gene that codes for monoamine oxidase type A (MAO_A) knocked out showed increased aggression, as did mice which lacked one of the sub-types of serotonin receptor. The MAO_A knock-out mice had increased levels of serotonin and decreased levels of 5-HIAA as pups, but by the time they were adults, the levels were normal (Mathews & Freimer, 2000). This implies that it is not the measurable concentration of serotonin which is important, but the altered concentration during early development.

Prenatal circumstances can be important as well. Female foetuses that are positioned between two male foetuses show greater interfemale aggression in later life, than do female foetuses positioned between two other females. The greater aggression is due to androgenisation in the female foetus.

There are some subtle genetic differences in fighting behaviour. Mice can be divided into prompt attackers and late attackers. The prompt attackers set about an intruder almost as soon as they hear it, whereas the late attackers wait before they take on the intruder. The prompt attackers are probably at an advantage in established communities, but in individuals or groups that are migrating or moving around widely the late attackers may be more successful because they expend less energy in random attacks (Monaghan & Glickman, 1992).

5.2 Overcrowding and Confinement

5.2.1 Overcrowding

Aggression is a problem in farmed chickens, pigs, turkeys and trout. These are naturally social animals. Chickens would normally live in small family groups with one dominant male and up to twelve hens plus immature offspring. On farms, layer flocks are single-sex and considerably larger than the normal family group. This can lead to problems with social stability, particularly if there is overcrowding.

Aggression in chickens occurs as threatening attacks (rushing at an opponent, sparring with the feet, standing over the opponent with the neck extended), chasing and pecking at the head and neck. During fights the opponents aim with the beak at parts of the body that are sensitive. They often try to peck each other's combs. When a bird gives in, it crouches with its head tucked down, often with its eyes closed. The victor stands over the victim and reinforces its dominance with a hard strike to the top of the head. This type of fighting is not necessarily a prelude to cannibalism. It is a way of enforcing the hierarchy within the flock. However, if it leads to a bird being wounded, the blood may draw other birds and cannibalism can then set in.

Fighting is often avoided by one opponent cowering or walking away, and by avoiding direct eye contact or not staring at the potential opponent. It is more difficult to express these avoidance behaviours when there is **overcrowding**, and this, plus lack of environmental complexity, may be why serious outbreaks of aggression and cannibalism occur in overstocked perchery and deep litter systems.

Territory may be important in hens kept in large flocks. These birds tend to organise themselves into subgroups. In addition, hens probably have a 'personal' space. If that space is encroached upon the bird may either move away or repel the bird that is getting too close, and this could lead to fighting, wounding and then cannibalism. High stocking densities will inevitably lead to more of these activities through competition for space.

Some of the worst effects of overcrowding have been in monkeys. In the 1950s primates were used for vaccine testing and production, in particular for poliomyelitis. Laboratories held up to 3000 primates which were imported into the USA from Asia and Africa. 'Gang cages', holding up to 300 monkeys, were introduced as a way of cutting down on the cost of vaccine production, but they made it more difficult to control enteric disease and tuberculosis. In addition there were problems with aggression. Some species of monkey exert rough and brutal methods when expressing social dominance. This leads to fear of the dominant animals amongst the subordinates, to the point of being terror-stricken. In the gang cages the weak or sick were often killed by the dominant individuals, and the subordinates were in danger of starving if the supply of food was limited or was controlled by the dominant individuals. At one unit of Cercopithecoids, mortality from fighting reached 30%.

Sometimes the cure for aggression has been worse than the vice itself. In Egypt a biting horse used to be trained out of biting by tormenting it and then present-ing it with a leg of mutton that had just been removed from a fire. The scalding to its mouth taught the animal to be selective in the things it bit.

5.2.2 Confinement

Depending on the design of the system, confinement in a **cage environment** (Plate 1) can cause the following types of suffering or compromise:

- discomfort to the feet from standing on wire;
- uncomfortable lying surface if there is no bedding area;
- inability to exercise, explore, forage, roost or roam;
- boredom, frustration, depression or despair from an unrewarding environment;
- limited social interaction;
- fear when threatened and inability to escape.

There are other impositions which are quite subtle. For example, nesting behaviour may be thwarted. The hen normally vocalises when she is about to lay an egg. In Jungle Fowl, this nest-call is used to recruit the cockerel to lead her to a potential nest site. In the cage situation, nest-calling is followed by a great deal of pacing, which is thought to be a sign of frustration (Wood-Gush, 1973).

In some species, confinement can cause frenetic, almost neurotic, behaviour. Foxes kept in cages for fur production show a remarkable amount of activity, some of which is stereotypic. They pace within the cage along the same route, often at high speed which makes it seem almost frenzied.

In psychiatric medicine it is well recognised that keeping prisoners in **solitary confinement** introduces a risk of depression (Andersen *et al.*, 2000). Depression seems to occur in some animals kept in isolated confinement. Pigs kept in isolation became withdrawn, lying against the wall, refusing to move except under duress, and they were less interested in their environment and feed, whereas pigs kept as pairs or group housed had normal behaviour.

The stress of isolation can precipitate heart disease (Ratcliffe *et al.*, 1969). Post-mortem examination after slaughter at about 14 months of age showed that **arteriosclerosis** was most advanced in confined, socially isolated female pigs. Arterial lesions were less pronounced in pigs kept in pairs, and least advanced in the grouped animals.

Social isolation is not the only cause of arteriosclerosis in animals. In fact, stress from social pressures has caused the same lesions. There was a case in 1948 at Philadelphia Zoo, when it was decided to keep many species in family groups instead of individually in cages. With the sudden change, conflicts arose, there were injuries, breeding failure and a rising number of premature deaths. Many of the premature deaths were due to coronary heart disease, arising from arteriosclerosis and ischaemic necrosis, and this was ascribed to mixing stress and to holding incompatible animals in the same pen.

5.3 Discomfort

Discomfort leads to suffering if it causes long-term physical or mental irritation. Examples include protracted or inappropriate:

- itching;
- abrasion against a cage or pen surface;
- surfaces to walk on;
- glare from the sun;
- loud noise.

An **itch** is a poorly-localised, usually unpleasant sensation which provokes scratching. A **tickle** is an itch-like sensation which only lasts for as long as the stimulus is applied. A **prickle** produces an urge to scratch and it originates from activation of nociceptors. An itch can be produced by chemical, mechanical, thermal or electrical stimuli and it can occur when the skin is injured by burning, freezing and some types of mechanical injury. Scratching can provoke satisfaction when it relieves the itch, but when severe it can lead to self-mutilation. Itching is an unpleasant consequence of obstructive jaundice, ectoparasites and some forms of worm infestation.

At one time it was thought that itch and pain shared the same nerve pathways, but it is now appreciated that the two are independent. Signals from the itch receptors are transmitted along unmyelinated C-fibres which enter the dorsal horn of the spinal cord and synapse with secondary neurones which themselves cross to the contralateral spinothalamic tract and ascend to the thalamus. The anterior cingulate cortex is involved in itch registration at the conscious level. **Central itch** is an itch which is perceived in the skin but actually originates in the central nervous system. This occurs with some forms of drug-induced itching.

Flies are a common cause of itching and discomfort amongst livestock. Tail-flicking, foot-stamping and continuous movement are obvious signs of this irritation in cattle. Horses wander about restlessly, ignoring feed, or stand head-to-tail to gain the benefit of tail whisking from other horses. Mosquitoes and biting midges attack cattle particularly during the two hours that follow sunset. They attack the legs and underside and it was estimated in one study in Queensland that cattle lost about 150 ml of blood each night during the months of December to March (Standfast & Dyce, 1968). Buffaloes wallow as a way of avoiding flies, and, given the chance, horses will stand in smoke on the lee side of a fire.

Stock often loaf in the shade even in the cooler times of the day. One reason is to avoid **glare** from the sun. Sun-glare might be a minor discomfort, but snow-glare and snow blindness are more serious. In the past, in the Russian steppes, cattle were fitted with head gear that had smoke-stained shields, to help control snow blindness.

Inappropriate **noise** can cause:

* annoyance and interruption of normal activities;
* sleep interference;
* fear and exaggerated startle reactions;
* ear pain and headaches.

It has even jeopardised survival in disease states. For example, 120 dB applied for three hours a day for six to eight days has resulted in raised mortality from encephalitis when mice were inoculated with vesicular stomatitis virus (Chang & Rasmussen, 1965). Some cases of hypertension and ischaemic heart disease in people have been put down to chronic exposure to irritating noise.

Sounds which exceed about 130 dB are painfully loud for humans – 140 dB would correspond to the noise alongside an aircraft jet on an aircraft carrier. Noises in the 90–100 dB range are very annoying – an example would be the noise from a riveting machine. When 90 dB is experienced for eight hours or more there is a risk of hearing damage. Noise is annoying or intrusive down to levels of about 60 dB, and 10 dB is just audible. Not all animals, however, avoid a noisy environment. For example, some insectivorous birds favour visiting noisy waterfalls when feeding, mice often inhabit industrial milling plants, rats live in Metro subways and gulls, starlings and crows are common at some airfields. Birds and rabbits that were familiar with the noise of the Concorde aeroplane seemed to pay little attention to its take-off or landing.

Various high-frequency and explosive noises are used as animal repellents. The high frequencies are barely audible to the human ear, but cause an alerting or flight response in many species of animal. Fish may respond with a brief bradycardia when they experience the noise of a ship above them. If the ship is emitting air gun discharges as part of a geophysical survey, the fish tend to move to deeper water and cluster together. Alarm behaviour occurs if they are close enough to the ship to experience more than 180 dB. Typically, the distance between a fish and the seismic vessel would be 300 m for a startle response to occur, and 5.5 km for an alarm response (Pearson *et al.*, 1992).

Exercise

The focus in this chapter is on the forms of suffering that occur during competitive and endurance exercise in horses, greyhounds and migratory birds.

6.1 Overexertion

Overexertion and other forms of inappropriate exercise can lead to the following types of suffering:

- muscular and skeletal injuries;
- muscle soreness following exercise;
- distress from metabolic disorders;
- exaggerated hyperthermia.

Signs of **overexertion** in horses include:

- slow recovery of heart rate;
- shallow rapid respiratory rate;
- gulping breaths;
- persistent elevated rectal temperature;
- dehydration;
- depression;
- muscle tremors and twitching;
- muscle cramps or tying-up;
- thumps (breathing in synchrony with the heart).

Muscle soreness following strenuous or unaccustomed exercise arises from stretching or tearing of muscle fibres. The generation of free radicals during exercise increases the likelihood of this type of damage through membrane damage, as does exercise which involves contraction of fibres whilst the muscle is in an extended state (eccentric contraction). The free radicals cause myofibril injury through lipid peroxidation. Muscle soreness is often delayed, being at its worst between one and two days after the exercise.

The metabolic disorders occurring with overexertion can come about in one of two ways. Either there is a progressive depletion of oxygen during steady exertion, such as a chase. Or, there is a massive burst of activity which depletes oxygen in a short space of time. In both situations, the subsequent anaerobic metabolism results in **fatigue**. The predominant metabolite which provokes the sense of fatigue has not been identified, but it is one of the end-products of anaerobic metabolism (H^+, K^+, lactate or phosphate), all of which can influence afferent activity in sympathetic pathways leading to the brain.

Fitness is important in allowing the development of **second wind**, which helps to limit suffering from overexertion. During second wind, breathing becomes easier, performance requires less effort, and taking exercise becomes more comfortable. This switch is accompanied by a rise in rectal temperature by about $0.5°C$, and it occurs earlier under warm rather than cold conditions (Berner et al., 1926). Just before the sensation of second wind, respiration rate rises to a maximum; afterwards tidal volume falls to a more or less constant value.

A metabolic disorder that is associated with exercise in horses is **Monday morning disease**, or **acute azoturia**. This occurs during vigorous exercise after a period of rest, and used to be common in draught horses that had a rest day on Sundays. It is associated with high levels of muscle glycogen at the start of exercise, leading to high blood lactate levels and muscle stiffness, especially in animals with compromised livers. The metabolic acidosis causes blowing and in severe cases there is sweating and myoglobinuria. The gluteal muscles are usually tied-up, and if this causes excessive pressure on the sciatic and crural nerves, there can be neuropathic atrophy of the muscles served by those nerves.

Heat stroke can be a risk in competitive racing or in prolonged exercise under hot conditions. In humans, the marathon runner becomes emotionally unstable as heat stroke sets in. He is irritable, sometimes aggressive and may display hysterical weeping. When disorientation develops, the gait becomes unsteady and the eyes have a glassy stare. Judgement is affected, and it has been known for competitors to run the wrong way round the track at the stadium. The physiological complications in this condition are circulatory collapse and metabolic acidosis. These impose localised hypoxaemia, acidosis and hyperthermia, which together act to compound the problem. If the circulatory shock is severe, there is a risk of renal vascular shut-down and kidney damage.

6.2 Endurance Riding

Endurance exercise used to be an everyday occurrence in horses. In the past, Pony Express horses used to run at 16 km/h whilst covering about 20 km. Modern endurance rides can be up to 40 km, and, although the aim is to complete the ride without overtaxing the horse, weight losses of 10% can occur. Under warm conditions, body weight loss can be as high as 1.5% per hour, and there have been deaths from overexertion. These deaths are normally avoided by eliminating overstressed animals during the event, and by judging contestants on their ability to control overexertion.

In competitive trial rides (CTRs), contestants travel a specified course and distance within a time limit, and judging is based on the physical condition of the horse during and at the end of the event. In endurance rides, there is also a specified course, but the fastest horse wins, provided it finishes in satisfactory condition. In CTRs the rate of recovery of heart rate and respiration rate during rest periods and at the end of the ride are monitored and used for determining whether a horse can continue. Exhausted horses have extremely shallow and fast breathing and are eliminated. This is an abnormal physiological response for the fit horse, which normally has a large ventilatory reserve. High respiration rates mainly develop when there is exercise-induced hyperthermia. Hypochloraemia from loss of chloride in sweat, hyperkalaemia from release of potassium from muscle and hypoglycaemia may occur.

Thumps are due to electrolyte imbalance, which causes synchronisation of the breathing rhythm with the beat of the heart. Breathing rhythm is controlled by activity in the phrenic nerve which innervates the diaphragm. The phrenic nerve passes alongside the heart, and, if the animal has experienced excessive loss of K^+, Ca^{2+} and Mg^{2+} through the sweat and has elevated levels of lactate from exertion, the phrenic nerve becomes sensitised. The nerve responds to electrical activity in the heart, and there is ephaptic relay of heart-beat signals to the diaphragm via the nerve. The rhythm is seen as twitching in the flank or can be felt by hand as a thumping at the flank. It sometimes gives the impression that the animal has hiccups.

Hyperthermia can be corrected by soaking the neck, chest and legs with water. Excessively rapid cooling can lead to **tying-up**, chilling and shock. Signs of tying-up are refusal to move, limb stiffness when moving, pain from muscle cramps, sweating, pawing at the ground and attempts at rolling, and there are also elevated heart and respiratory rates in response to pain.

6.3 Horse-racing Injuries

Serious **injuries** incurred during horse-racing are referred to as being either fatal or catastrophic. In fatal injuries, the horse dies during the event or has to be euthanased at the track. A catastrophic injury includes fatal injuries as well as those cases where the horse is unable to race again within six months. In a study of 216 race-track injuries in Kentucky, 87% were catastrophic and 43% were euthanased at the track (Cohen *et al.*, 1997). Most (72%) of the injuries occurred when racing conditions were 'fast', and catastrophic injuries were more common during hurdle and steeplechase racing. Male horses were more prone to catastrophic injuries (Table 6.1).

Traumatic disruption of the tendons, ligaments or bones in the lower foreleg is the single most common form of injury (Bowman *et al.*, 1984; Cohen *et al.*, 1997). It results in severe, non-weight-bearing lameness with abnormal dorsoflexion at the fetlock joint. Usually, either the sesamoid ligaments, the third metacarpal, the proximal sesamoid bone or branches of the suspensory ligaments fail (Figure 6.1).

Table 6.1 Fatal injuries during competitive horse-racing (after Bailey *et al.*, 1998).

Type of race	Death rate (deaths/1000 starts)
Flat	0.6
Hurdle	6.3
Steeplechase	14.3

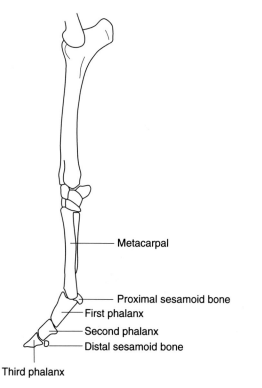

Metacarpal

Proximal sesamoid bone
First phalanx
Second phalanx
Distal sesamoid bone

Third phalanx

Figure 6.1 Bones of the horse's foreleg.

Situations which increase the risk of these injuries include uneven ground, pot-holes, stones, steep camber, slippery conditions, ground that is alternately hard and soft, excessively soft ground causing fatigue and lack of fitness in the horse. When fatigue sets in, the fetlock tends to drop close to the ground, predisposing the ligament or tendon to overstretching. Rupture of a whole tendon causes the fetlock to drop well below its normal position and, typically, the horse is in pain and distress, especially when swelling starts. A light strain in the tendons or ligaments can be detected from the presence of heat and pain on palpation.

Normal tendon repair starts to occur once fibroblasts have accumulated at the injured site. The fibroblasts form new collagen, which at first is laid down in a disorganised manner. Light exercise places strain on that collagen which helps to align the filaments in an appropriate orientation. This exercise has to be gentle, otherwise there is a risk of re-injury.

Concussion injuries can develop in the third carpal bone, the shin and at the hock especially when training on hard ground. Short-term injuries include sesamoiditis and sore shins. The sesamoid bones in the fetlock are subjected to a great deal of strain during training and racing, and they are prone to injury from repeated concussion. Shin soreness is a common problem in young horses, involving inflammation of the periosteum, sometimes with a micro-fracture in the cannon bone. Deformities can develop if there is long-term concussive injury, and these include ringbone, navicular disease, pedal osteitis, sidebone and spavin (Gray, 1994). In trotters, there is a risk of sprain of the plantar ligament of the hock.

All these conditions are painful. Conditions that predispose to them include hard ground on the far side of a fence, inappropriate camber on a turn and trotting on hard tracks. Trotters have a particular gait that affects the lower parts of the legs. A study in Norway showed that 318 out of 753 trotters had osteochondrosis of those joints, and it was an important cause of lameness in this type of horse (Grøndahl & Engeland, 1995).

Abnormal pressure on the spinal nerves can cause **tying-up**. The main complaint is a slight defect in the gait. The pressure usually occurs in the caudal thoracic and lumbar regions, and this can be narrowed to within three vertebrae by examining the horse's spinal reflexes. Normally, when a pencil is stroked along the side of the thorax and abdomen, there is a reflex contraction of the underlying muscle and a localised exaggerated response helps to pinpoint the dermatome which is causing pain (Steel, 1969). The precise point at which spinal nerves are being pinched can then be tested by applying deep pressure over the spine cranial to that dermatome, watching for a painful reaction.

Race-track authorities in various countries are putting more effort into minimising the risks of serious injury during events. A study in the United States indicated that the strongest predictor of injuries was **pre-race physical inspection** of the horses. Abnormalities of the suspensory ligaments were detected in 29% of horses that subsequently developed suspensory apparatus damage during the race

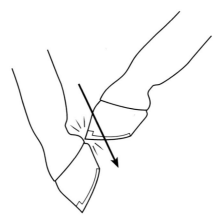

Figure 6.2 Overreaching.

(Cohen *et al.*, 1997). However, this approach is not perfect, as it was found that some horses (about 12%) with ligament abnormality were not injured.

Analysis of videotapes of racing accidents has been helpful in determining events that lead to an injury. A change of lead limb was a common sign of imminent trouble. Stumbling, oblique movement across the track and physical interaction with another horse often preceded an injury because they imposed abnormal mechanical stresses and strains on the ligaments. Injuries were more common in the home stretch, and this coincided with greater **use of the whip**. Whether it was the whip or tiredness that was to blame is not clear. Scientists in Japan claim that the whip could be a predisposing cause, whereas researchers in the USA claim that the whip had a protective effect against injuries (Cohen *et al.*, 1997).

When poorly-performing racehorses were examined after a racing event it was found that the more common injuries developed from overreaching (Figure 6.2), cross-firing, scalping, speedy cutting and interfering (Knight & Evans, 2000). Cross-firing is contact between the inside of the diagonal fore- and hind feet; overreaching is contact between the hind foot and the ipsilateral forefoot; scalping occurs when the toe of the forefoot strikes the ipsilateral hind foot; speedy cutting is a form of overreaching where the outside wall of the hind foot strikes the medial wall of the ipsilateral forefoot; and interfering happens when a moving foot strikes the opposite leg. The degree of banking on bends in the tracks is thought to be important in influencing the incidence of these injuries.

6.4 Greyhound Racing Injuries

It has been said that most racing Greyhounds have toe injury and some degenerative joint disease by the time they are retired. Their build, their desire to run and

Table 6.2 Leg injuries causing lameness in racing Greyhounds.

Main injury sites			
Nearside foreleg	223	*Offside foreleg*	162
Shoulder	52	Shoulder	59
Knee or carpus	23	Knee or carpus	31
Flexor tendons	12	Flexor tendons	9
Toes	136	Toes	63
Nearside hind leg	64	*Offside hind leg*	104
Muscle	22	Muscle	56
Track leg region	20	Track leg region	0
Hock	1*	Hock	31
Toes	23	Toes	17

* resulting from a severe collision

the strains of competitive racing lead to injuries in bones and joints of the feet and the leg muscles that accumulate during their racing career, whereas, in pet dogs most of the bone and muscle injuries are externally induced (Table 6.2).

Bone injuries in Greyhounds often occur on their left side. This is because on most tracks the dogs race anticlockwise. This places greater loading on the nearside limb at the bends. Injuries to the two innermost toes of the left forefoot are particularly common, as this site acts as a pivot on the turns whilst taking much of the weight. Good racing dogs tend to contact the ground with the right forelimb first, and this helps to force the dog into the bend and relieves some of the torsion otherwise placed on the left foot. Dogs with this running pattern are called 'railers'. Non-railers are more prone to fractures of the carpus and tarsus. Being pigeon-toed in the forefeet and splay-footed in the hind legs gives added cornering advantage (Davis, 1967).

Fractures of a solar sesamoid sometimes occur in the paw, and it can be painful when the bone fragment moves out of position or is subjected to direct pressure. The fracture is thought to occur when the running dog springs forward using the forefoot as a lever (Davis *et al.*, 1969). If a dog is forced to stop or change direction suddenly, there is a risk of injury to the stopper pad on the sole of the foot. More common injuries are sprung toes, where the phalangeal joints are dislocated because of rupture of the interconnecting ligaments and fatigue fractures in a metacarpal in the left foot. The risk of dislocation of a phalangeal joint can be reduced by ensuring that the toenails are not too long. Fractures of the accessory bone can occur when the dog is travelling at top speed round a bend. As with racehorses, track maintenance is important in preventing injuries.

It is generally recognised that the faster dogs are more prone to muscle injury. Sometimes the force of contraction in the *triceps brachii, gracilis, gastrocnemius* or *rectus abdominis* muscles causes a fascia to split open, and the belly of the muscle protrudes as a hernia. Sprains occur in the pectoral muscles if the forelimbs splay, and the *infraspinatus* and *supraspinatus* when dogs race on hard ground.

6.5 Migration

Some of the most impressive forms of long-distance exercise are migratory flights in birds. They have to sustain non-stop flights for 50–100 hours when crossing the oceans. During these flights they use body fat as their main energy source. When fat reserves fall to below 5–10% of dry body weight they use body protein stores, in particular breast muscle and proteins in the digestive tract (Schwilch *et al.*, 2002). Flight performance deteriorates once this stage sets in, and the birds' chances of making it decline rapidly. Although body fat is essential for migratory success, excessive body fatness at the start of the journey can be a hindrance for some species.

In many species, the energy needed to complete the journey exceeds the amount of energy that can be stored in their bodies. These species, which include several warblers (*Acrocephalus* sp.), make stopovers to replenish their body reserves, and the success of the overall journey depends on their ability to replenish their energy stores at the stopover sites. Some species fit in a moult during the migration period, whilst others delay the start of migration until the moult has been completed, and this can jeopardise survival if they are insect-feeders and winter comes early. One can only speculate about the suffering that occurs in those birds that fail to make the journey.

Cold

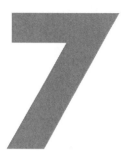

Cold causes suffering when it is prolonged or severe. It causes discomfort, misery, debilitation and in some instances pain. Some easily recognised situations are:

- hypothermia in newborn animals;
- hypothermia in underfed, diseased or sick animals;
- post-shearing mortality in sheep;
- hypothermia during unexpected blizzards;
- cold exposure when adrift in water;
- hypothermia in the extremities under wet conditions;
- frostbite and chilblains;
- reperfusion pain;
- disturbance of hibernation.

7.1 Cold Discomfort and Pain

The **discomfort** associated with cold can range from a chilly feeling that is irritating to cold-induced pain. During immersion in cold water there is initially a period of physical arousal and often excitement. This is followed by a period when the skin becomes livid and pale, blood is centralised to the internal organs, metabolism is slowed and there is limb and body **stiffness**. The rigidity is due to muscle stiffness and increased viscosity of fluids at the joints. Movement of the limbs becomes clumsy, and the extremities are often numb.

Arthritis-like **joint pains** can develop, and in severe cases the muscle rigidity can inhibit breathing. According to reports from Dachau, it was as though the chest was encased in an iron band (Gagge & Herrington, 1947). Breathing is stertorous, expiration is difficult and more prolonged, and there may be foam at the mouth. As body temperature decreases further, the rigidity suddenly ceases and, at this stage, death is usually imminent. Blood pressure and heart rate fail, leading to cerebral ischaemia, somnolence and ultimately coma. Death occurs from heart failure.

In some reports of severe cold exposure there have been early periods of numbness and a sense of intoxication. The subject eventually fell asleep or lapsed into unconsciousness. In other situations, there has been a period of initial discomfort which was related to skin temperature. As hypothermia sets in, the discomfort is more related to deep body temperature and to the gradient between deep body temperature and skin temperature, plus the presence of shivering (Marcus & Belyavin, 1978). Slow chilling can be painless, but pain is more likely with rapid chilling, and to begin with it is often an unbearable pain in the fingers or toes.

The nature of the pain changes as exposure progresses. For example, when a hand is plunged into ice-cold water the pain rises to a maximum in about a minute and thereafter fluctuates in intensity. As the hand cools, it acquires a nauseating ache, combined with paraesthesias, which alter in severity as periods of vasoconstriction alternate with periods of cold vasodilatation. The pain is temporarily relieved during the vasodilatation phase. However, when full circulation is re-established **reperfusion pain** sets in. The nerve fibres responsible for cold pain are particularly resistant to hypoxaemia.

Failure of sensory nerve function during chilling has been studied by cooling the superficial ulnar nerve at the elbow. The first effect was a loss of sensation to light touch and to cold. This was followed by impairment of motor power in the lower arm and hand. Then paralysis of vasoconstrictor nerve fibres set in, and finally there was full analgesia. The ability to feel pain persists for longer than other sensory faculties.

7.2 Skin Freezing and Chilblains

Freezing of the skin causes a pricking sensation which is not particularly painful at the outset (Lewis & Love, 1926). However, if the skin freezes in a draught of cold air, there is a stinging pain. Pain is first felt at the time the skin develops freezing burn (white powder-like surface). At this stage, supercooled water is being transformed to ice, and there is a sudden small rise in skin temperature (Beise *et al.*, 1998).

When thawing begins, the area surrounding the frozen skin develops a bright red flush, and an inflammatory response develops, with itchiness. The area becomes hyperalgesic without spontaneous pain. If the skin was frozen for a long period, a prominent wheal, which may develop into a blister, forms. Blistering can be associated with hair or claw loss, and in humans there is a severe burning pain. In time the wheal subsides leaving an area of skin which is tender for four to five days. If subcutaneous oedema occurs from freezing or severe chilling, the swelling in the region can be painful when it is rewarmed. Pain can be a sequel to cryosurgery of the skin (Zouboulis, 1998).

In **freeze branding**, the aim is to destroy the melanocytes in the skin that are responsible for hair pigmentation. The injured area produces white hair instead.

If the animal has a light-coloured coat, the usual procedure is to apply the freeze branding iron for longer. This causes more intense freezing and necrosis of the follicles, leaving a hairless brand mark. When the iron is applied, the skin is indented and frozen in the shape of the brand. Within a few minutes of removing the iron, the skin warms up and there is marked reddening followed by swelling of the skin. If the subcutaneous tissues freeze as well as the skin, blood clots form in the subcutaneous vessels, and on thawing the tissue becomes necrotic. During the following weeks, hair and necrotic skin peel off leaving a legible mark, and, from six to ten weeks, white hair growth is evident. Freeze branding causes less severe damage to the skin than hot-iron branding. Both procedures cause pain. Hot-iron branding is painful initially whereas freeze branding causes a delayed pain.

In **frostbite** the skin does not actually freeze. Instead there is a gradual cooling of the affected part and a painful tingling sensation (Lorrain-Smith *et al.*, 1915). The pain gives way to numbness, discomfort, inability to move and a heavy feeling in the affected regions. The frostbite can vary considerably in appearance, from a mild redness to black, dry tissue. An aching burning pain becomes noticeable during recovery when sensation starts to return. If gangrene sets in, there will be pain in the early stages if the part is touched, especially proximal to the gangrene.

Immersion foot is the name given to a mild form of frostbite that develops when the foot is immersed for long periods in cold (e.g. 5°C) wet mud, snow or water whilst there is limited movement or exercise. It is a vasoneuropathy which is accompanied by swelling of the feet, and the colour in the skin changes from an initial redness to a pale sickly yellow, followed by a blue or black mottling. In the rabbit, the fur on the foot protects the animal from developing immersion foot when kept in cold wet mud. Without that fur, oedema develops in the subcutaneous connective tissue from impaired venous drainage, there is secondary deposition of fibrin and eventually collagen breakdown. The animals show obvious signs of reperfusion pain when the feet are warmed up. In humans this takes the form of severe aching, throbbing pains in the swollen regions, interspersed with shooting pains that feel like sharp stabs (Ungley & Blackwood, 1942). These pains are accompanied by allodynia and may be worse at night or when warmth is applied. If gangrene occurs it is superficial, whereas with frostbite it is deep.

Chilblains are caused by sudden external warming of cold tissues, which increases metabolism of the tissues before perfusion by the bloodstream has been reinstated. There is a localised oxygen deficit coupled with inadequate removal of end products of metabolism, which causes tissue necrosis.

7.3 Hypothermia

When environmental temperature drops below the animal's **lower critical temperature** (LCT) it experiences cold stress, and metabolic heat production is increased

Table 7.1 Lower critical temperature (LCT) and the increase in heat production per degree fall in temperature below the LCT (ΔHp) in sheep.

Life stage	LCT (°C)	ΔHp (W/m²/°C)
Newborn lamb	27	4.8
Growing lamb	4	2.5
Ewe late pregnancy (shorn)	2	2.9
Ewe lactating (shorn)	–8	2.9
Ewe late pregnancy (not shorn)	–46	1.2
Ewe lactating (not shorn)	–70	1.2

to maintain body temperature. Table 7.1 shows the lower critical temperatures for different types of sheep, and it emphasises the susceptibility of the newborn lamb compared with the adult ewe. The table also shows the extra heat that the animal produces for every degree that the temperature falls below the animal's LCT, and it is clear that energetically the newborn lamb is particularly disadvantaged. The newborn calf is in a better position, as its LCT is about 8°C.

7.4 Sensitivity to Cold

Animals and humans are particularly sensitive to cold when they are ill. Sensitivity to cold is also influenced by previous experience or acclimation, and exercise can offset some of the cold-induced discomfort of hypothermia, independently of any effect of the exercise on body temperature. Instead, it is partly psychological (Marcus & Redman, 1979). Excessive exercise during hypothermia can, however, result in bronchial haemorrhages.

Some people are able to shiver in their sleep. This allows them to maintain body heat production without disturbing the sleep pattern. When an animal shivers, it often starts as a shudder during inspiration. The primary motor centre in the caudal hypothalamus then takes control and a more persistent shivering sets in. **Shivering** also occurs during recovery from anaesthesia because of disturbance in the central control of this behaviour, and not necessarily related to cold perception or a low body temperature. Adrenaline can also induce shivering, and this combination is seen following trauma or during fear. When animals emerge from hibernation there is often violent shivering.

7.5 Hypothermia and Cold Survival

In most domesticated mammals, if core body temperature falls by more than 2°C coordinated movements start to deteriorate, physiological functions are affected

Table 7.2 Degrees of hypothermia.

Degree of hypothermia	Core body temperature (°C)
Mild	32–35
Moderate	28–32
Severe	20–28
Profound	14–20
Deep	<14

and there is a risk of loss of consciousness. Hypothermia of more than 5°C can result in death. However, some wild birds and mammals can maintain normal activity and withstand body temperature falls of 14°C. In humans, hypothermia is defined as a core temperature below 35°C, and this definition suits many other mammals. The degrees of hypothermia are shown in Table 7.2.

Death during hypothermia is usually from cardiac arrest. At 32°C, cardiac conduction disturbances become apparent, and at 28°C serious dysrhythmias occur (Gentilello, 1995). Below 28°C, heat production and conservation mechanisms fail and at 20°C the heart is likely to stop beating. The chance of surviving a period of **cardiac standstill** varies with species. For example, rabbits are less likely to survive than hamsters.

Provided the cold episode is not too long, there should not be any lasting neurological disturbances (Smith, 1959). When people have experienced immersion in water at 1°C, death usually occurred if the exposure lasted for 60 minutes, but exceptional cases survived four hours' exposure (Gagge & Herrington, 1947). There was a well-publicised case of a two-and-a-half-year-old girl who fell into a creek near Salt Lake City and survived complete submersion in 5°C water for over 66 minutes. Her rectal temperature fell to 19°C. During severe cooling, the lungs remain functional whilst heart activity is suppressed, and there is greater reliance on anaerobic metabolism.

Some examples of species variation in resistance to cold are shown in Table 7.3. The insulation provided by fur or feathers contributes to this variation. The importance of feather insulation was demonstrated in a study where feathered pigeons survived fasting at −40°C for 2 to 6 days, whereas featherless pigeons died within 20–30 minutes.

Life under Antarctic and Arctic conditions requires special survival features. Polar bear cubs (*Ursus maritimus*) would normally die within two hours of being exposed to −45°C that occurs in the far north. They are born in a relatively under-developed short-furred state, and depend on sharing body warmth with the mother in a snow den. The den, which is dug out by the mother shortly before parturition, stays at or slightly above 0°C. Semi-aquatic mammals such as the polar bear depend on an **underfur** which retains water as a stagnant layer to withstand chilling by water. In harp seals this water layer is about 2 mm thick, and in polar bears

Table 7.3 The lowest ambient temperature at which selected species can maintain normal body temperature for one hour.

Species	°C
Duck	−100
Goose	−90
Pigeon	−85
Rabbit	−45
Rat	−25
Guinea Pig	−15

10 mm. Fish adapt to seasonal cold with cellular changes in membrane fluidity, enzyme activity and the substrates used in providing energy.

If a newborn animal, such as a rodent pup, which lacks fur and subcutaneous fat, cannot see or hear and has limited thermoregulatory and locomotor ability, is separated from the nest, it will cool rapidly. This is dangerous, and an unusual defence mechanism has evolved to protect against this hazard. By reflex, its laryngeal fold constricts. This causes air that is exhaled under pressure to produce an involuntary ultrasound noise of about 40 kHz. The mother is particularly responsive to this ultrasound call and it allows her to rescue the pup without alerting predators.

When a chick gets cold it shuts down its heat production and its respiration. This increases its chance of survival by conserving energy and oxygen. The young chick that falls to the ground from its nest in a tree soon becomes hypothermic. Seemingly-dead chicks found in this situation have revived when re-warmed.

The risk of mortality from cold exposure is greatly increased if there has also been trauma or if the animal is diseased. For example, cold stress was found to increase mortality from encephalitis in mice infected with West Nile virus, by reducing lymphoid organ function and increasing the levels of the virus in the brain and spleen (Ben-Nathan & Fenerstein, 1990). In general, when cold stress is sufficient to cause weight loss, the animal's immune responses are likely to be compromised.

7.6 Cold in Combination with Starvation

Starvation adds to the misery of hypothermia. There are the conflicting demands of using more energy to keep warm, sparing energy reserves for extending survival and expending energy in obtaining feed. These balances are critical in the newborn, which, under cold conditions, is prone to rapidly-developing hypothermia, especially if it does not obtain an early feed when it is born. When resuscitating a comatose hypothermic newborn animal the procedures that should be followed are

Table 7.4 Estimated net energy costs of daily activities to cows grazing winter range.

Activity	Mean daily range ± sd	Energy expenditure (kcal)	% of total activity cost (%)
Grazing	9.5 ± 0.6 hours	2525	59
Standing	1.7 ± 0.9 hours	88	2
Ruminating	8.9 ± 1.0 hours	725	17
Walking	6.3 ± 2.1 km	965	22
Lying	12.2 ± 0.9 hours	–	–

first to dry the animal, then to feed it by stomach tube or by intraperitoneal injection of glucose, and then to warm it gradually. If the animal is warmed abruptly before receiving a supply of energy from milk or glucose, and if it is still wet when it is warmed, it is likely to die from shock.

Under winter range conditions, when mean daily air temperature ranged from −24 to +5°C, beef cows have focussed their behaviour on heat conservation at the expense of feeding, even when consuming sub-maintenance amounts of feed. On cold days they spent more time standing whereas on warmer days they were foraging (Malechek & Smith, 1976). Distance travelled each day was inversely related to wind speed. This strategy of forgoing feed is not as drastic as might be imagined (Table 7.4). The energy saved from not walking and not grazing can be substantial, but the added discomfort or lack of satisfaction from not feeding would presumably be strong.

Birds of prey, such as the barn owl (*Tyto alba*), undergo prolonged periods of fasting during the winter because of food scarcity, and there can be high mortalities during severe winters. Other raptors, such as the snowy owl, adapt by lowering their body temperature by as much as 8°C when fasting during the winter.

Snow makes feeding difficult for grazing species. Feral horses manage this by moving to the edge of woodland or exposed areas where snow depth is less, and by pawing or pushing the snow away with the muzzle.

7.7 Cold-induced Analgesia

The deep body temperature at which **cold narcosis** develops varies with species. As the body cools, there is progressive loss of voluntary and reflex activity, with cerebral functions disappearing first and reappearing last on re-warming (Smith, 1958). The effect on brain function is due to a combination of chilling, reduced blood flow to the brain and reduced intracranial pressure.

The peripheral numbness that develops during prolonged cooling is due to failure in afferent neurotransmission. In the cat's sciatic nerve, conduction completely fails at temperatures below 8°C, and at 8–15°C action potentials are reduced. This blockade of sensory activity is the basis for **refrigeration surgery**, which has been used when amputating limbs during wartime. Blood flow to a limb is arrested with a tourniquet and the limb is then chilled for about three hours with ice or snow packs (Mock, 1943). At this stage the sciatic nerve can be picked up and crushed with artery forceps and then cut without any sense of pain. Amputation of the limb can follow. Cold-induced loss of afferent signals also probably explains why rapid freezing of tissues is a relatively painless experience, at least until thawing sets in. Amphibians can show neural responses at temperatures well below 8°C, and so refrigeration analgesia is less likely to provide a surgical plane of analgesia. Natural hibernation does not produce a surgical plane of analgesia, unlike refrigeration analgesia.

In reptiles, hypothermia used to be recommended as a restraining method for general surgery. However, necrotic changes have been reported in the brains of snakes and turtles following hypothermia, and anaesthetics have replaced hypothermia as the preferred method of restraint.

Heat and Burns

8

Excessive heat is an obvious cause of suffering in the following situations:

- when an animal has difficulty with thermoregulation;
- exercise in combination with heat exposure;
- sunstroke;
- burns and scalds;
- heat-induced pain.

It is particularly unpleasant when accompanied by pain or dehydration.

Heat stress is common in arid parts of Australia and Africa. In the central outback of South Australia and the Northern Territory, air temperature in the shade rises above 50°C, and sand temperatures of 84°C have been reported. It has been estimated that the radiant heat load absorbed per day by a 10 m × 20 m piece of ground can be equivalent to the energy of one of the early nuclear bombs. The heat loads are immense, and there is a strong risk of death from heat stress in unprotected animals.

8.1 Heat Stress

The initial feelings in humans accompanying sunstroke are a sudden languor especially if fatigued by exercise. Often the head feels as if it is burning hot, and the face can become dark and swollen. Breathing may be painful, and the feet and hands seem cool. There may be a headache or dizziness, which, as heat exposure gets progressively worse, is replaced by delirium, convulsions and then coma.

Besides the discomfort of hyperthermia, heat stress can lead to:

- diarrhoea;
- tachycardia and increased cardiac output;

- increased susceptibility to infections, and in particular to respiratory tract infections. This may be partly due to increased interleukin-6 release, which normally reduces immune responses by controlling the levels of other cytokines;
- shunting of blood away from the viscera and towards skin and muscle. If this leads to gut ischaemia, the gut wall may become more permeable to endotoxins present in the digestive fluids, and an endotoxaemia may develop. An endotoxaemia can compromise the hyperthermia further by causing a fever;
- production of heat shock proteins that induce a transient state of tolerance to the cytotoxic effect of further heating;
- reduced lactation;
- reduced foetal growth, abortions and embryo resorption;
- teratogenic effects such as limb deformities and retarded CNS development, including hydranencephaly.

If heat stress is superimposed on dehydration, the human or animal has the conflicting needs to dilate its peripheral blood vessels to allow heat dissipation, and vasoconstriction to compensate for lowered blood volume. If vasodilatation does occur, there is a risk that blood pressure will collapse and the subject will faint. In humans, **heatstroke** that develops in this way has been known to cause lasting mental debilitation from cerebral hyperthermia. If the subject is exercising at the time of heat stroke, there is often a respiratory alkalosis plus lactic acidosis, whereas in non-exertional stroke there is a respiratory alkalosis. Heat stroke often coincides with an intravascular coagulopathy, which can be fatal.

In humans and pigs, if skin temperature rises to 47°C, there is complete epidermal necrosis within 35 minutes. Death from being trapped in conditions as hot as this can be rapid. It has been estimated that fatal exposure for a dog trapped in a car that is parked in the sun can be as little as 20 minutes (Gregory & Constantine, 1996).

8.2 Heat Intolerance

Some subjects have a low **heat tolerance**. This is due to one of four types of physiological reaction:

(1) *Insensitivity to adrenaline* In the horse, sweating is activated by adrenaline, and it is obvious from the patches of dampness on the skin and from tracks that appear on the skin over the lymphatic vessels. If a horse is exercised when it has developed sweat-gland insensitivity to adrenaline, death can occur from hyperthermia (Evans, 1966). This has happened when racehorses have been transferred from a temperate to a tropical climate for a competition.

(2) *Adrenal exhaustion* This is similar to insensitivity to adrenaline, but is due to catecholamine deficiency rather than insensitivity. Previous heat exposure

depletes the adrenal medulla of its reserves of adrenaline, and, when a fresh challenge occurs, the subject cannot cope. In humans, the signs are hypotension, fatigue, exhaustion, apathy, depression, lack of concentration, confusion, hypoglycaemia and ataxia (Sulman *et al.*, 1977).

(3) *Serotonin overproduction* Subjects that release excessive amounts of serotonin under hot conditions can be irritable or aggressive, and develop sleep disturbances, headaches, tension, palpitations, nausea, vomiting, anorexia, dyspnoea, flushes, with sweat or chills, vertigo, tremor and polyuria.

(4) *Intermittent hyperthyroidism* Many of the signs are similar to those in serotonin overproduction, but there are, in addition, over-activity, diarrhoea, increased appetite, weight loss and skin reactions.

8.3 Some Species Differences

Animals that are heavily insulated by fur or fat can have problems with dissipating excess heat. The **whale** manages this through a series of rete in its flukes and flippers, which act as heat exchangers between its bloodstream and the sea. The well-insulated **pig** with its thick layer of subcutaneous fat depends on seeking shade and wallowing to keep cool. It does not sweat, except at the end of its nose, which develops beads of sweat when it gets hot. At about 38.5°C the pig becomes drowsy, and open-mouthed panting sets in when rectal temperature reaches 39.2°C. Above this point there is a lot of salivation, and the animal can lose as much as half a litre as dribble falling from its mouth per hour. The frequency of the panting can climb to 280 breaths per minute, but heart rate does not usually exceed 100 beats per minute. Breathing becomes laboured when rectal temperature reaches 41.1°C, the pig is very restless, and if water is provided it drinks avidly and endeavours to roll in spilt water. It cannot survive rectal temperatures much higher than 41.6°C.

Physiologically, **dogs** are also relatively sensitive to heat stress, and rely on panting and drinking to keep cool. Open-mouthed panting starts at a relatively low temperature, often within the normal body temperature range. This is followed by salivation and the tongue hangs out of the mouth. When rectal temperature reaches 40.5°C, equilibrium starts to break down and uncontrolled hyperpyrexia may develop. The dog starts to bark and becomes excited, and at 42.8°C it becomes ataxic, the abdomen may be swollen from swallowing too much air, and the dog is likely to collapse. Access to drinking water can be critical for survival.

Sweating is an important method of heat loss for **cattle**. Sweating is provoked by autonomic nervous activity. In general, newborn calves are more heat tolerant because they sweat more than older cattle (Bianca & Hales, 1970). Calves that sweat least tend to pant the most, and calves that are inherently unable to sweat are seriously compromised during heat stress. Advanced cases of heat stress have been found sitting in sternal recumbency with the head lolling on the ground, tongue protruding whilst panting rapidly, and seemingly unaware of what is going on about them (McQueen, 1972). Dairy cows are reluctant to drink water that is warmer than 28°C, and this can compromise thermoregulation (Stermer *et al.*, 1986).

Sheep rely on taking shade to get out of the glare of the sun and panting for keeping cool. Thermal discomfort is thought to occur once rectal temperature exceeds 40.5°C (Lowe *et al.*, 2002). In the absence of exercise, catecholamine secretion does not increase until rectal temperature exceeds 42°C, by which time the sheep may be *in extremis*. In hot sunny climates, underfeeding and shearing reduce heat tolerance. This is an unfortunate combination, as in practice shearing is often done at the beginning of the hot season when undernutrition can occur if there is a drought.

The **cat** has a limited ability to sweat, most of the sweat glands being in the paws. Its fur also limits radiant, conductive and convective heat loss. Instead, it depends on evaporative heat loss through panting. At first the panting is through the nose, but when rectal temperature approaches 39.4°C, it breaks into open-mouthed panting. It may also spread saliva on its fur to encourage evaporative heat loss from its coat, and this increases the demand for drinking water.

Unlike the cat, the **rabbit** does not lick its fur when it gets excessively hot. It lies outstretched, dribbles and pants, and panting rates of 700 breaths per minute have been recorded. It is obviously distressed when rectal temperature reaches 41.5°C, but it can still stand and carry out normal movements.

Chickens rely on drinking and panting to relieve hyperthermia. They also spread their wings to increase their effective radiating surface and to expose the less densely-feathered parts of the body. They do not sweat. Panting is not particularly efficient in controlling temperature rise, because the evaporative surface in the upper respiratory tract is limited in size. Instead, they depend on drinking. The water settles in the crop which lies against the carotid arteries, and so it cools blood flowing to the brain. In addition, they may dip their heads in open water if it is available. Keeping the head cool, seems to be a priority and a preoccupation. Their normal body temperature is higher than that of most mammals, and the upper temperature they tolerate is correspondingly higher. The terminal stages are obvious from ataxia, deep sighing breathing and collapse.

8.4 Pain

Heat and pain have separate neural pathways. Very brief stimulation with a hot object can give rise to pain without recognition that it was hot. If the contact is maintained and the warmth is detected, the experience becomes recognisable as heat pain. Heat, or 'burning', pain, however, is not solely due to a high temperature. It can occur with other types of stimuli, such as solid carbon dioxide.

The pain associated with burns is often a continuous pain. This was vividly described by Lewis and Hess (1933) when they applied molten wax to their own skin. The burn produced slight blistering, and there was an interval of 10–60 seconds or more before they began to feel any pain. The pain developed gradually and continued for an hour or more. Its intensity was continuous, but there was also a slow fluctuation above a background pitch. The threshold for continuous thermal pain and for thermal injury of the skin were approximately the same (45°C). However, thermal injury was more dependent on the duration of exposure at the critical temperature. Severe burns developed a tenderness that lasted for days.

The pain threshold for heat pain in humans usually lies at 43–47°C skin temperature. There have been reports of pain sensation at skin temperatures below this range, but they were very brief, wearing off in two to six seconds (Hardy & Stolwijk, 1966). The pain threshold may be higher in some animals. In the sheep's ear, it is usually 52–56°C.

8.5 Burns and Scalds

Burns can be caused by flames of a fire, contact with hot materials such as ash, branding irons, scalding water, corrosive chemicals or by electricity, lasers and radiation. Death in burns victims can develop from temperature-induced brain or heart failure, hypovolaemic shock, acute renal failure, metabolic wasting or infection.

Burns are produced intentionally during hot-iron tail docking, with disbudding horns, hot-iron branding, firing in horses and Greyhounds and beak trimming. In Australia, mouse plagues are sometimes controlled by burning them en masse with flame-throwing equipment. In addition, cauteries are used routinely under anaesthesia during surgery for removing growths. When a **hot-iron brand** was applied to the hindquarters of calm dairy cows held in a headbail, the animals reacted by jumping away and kicking at the person applying the branding iron. With freeze branding, the typical response is lowering of the back and alternate movement of the hind legs, without kicking. Hot-iron branding caused an increase in plasma cortisol, and the initial heart rate rise was greater than with freeze branding (Lay et al., 1992). There was no vocalising with either hot iron or freeze branding. These physiological changes suggested that the initial effects of hot iron branding were more unpleasant than those of freeze branding.

Accidental burns occur during **bush fires** and barn fires. Wildlife is inevitably caught up in bush fires. The animals that are most affected are snakes, young rabbits, rodent pups and ground-nesting chicks. During the fire, adult mice often shelter underground in holes, whilst some lizards escape by climbing trees. The season when the fires occur is critical. If they occur during the nesting and brooding season losses will be high. It has been estimated that during a planned prairie regeneration fire in Omaha up to 522 young western harvest mice were burned alive and 38 ring-necked pheasant nests containing a total of 336 eggs were destroyed within a 23 hectare area. A young cottontail rabbit was found afterwards, badly burned and screaming (Erwin & Stasiak, 1979).

When sheep have been caught in bush fires the wool has helped to protect them from burns. The worst affected areas have often been the bare areas of the belly, crutch, legs and sternum, but in recently-shorn animals the damage is more extensive. From experience in South Australia it has been concluded that burns to the feet alone were not as serious in terms of survival as they might first appear. They could be treated even when the hooves were shedding, simply by providing a soft paddock and access to feed and water without the need for too much walking (Willson, 1966). Salvage or culling was recommended where there were any of the following signs: burnt udder, teats, vulva or pizzle in breeding sheep; third-degree burns or oedema under the body, in the axilla and inguinal areas; and severe burns to the eyelids and/or lips. Dairy cows were prone to burns on the udder and teats. The skin in this region is relatively thick and so it tended to turn black and hard, but weeping of plasma was not pronounced. After a few days, the skin became leathery, cracked and started to slough. The animal should be slaughtered before this stage. If it is allowed to go further there is a chance that the teat orifices become occluded as the skin heals.

Barn fires are a particular hazard in broiler-chicken farms because of the combustible wooden construction and litter, and because the birds are not inclined to move when the doors are opened to allow them to escape. Once a fire starts, it is difficult to control. In most cases the birds probably die from lack of air and smoke inhalation. In survivors, leg and foot damage is to be expected if the bedding caught fire.

In the Arabian Peninsula, North Africa, India and Pakistan, fire branding is a traditional way of treating certain animal diseases and disorders (Manefield & Tinson, 1996). Various burn patterns can be seen in camels between the head and tail as part of the therapy system. Severe cases of periostitis in the metacarpal bone have been known when the burns have been applied too deeply, and reduced flexion of joints from subsequent fibrous reactions has restricted mobility in other cases.

The initial effects of burning are unquestionably painful. However, the lasting experience of **pain** depends on the depth of the burn. When there has been a full-thickness skin burn there is seldom any complaint of pain in humans, because the nerves in the skin have been destroyed (Muir et al., 1987). Pain perception can be present in partial-thickness burns, and this can be tested by pricking with a sterile pin or needle through to the subcutaneous fat. This type of burn can lead to insomnia, and the subject may be hyperactive or even manic. Burn patients have an elevated metabolic rate (Wilmore et al., 1975), and in some cases their hyperactivity could be due to distress associated with their hyperthermia. Morphine provides pain relief and acts as an anxiolytic.

Table 8.1 Clinical features of partial and full thickness burns.

Depth	Colour*	Blisters	Capillary refill	Pain following the burn
Superficial, partial thickness	Pink	±	Present	Present
Deep, partial thickness	Red/pale	±	Absent	±
Full thickness	White	Absent	Absent	Absent

* in non-pigmented skin. ± can be present or absent.

Table 8.2 Four degrees of tissue burning.

Degree of burning	Tissue appearance
First	Hyperaemia and redness
Second	Hyperaemia and blistering
Third	Necrosis of the skin layer
Fourth	Charring and blackening

Both the depth and the area of a burn are important in terms of survival and recovery of a body part. In terms of the depth of a burn, there are three **degrees of burning** (Table 8.1). Partial thickness burns can be recognised from local erythema, oedema and exudation, as well as painful responses to pressure. In partial thickness burns the hair cannot usually be pulled out, whereas hair comes away in full thickness burns.

In terms of overall tissue-damage, there are four degrees of burning (Table 8.2). These are also helpful in diagnosing the severity of a burn, but they need to be considered with the depth and the size of the burn (Table 8.1).

Skin burns can lead to **dehydration**. If the epidermis blisters and is removed, the evaporation rate from the surface increases about eightfold. The size of the area of a burn is of course critical in influencing the total amount of fluid loss. When more than 10% of the body surface area is affected, the animal should receive prompt intravenous fluid therapy. The single best indicator of the adequacy of the fluid therapy is the subsequent output of urine. Most animals die within ten days if the burns exceed 50% of the surface area.

The physiological events leading to **fluid loss** from burnt tissue are as follows: the polymorphonuclear leukocytes, mast cells and endothelial cells initiate an inflammatory response at or near the site of a burn. In the early stages, histamine released from mast cells is largely responsible for the oedema and plasma-protein leakage from the wound. Kinins assist vasodilatation and stimulate pain if nerve receptors are not damaged. Leukocyte and platelet recruitment results in prostaglandin release, which also increases capillary permeability, and vasodilatation is reinforced by nitrous oxide release from endothelium. Vasodilatation occurs in the undamaged tissue around the burnt areas and there is intense hyperaemia. Plasma escapes from the bloodstream into tissues near the burn and leaks onto the surface to form blisters or a weeping wound. The weeping can persist for up to 36 hours, and, if the flow is not arrested or compensated for, there is a strong risk of circulatory collapse.

This gives rise to secondary shock, which is called **burn shock**. The plasma leakage also causes haemoconcentration, at first locally, but later generally. There is a feeling of 'slow burning' near the wound, and intense thirst. The more severe the burn, the higher the rate of fluid loss, and the greater the fall in blood volume. If there is muscle injury, myoglobin is released into the circulation, and is subsequently excreted in the urine. Urinary myoglobin output is directly related to the degree and, in particular the depth, of muscle injury from the burn.

In severe cases of hypotension, renal perfusion may collapse and sustained hypoxia results in kidney cell damage. If there is hypoxia from secondary vasoconstriction in the gut wall, fluid absorption from the intestines will be impaired. The subject, by this time has a keen thirst, but attempts at drinking may result in vomiting. A vicious cycle is set up in which the defence mechanism which is helping to compensate for the fall in blood volume is instrumental in preventing the subject from restoring blood volume by absorption from the gut (Muir *et al.*, 1987). Anaemia can also set in, because of direct destruction of red blood cells.

Besides drinking more fluid, there are two other compensatory mechanisms for the oligaemia (reduced blood volume) associated with burns:

(1)   Fluid shifts from the extracellular space in undamaged parts, secondary to an osmotic gradient.
(2)   There is vasoconstriction of the splanchnic bed and the skin, under the influence of circulating catecholamines and the renin-angiotensin system.

Two methods may be used to check or control the weeping from the wound. Pressure can be applied over the surface, or the surface may be coagulated chemically with a protein denaturing agent. However, if a denaturant is used, there can be a risk of absorption of the chemical leading to liver damage.

Burns can lead to death in four ways:

(1)   *Primary shock* This is cardiogenic shock, with a lowered blood pressure and a weak fast pulse. The subject is cold but may be sweating, and fear increases the shock effect.
(2)   *Secondary shock* This is hypovolaemic shock due to loss of plasma as exudate from burnt surfaces. This is the most common cause of burn deaths, and can occur within two hours of the injury.
(3)   *Toxaemia* Pathogens or toxins may be absorbed by the burnt area leading to septicaemia and eventually death.

(4) *Failure to eat and drink* Burns to the muzzle affect the animal's ability to eat and drink, and, during a bush or grass fire, the legs, feet and belly are burnt, making walking and foraging more difficult.

People with major burn injuries have substantial suppression of their cellular immune system, including lowered lymphocyte blastogenic responses, defects in mononuclear phagocyte and polymorphonuclear leucocyte function, increased T-cell suppressor activity, impaired IL-2 synthesis and reduced activity of granulo-cyte macrophage colony-stimulating factor (Molloy *et al.*, 1995). This is helpful in allowing successful skin grafts, but is a menace in terms of the risk of infection.

There is a high risk of infection in burn wounds if they are not managed appropriately. In severe cases this can lead to septicaemia. The signs associated with septicaemia include anorexia, reluctance to drink, mild confusion and disorientation and fluctuations in body temperature, white cell count and blood glucose. There may be rapid development of septic shock accompanied by hypothermia and hypotension. There is increased risk of spontaneous abortion in pregnant animals that experience burns.

One sometimes hears of animals maliciously being set alight with **burning petrol**. Burns produced by petrol are often extensive and deep. The petrol soaks into the animal's coat, and once alight it is difficult to extinguish. In hairless animals and humans the exposure to heat is short lasting, but it may be long enough to destroy the thinner skin in exposed parts. Incendiary devices such as flame-throwers and incendiary bombs, not only burn the animals alive, but the gases that are released are liable to produce lung lesions resembling corrosive bronchitis in those that survive. The chemicals in the gases cause extensive oedema, and, in wartime incidents in humans, it has been known for the face to swell to two or three times its normal size.

If the flame or hot gases reach the larynx and upper trachea, airway obstruction due to laryngeal oedema is inevitable. The oedema can compromise the patency of the airway, and lead to poor oxygenation. In cases of smoke inhalation, respiratory complications may not be seen straight away. Chemical toxicants in the smoke, together with soot, adhere firmly to the mucosal layer of air passages. The toxic agents can include P_2O_5, SO_2, NO_2, acrolein, formaldehyde and acetaldehyde, and, in the presence of water, they form corrosive acids and alkalis which damage the mucosa and are toxic when absorbed (Chu, 1981). Laryngitis, tracheitis, bronchopneumonia and pulmonary oedema may be delayed by four to eight days. A disseminated intravascular coagulopathy can also accompany severe burns.

Electrical burns are partly due to the heating effect of the current, but there is additional damage from electroporation. Electroporation is a form of cell-membrane breakdown, probably due to perforation at the entry and exit sites. At the time of an electrical burn, there can be puckered circular or punctate marks depending on the shape or form of the electrode that was applied. Histological examination of the fresh burn can be used to distinguish electrical from thermal injury in skin. If the current tracks along blood vessels, thromboses can develop. In practice, the severity of an injury depends on the voltage, skin thickness and wetness, and the duration of contact. In accidents involving very high voltages, part of a limb may be lost, with the edges of the wound flared, giving the impression of an internal explosive effect.

Lasers are used in a number of surgical procedures for cauterising tissue. The severity of laser burns depends on the wavelength of the laser emission, power, duration of exposure, direction of the beam and skin colour. Most lasers heat from the outside, penetrating inwards. They vaporise and coagulate the skin or surface tissue. Carbon dioxide lasers produce a sharp pricking burn. Argon lasers are more likely to create spreading damage with scarring, whereas tuneable dye lasers can be set to deliver a selected wavelength for a limited duration, so the damage is much more controlled.

Chemical burns are not common in animals. Dogs that have been exposed to caustic chemicals tend to lick their feet if they are irritated, and this can cause mouth and muzzle burns. It has been known for their toes to be corroded to the bone from treading in caustic chemicals. Ducks and swans have been known to ingest phosphorus from the sediment of contaminated lakes on an artillery training range (Racine *et al.*, 1992), and during World War II horses and cattle died from eating phosphorus-contaminated pasture. The horses died within 24 hours of showing signs of renal colic (Blount, 1944). Other chemicals that cause burns and have been used during wartime include dichlorodiethylsulphide (mustard gas), lewisite and cordite. Mustard gas and lewisite cause irritation and burns that blister. When inhaled, mustard gas causes necrosis of the respiratory mucosa, which, if not immediately fatal, can be followed by pneumonia, abscess or gangrene of the lungs.

At one time caustic soda mixed into molasses was used for killing rats. It was spread on a board which was placed in their normal path. The sticky paste stuck to their feet. The rat then licked its feet, and death was from the internal burns. In New Zealand, a **chemical branding** compound based on potassium hydroxide and barium sulphite was used for branding livestock. Potassium hydroxide is still used to cauterise horn buds in calves, but this carries a risk of inflicting chemical skin burns in other calves in the same pen, and the fluid has been known to get into the calves' eyes. It is used because it is a highly convenient disbudding method, but is falling from favour because of these hazards. Phenols and cresols have been trialled as an alternative to surgical methods for mulesing sheep (Morley, 1949). Again, great care is needed in handling, applying and avoiding the spread of the chemical. Chemical mulesing with quaternary ammonium compounds has been compared with the surgical method in terms of the plasma cortisol response, and the conclusion was that the quat' caused a delayed discomfort and pain, but whether or not it is more protracted is not certain (Chapman *et al.*, 1994).

Asphalt tar, used in road surfacing, is heated to about 230°C to keep it liquid. If the liquid tar is spilled or poured on skin, it rapidly cools, but the retained heat is sufficient to produce a second-degree burn. Removal of the tar once it has set can be very difficult especially when it has congealed with hair or feathers. Organic solvents have to be used.

The main cause of **sunburn** is ultraviolet radiation of wavelengths 290–320 nm (ultraviolet B). The short-term response is a transient erythema and increased dermal vascular permeability. This is followed by a more persistent erythema which starts about four hours after the exposure, and may last for 24 hours. In extreme cases, there are oedema and blistering in the skin, destruction of the superficial sebaceous glands and the distal portion of the sweat glands and there may be fever.

Sunburn is a significant problem in recently-shorn sheep, pigs kept outdoors, and in livestock that have a photosensitisation disorder such as facial eczema. In some situations squamous cell carcinomas can develop, for example in the vulva of short-tailed mulesed sheep (Vandegraaff, 1976). These tumours rarely develop in sheep if the tails have been docked so that they cover the perineal region. The risk of sunburn in chemically defleeced sheep has been a hazard that has checked the development of this method as an alternative to manual shearing (Chapman et al., 1984).

Thirst and Hunger

This chapter considers the disorders and suffering associated with thirst, overhydration, osmotic stress, hunger, underfeeding, force-feeding and overeating.

9.1 Thirst and Dehydration

Thirst is a very strong drive, and a powerful form of suffering. There is a **dry-mouth sensation,** a longing for a drink, and the dehydration ultimately leads to dizziness and collapse. The dry-mouth sensation contributes to the sense of thirst, along with osmoreceptor activation in the circumventricular organs of the brain and sodium sensors within the blood–brain barrier. When thirst is not satisfied, it dominates our thoughts and behaviour, and we put great effort into getting a drink. If it cannot be satisfied, we despair and lose self-control. The conscious perception of thirst probably emanates from the posterior cingulate cortex of the brain (Denton *et al.*, 1999).

The importance of dry-mouth sensations may be different for ruminants. This is because they produce saliva even when they are dehydrated and thirsty. Presumably osmoreceptors and sodium sensors play a more important role than dry-mouth sensations in initiating thirst.

When we take a drink, our thirst is quickly satisfied. Satisfaction comes long before water is absorbed by the gut. Satiation occurs from wetting the mouth. It can be produced by gargling without drinking, cooling the mouth, swallowing, immersing the body in water and by stomach distension. Rapid satiation of thirst carries high survival value for animals, as it helps limit attendance at waterholes.

Thirst can develop from loss of body water (symptomatic thirst) or from inappropriate activation of the thirst mechanism whilst normally hydrated (pathological thirst). Symptomatic thirst can be caused by:

- lack of access to water or milk;
- severe diarrhoea;

- severe vomiting;
- diabetes insipidus;
- certain forms of chronic renal failure;
- sodium depletion;
- surface burns.

Pathological thirst can be caused by:

- compulsive water drinking;
- oversecretion of renin;
- onset of oedema in congestive heart failure;
- hypokalaemia or hypercalcaemia.

Dehydration caused by fluid deprivation can produce a sense of exhaustion, because of poor tissue perfusion from a reduced blood volume. The body attempts to compensate by raising the heart rate and overbreathing, both of which may already be challenged if there has been forced exercise. In the absence of exercise, dehydration-induced exhaustion causes depression, mental instability and reduced work performance in people.

Animals that become hot and dehydrated, and develop a **sodium deficit** through sweating, sometimes experience difficulty in rehydrating. Their sodium deficiency can suppress their drinking drive, and they need to restore sodium balance before their normal water appetite recovers (Nose *et al.*, 1985).

Animals that are adapted to arid conditions have three survival strategies when managing a water shortage:

(1) reduced rate of water loss – lower volumes of a more concentrated urine, drier faeces and less sweating;
(2) storing water when it becomes available – for example the camel retains water in its forestomachs;
(3) continue to feed, even in the absence of water.

Reptiles survive **water deprivation** by having a relatively impermeable skin, which prevents water loss, and by concentrating their urine into a uric acid paste. The advantage of excreting uric acid is that it has low solubility and, on precipitation, its osmotic effect is removed allowing resorption of water (Chew, 1961). Reptiles living in salt deserts are, however, particularly challenged, and they rely on protection from shade. Desert birds are more dependent on drinking water than are rodents. They are often active during the day, they pant to keep cool and so lose water through respiration. The desert rodents instead can survive for longer just on their metabolic water. In some mammals, there are surprising adaptive differences within species. For example, the black Moroccan goat loses water at about one third the rate seen in European breeds when heat stressed.

Dehydration can be a common problem in horses working in hot climates if they are given insufficient water breaks. In sheep, withholding water was used in South America as a crude way of treating animals for gut parasites. Water was withheld from sheep for up to 60 hours, and then they were dosed with 250 ml 2.5 M sodium chloride. Two hours after the salt load, they were allowed to drink normal water. Too much salt water was apt to kill the animals, and no doubt the survivors had a very keen thirst.

Sheep can survive long periods without drinking water, but their thirst is very obvious. In the mornings they move rapidly over the pasture mouthing the vegetation to gather the dew and water produced by leaf guttation (excretion of drops of water by plants through hydathodes). They may also move along fences licking water off the wires. Cattle and horse herds have been known to survive on remote islands where there has been no supply of fresh water from pools or creeks. It was presumed that they survived on moisture obtained from the plant material they ate.

Dehydration can be a problem in broiler chickens. In broiler sheds, the height of the nipple drinker beams above the floor is raised periodically to prevent the birds from knocking into the drinkers as they grow. Raising the drinkers is recognised as good practice, as it helps to minimise water spillage onto the litter and the subsequent risk of ammonia fouling the atmosphere and of hock burn. However, it also means that birds that are lame, and any undersized birds may not be able to reach the raised drinkers. Death from dehydration is a problem in flocks where these birds are not removed and culled.

Newborn calves experience the combined effects of starvation and dehydration if they are slow to learn how to feed, or they are sold through a market, are anorexic, develop **diarrhoea** which impairs absorption or are intentionally starved as part of a treatment schedule for diarrhoea. Calves can tolerate dehydration quite well because they are able to concentrate their urine. In general, the maximum tonicity of urine in dehydrated animals is limited to double that present in its plasma, but in the calf it can be fourfold higher (Dalton, 1967).

Diarrhoea develops if the colon is unable to absorb sufficient water to form a firm stool. The maximum amount of water that can be absorbed by the healthy human colon is about six litres per day. When this limit is exceeded, or when the entry rate of fluid into the colon is too fast, the colon becomes overloaded and the faeces start to act as a drain on body water (Hammer & Phillips, 1993). This balance is probably more delicate in the case of cattle because of their relatively short colons. When cattle develop dehydration their red blood cells become more fragile. This increases the risk of haemolysis and haemoglobinuria when they rehydrate.

Amphibians such as frogs and toads are prone to dying from dehydration when on dry land because of evaporative loss through their skin; however, they can rehydrate rapidly by absorption of water through the skin when placed in water. This is achieved by **cutaneous drinking** which involves pressing the belly against wet

materials such as grass or litter. Cutaneous drinking occurs when the animal antici-
pates dehydration, and it is stimulated by angiotensin-2. In the absence of cutaneous drinking, their main protection against dehydration is the large reserve of
water in their urine which is resorbed through the bladder wall (Barker Jørgensen,
1994). Only a few frog species rehydrate by actively drinking through the mouth,
and they are mainly arboreal frogs. One curious behaviour amongst frogs and
toads is mouth wiping, which occurs when they are placed in hypertonic salt solutions. It is as if they are trying to remove an irritant from their lips and nose.

9.2 Overhydration

Compulsive water drinking can be a sign of frustration or anxiety. It occurs in laboratory rats when they receive their feed in small amounts intermittently. For
example, if the feed is delivered as one pellet every 60 seconds for 30 minutes they
drink three to four times more water. This **polydipsia** can be attenuated by serotonin re-uptake inhibitors such as fluoxetine and clomipramine, but is not affected
by neuroleptics such as haloperidol or diazepam (Woods et al., 1993). It is due
either to thwarting of the normal feeding drive or to overexcitement during the
delivery of feed, which overflows into an interim activity such as drinking. Rats
that develop this form of polydipsia have a higher than normal metabolic rate.
Polydipsia is also seen in broiler breeder hens that have their feed restricted
(Hocking et al., 1996). A potential metabolic consequence of polydipsia is hypona-
traemia through overloading of water excretory capacity.

The gut has a remarkable capacity to manage excessive amounts of fluid. When
water has been infused into the rumen of sheep at up to 12 litres per day, the
rumen wall absorbed most of the water (Harrison et al., 1975). Similarly, cows
given 18 litres of water intraoesophageally in a 3–7 minute period, seemed to
handle it adequately (Dalton, 1964). Normally, a non-lactating cow would drink
this amount in one day. Water intoxication has been observed in unweaned calves,
and the signs are haemoglobinuria, colic, arrhythmia, salivation, lethargy and mild
ataxia (Kirkbride & Frey, 1967).

9.3 Osmotic Stress

We have no conception of what a fish or crab feels when it experiences osmotic
stress. However, judging from its behaviour it is unpleasant. When marine lobsters
are killed for meat consumption by 'drowning' in fresh water, they show considerable struggling before they die, and many onlookers consider that this is an
inhumane death.

Several physiological strategies are used for protecting against osmotic stress.
When a salt-water fish enters fresh water there is rapid loss of Na^+ and Cl^- from

the gills which results in demineralisation. Some species, such as the flounder (*Platichthys flesus*) guard against this by actively reducing Na$^+$ efflux by up to 90%. Elasmobranch species, such as shark, skate and ray, combat the high osmotic stress associated with living in salt water by maintaining high tissue concentrations of urea. Normally urea is excreted via the gills, and these species reduce elimination by this route in order to maintain osmotic balance. Several attempts have been made to farm euryhaline species in brackish inland water reserves. Experience has shown that it is critical to establish the right osmotic strength.

Physical and emotional stressors, such as capture and transport, can upset osmoregulation even when the water is maintained at the right osmotic strength, and high water temperatures add to the stress effect (Hattingh & van Pletzen, 1974). Osmotic stress also occurs when freshwater fish move into estuarine or salt water. This happens when Atlantic salmon (*Salmo salar*) smolts migrate seaward, and it is responsible for large losses from predation (Järvi, 1989). During osmotic imbalance, the smolts show reduced shoaling behaviour and sluggish reactions in the presence of a predator.

9.4 Hunger

Some of the early studies on hunger were conducted on an American named Fred Hoelzel (Carlson, 1918). Fred was an unusual person. He was in the habit of voluntarily fasting himself for one or two weeks at a time, except for eating wads of indigestible cotton fibre to stave off the pangs of hunger. He noted that once he was well into a fast, a foul-mouth sensation developed, with coating of the tongue. This suppressed his appetite for food, and it overrode or displaced the pleasant memories of eating.

Appetite is a mild form of hunger, and is strongly linked to recollection of the taste and smell of food. This advances into a sense of mild hunger, which is initially an enthusiasm for food, but develops into an aggravating empty sensation and then a dull ache in the lower thoracic and epigastric regions. The hunger grows further into an uncomfortable pang that is less localised and more intense. The unpleasant sensations associated with longer-term starvation, besides foul-mouth tastes, are hunger pangs, a feeling of being 'sick in the stomach', hot flushes, headache, weakness, difficulty in sleeping and a general disinclination to perform physical or mental work.

In non-obese subjects, hunger pangs coincide with gastric **hunger contractions**. During advanced starvation the contractions become erratic, and they involve almost the entire abdomen. The hunger contractions can disturb the normal sleeping pattern, but, if there is a fever, they are reduced or absent. When a monogastric animal dies from starvation, the stomach is often in a state of strong tonic contraction, and the faeces may be replaced by a semi-liquid bile-stained mucus.

9.5 Underfeeding

Starvation is a particular hazard for newborn animals. Failure to learn how to eat
or drink can be a problem in chicks, and, in particular, turkey poults. If they have
not learnt how to feed by the third day of life their chances of survival are poor.
Piglets die within 30 hours if they do not get a feed. However, the calf is relatively
resilient, and has survived for over ten days without either food or water, provided
it gained passive immunity from a colostrum meal once it was born. The calf's
better survival is thought to be due to its more mature renal function at birth
(Dalton, 1967).

During the first four days of starvation, calves are robust and jump to their feet
when approached, but thereafter they become less interested in sucking or other
activities (Goodwin, 1957). This loss of activity and responsiveness occurs in most
species. In laboratory rats it sets in two or three days before death, and they remain
curled up in a ball before becoming comatose. Newborn lambs become comatose
in about eight days when air temperature is around 21°C.

Weaning can be a time when animals experience insufficient food and fluids,
especially if the separation is too early. In puppies there has to be a transition from
sucking to chewing behaviour, and this develops once there has been sufficient
mechanical stimulation of the teeth ligaments. This stimulation enhances maturation of the masticatory centre in the brain (Iinuma et al., 1994). In cattle, fence-
line weaning is a preferred farming practice because it is less stressful for the cow
and calf. In this system the cow and calf can see each other through a fence, and
visual contact makes for quieter behaviour provided weaning is not too early. The
reverse seems to be the case when practising early weaning in farmed mink, where
complete separation is less stressful for the mothers than removal to an adjoining
cage (Heller et al., 1988).

The modern broiler chicken has been genetically selected for rapid growth and
efficient conversion of feed into live weight. This selection has also meant that
they have an **excessive appetite**. The physiological basis for the genetic increase in
appetite has not been established, but it could be due to an increase in expression
of neuropeptide Y or its receptors in the brain.

Unfortunately, the enhanced appetite has affected the survival of the female
parents (Mench, 1993). The broiler breeder hen has a voracious appetite, and its
abdomen tends to be overcrowded by its active reproductive tract, feed within the
gut and intra-abdominal fat. This can lead to prolapse of the vent, which in turn
leads to vent-pecking and cannibalism. In addition, full-feeding causes reduced
fertility and the birds are more prone to heart failure. Prolapse and infertility are
controlled by underfeeding the hens, which aggravates their keen appetite further.
They are either fed on a skip-a-day system or they are fed each day but with a
reduced amount. Typically, they consume their daily allowance in two hours, but
it can be less than 15 minutes.

Increased aggression is a common consequence of **frustration in underfed animals**. Broiler breeder hens are prone to attacking each other, becoming cannibalistic, or they can develop a compulsive polydipsia. Mild frustration can result in displacement preening, and more intense frustration results in escape behaviour, which develops into stereotypic pacing (Duncan & Wood-Gush, 1972).

In wild herbivores, the amount of time spent foraging can be restricted by predation pressure, short daylength in winter and inclement weather. This results in intermittent periods of feeding and fasting, and species that are able to respond by **eating faster** are at an advantage. In rodents, periods of feed deprivation arouse **food hoarding** behaviour. Females hoard more than males, and, in captive rodents, depriving them of opportunities for exercise increases the drive to hoard food.

Mortality from **anorexia** occurs amongst so-called 'non-starters' in some species of fish, and amongst some birds that have precocial chicks. Anorexia, without mortality, occurs in some dogs that have lost their owners, especially in dogs that were very attached to their owner. It has occurred when dogs have been quarantined or boarded, when there has been a change of home or when strangers have visited the house. In anorexia, there is a persistent repugnance for food. It has sometimes been broken by introducing another animal at feeding time.

During starvation or underfeeding there is a progression in the way body energy stores are depleted. First liver glycogen is mobilised, and it is usually depleted within 48 hours. However, birds have relatively little glycogen in their liver, and depletion is much quicker, especially in smaller birds. Then, body fat takes over as the main energy supply, and it is mobilised as free fatty acids (FFAs). If the animal develops hypoglycaemia whilst it is mobilising body fat there is a strong likelihood of **ketosis**. Body protein becomes an increasingly important source of energy as body fat reserves diminish. In some situations, fat animals are less able to mobilise their body fat as FFAs, and **body-protein breakdown** sets in sooner. The ability of the liver to store glycogen can increase if the animal becomes adapted to fasting, or to cold or exercise. This adaptation improves the animal's tolerance to cold.

9.6 Emaciation

In modern agriculture, the dairy cow and layer hen are at particular risk of becoming emaciated. The dairy cow usually produces over 6500 litres of milk in a year, and the hen lays about 300 eggs. Their appetites have to keep up with this strong demand, and, by the time cows reach the end of lactation and hens are at the end of lay, some of them have become extremely skinny. In New Zealand, about 34% of dairy cows were reported as emaciated when they were sent for slaughter (Plate 2). In other words, they had less than 5% body fat, which corresponds to a body condition score of less than four on the Australasian condition score scale (Figure

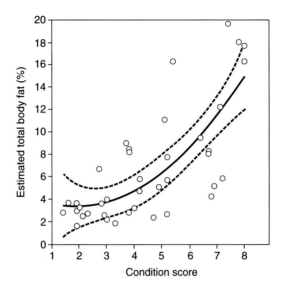

Figure 9.1 Relationship between body condition score and body fatness in dairy cows (courtesy of the *New Zealand Journal of Agricultural Research*).

9.1; Gregory *et al.*, 1998). In layer hen flocks, up to 9% of birds were severely emaciated by the time they reached the end of lay.

Emaciation is also a problem in neglected and ill companion animals (Figure 9.2). Whether these animals suffered depends on whether they became weak from the emaciation, and whether they experienced a persistent hunger and cold conditions.

Emaciation is also common during **droughts**. In Africa, emaciated cattle are often submitted for slaughter for processing into canned meat, and it has been known for them to collapse at the yards in the abattoirs, too weak to get up. Standard practice in Australia is to de-stock a property before a drought becomes too advanced. This allows the farmer to realise some value from the animals, even though it sets the farm back before it is restocked in two or more years time. Reliable long-term weather forecasts are extremely important in drought management.

In humans, the corresponding condition to emaciation is **marasmic kwashiorkor**. There are four psychological changes as marasmic kwashiorkor progresses. Initially there is frustration, which is followed by irritability. Then there is a stage of anger and aggression and finally apathy. During apathy, the individual wants to be left alone, seems to accept the prospect of death and there is resentment at being disturbed. These moods are quickly reversed during recovery, and loss of apathy is a good indicator of the start of recovery.

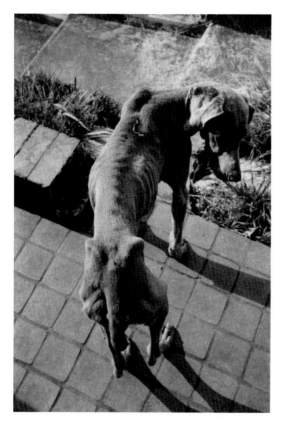

Figure 9.2 Emaciation in a Weimaraner dog (courtesy of Steve Coleman, RSPCA, New South Wales).

9.7 Inappropriate Diets

This section gives some examples of problems that may arise from eating an inappropriate diet. When animals are deprived of their normal feed they are prone to eating inappropriate materials. Broiler chickens may eat **wood shavings**, broiler breeder hens may become cannibalistic or eat dead penmates and horse, cattle and sheep may turn to less palatable and sometimes poisonous plants. There is sometimes concern that sawdust or wood shavings will cause impaction in the gut, but work done in calves showed that low levels of sawdust produced loose faeces, and it was only when sawdust was more than 25% of the diet that normal passage of stools was reduced.

Iron deficiency **anaemia** is a problem in white veal production. The calves are fed a low-iron milk replacer to encourage the production of white meat. The animals become clinically anaemic, they are weak and have poor walking ability. In humans the feelings associated with iron deficiency anaemia include: tiredness, breathlessness following moderate exertion, dizziness, headaches and palpitations.

There is often a learning phase in determining how best to feed a species that is not normally kept in captivity, a recent example of which is the capercaillie (*Tetrao urogallus*). With loss of natural habitat in Europe, some of these birds have been hand-reared and then released in regions where numbers have been depleted. Most of the released birds have died during the first few weeks after release. Part of the reason has been the high digestibility of the feed they were given in captivity. In particular, they had under-developed gizzards, caeca and small intestine, which failed to adapt quickly enough to the changeover to nutrient-poor feed sources (Luikkonen-Anttila *et al.*, 2000). The released birds either starved or succumbed to predation.

The digestive enzymes in the gut have evolved for the diets that are natural to a given species, and deviation from these diets can have drastic effects. For example, when orphan marsupials have been fed cow's milk they have developed osmotic diarrhoea. Many marsupials are **lactose intolerant**, as their milk contains no lactose and the gut has no lactase. Some marsupials also have low activity of the enzyme that metabolises galactose. Accumulation of galactose-1-phosphate leads to the formation and accumulation of a sugar alcohol in the lens of the eye. This sugar alcohol exerts an osmotic effect with resulting influx of water and electrolytes into the lens, and cataract formation (Stephens, 1975).

9.8 Forced Moulting

Forced moulting is used by some egg producers to extend egg production into a second laying period. In many situations it also helps to improve shell quality. The main method used for inducing a moult is to withhold feed temporarily. This causes the birds to stop laying eggs, shed their feathers and then resume laying after the pause in egg production. Sometimes feed is withheld for six days or more, and it has been withheld for as long as 12 days. Feeding recommences when the birds have lost about 30% of their body weight. Feed withdrawal causes a reduction in the release of luteinising hormone (LH) from the pituitary gland. LH is responsible for controlling ovulation, and so its reduction leads to failure in the shedding of eggs from the ovary.

9.9 Force-feeding and Overeating

Force-feeding is used in geese and ducks in the production of pâté de foie gras. A wet mash is introduced into the crop through a funnel that is inserted into the oesophagus. The birds go into torpor for a period of 3–5 hours following a feeding episode, but corticosterone levels do not show that there is a stress response. It should be noted, however, that in rats overeating is usually associated with reduced sympathoadrenomedullary and adrenocortical responsiveness, and it is questionable whether these are useful stress indicators in this context.

In recent years there has been an increase in the number of newborn calves that receive their first feed through a tube inserted into the rumen. This method of force-feeding developed from a need to get shy feeders started, but is now used more generally in calves. If the calf is too mature it objects vigorously to being intubated, and there is a fight in getting the tube inserted. This is undoubtedly stressful for those animals.

Cows that overeat during pregnancy can become overfat and are more prone to dystocia. Overeating and obesity are problems in dogs that are given too much food and limited exercise. In some dogs, overeating and **obesity** have occurred as a psychotic response to enforced socialisation with a puppy or kitten.

When the ability to taste and smell has been obliterated by **olfactory bulbectomy**, in species such as the hamster (*Cricetus cricetus*), which is highly dependent on its sense of smell, the animals overeat and become obese. It is as if the sense of smell and taste are important as satiety signals. Alternatively, it may be that they become mentally disturbed, and eating becomes a displacement behaviour.

Pain

10

10.1 The Value of Pain

Pain serves a useful function. It provides an incentive to protect the body from damage and it also helps limit harmful movement, for example in a fractured limb. It is closely linked to some of the neurohumoral responses that are necessary for inflammation, and it can modify psychological responses, which in turn help the subject cope with an injury. Being indifferent to pain, or being reared in a pain-free environment, is potentially dangerous.

When rats were reared in a restricted environment without pain, and were then given access to a lighted candle they showed reduced pain avoidance (Riesen & Zilbert, 1975). Similarly, when Scottish Terriers were reared in a pain-free environment, they had a poor ability to learn how to avoid painful stimuli. They also reacted wildly and aimlessly when hurt.

Some early knowledge or awareness of pain is a useful experience for animals. It is part of a normal learning process. At the other extreme, in many disease situations, continuous pain seems senseless. For example, when pain develops during terminal cancer it contributes nothing to survival. The pain is too late, and all it achieves is additional suffering.

People who are indifferent or **insensitive to pain** also have difficulty in avoiding dangerous situations. This has occurred in people with lesions of the parietal lobe of the brain, or frontal leucotomies. Instead of being painful, the stimulus is itchy or tingling. In cases where pain insensitivity has been congenital, the subjects have to be specially trained as children to respect and avoid things which cause those sensations, and to treat them as potentially damaging. These pain-insensitive people usually die young. Their lack of concern about pain often leads to self-mutilation or puts them into life-threatening situations.

One exception was a Canadian woman who lived to the age of 29 (Sternbach, 1968). She was intelligent, had a normal personality and possessed all sensory modalities except for pain. She could distinguish hot from cold, even at a fine level, but her corneal reflex was absent, she did not cough or gag when the pharynx was stimulated and she did not report any pain when exposed to electric shocks, muscle ischaemia or insertion of a stick up a nostril. During the course of her life she experienced extensive skin and bone trauma. She survived because of careful tuition and adapting her other senses to identifying otherwise life-threatening injuries. She died from bronchopneumonia.

Congenital insensitivity to pain occurs in animals, and is often accompanied by an inability to sweat (anhidrosis). This combination is due to a mutation in a gene contributing to the function of nerve growth factor (NGF) receptor. There is a laboratory animal model for pain insensitivity that is based on a genetic strain of mice, but, as an exception to the rule, it is not anhidrotic (Indo *et al.*, 1996).

In scientific discussions, the word **nociception** is often used as an alternative to the word pain. They both refer to the detection at some level of potentially damaging physical or physicochemical experiences. Nociception is used more by physiologists, for example when considering pain pathways in anaesthetised animals. In that situation there is no conscious perception of 'pain', but the peripheral pain pathways are active.

10.2 Pain Associated with Trauma

Not all forms of trauma are immediately painful. In a study of 138 patients attending an emergency clinic, 37% stated that they did not feel pain at the time of the injury (Melzack *et al.*, 1982). In most cases, pain developed within an hour of injury, but in others the delay was as long as nine hours. Pain from cuts and lacerations usually developed within an hour of the injury, whereas pain after sprains usually took more than an hour to set in (Table 10.1). If the injury was deep in the tissues, the majority (72%) of subjects experienced prompt pain. This occurred with fractures, crushes, amputations and deep stabs. In the fracture cases, where there was no immediate pain, there was an initial feeling of numbness instead.

There has been some confusion about which types of nerve damage are painful. Neurophysiological studies have shown that the barrage of **injury discharges** that

Table 10.1 Time to onset of pain after an injury (after Melzack *et al.*, 1982).

Type of injury	Time to onset of pain (min)
Fracture	5
Cut	13
Bruise	15
Laceration	21
Sprain	105

occurs when a nerve is severed lasts for up to four seconds. Thereafter the cut end of the nerve is depolarised and unresponsive to most stimuli (Wall *et al.*, 1974). However, when nerves close to the wound are stretched or stimulated without being severed or disabled, there is a period of increased activity that lasts for minutes. This activity is likely to create a sense of trauma or tissue disturbance and paraesthesia. It may or may not provoke pain, depending on circumstances and, in particular, whether or not functional pain receptors are in the field of activation. Typically, when deep structures are injured, the pain may be felt at a site which is alongside rather than within the damaged site. Persistent pain develops subsequently when the pressures associated with haemorrhage, oedema and inflammation develop, and when pain-receptor agonists, released from the injured tissue, accumulate at the wound.

The findings on injury discharges in severed nerves have important implications for the humaneness of slaughter without any stunning, such as religious slaughter (Plate 3). When the neck is cut there is likely to be an intense burst of impulses as the nerves are transected, but this activity will quickly subside (within four seconds), and the cut nerve ends will be inactive. Undamaged nerve terminals and receptors that are exposed at the wound would be responsive to stimulation, especially from cold drafts and mechanical effects. Whether any nociceptors are activated at the cut edges of the wound will depend on circumstances, in other words, on how the wound is managed and handled.

There have been some exceptional instances in experimental work where prolonged injury discharges have occurred following nerve section or injury. These cases may be explained by activity in small intact side branches which joined the damaged nerves above the point of injury (Horowitz, 2001). The normal endings of these side branches were evidently responding to irritation or blood seepage at the site of the wound.

In addition, **ectopic activity** has been seen after an interval of no activity. This happens after neuroma (nerve tumour) formation, and it would take days or weeks following the nerve injury before it started. The sprouted sections of nerve in a neuroma are hyperexcitable, and their activity adds to central sensitisation and neuropathic pain (Seltzer *et al.*, 1991), which develop from hyperexcitability of interneurones within the dorsal horn. There is also one situation where ectopic activity develops soon after nerve transection. The fibres that show this type of discharge seem to be those that were spontaneously active prior to the nerve damage. Blenk *et al.* (1996) observed this type of discharge within the first 15 minutes of nerve transection.

Many of the pain sensations that we describe for skin have a common physiological basis. When there is brief contact with a sharp piece of wire, or a hot wire or an electric current, or a hair is quickly tugged, the pain we feel has a **pricking sensation**. A blindfolded subject would have difficulty distinguishing the cause of such pain. Instead, the cause is identified from accompanying sensations. The hot wire is distinguished by warmth in the adjacent skin, and hair tugging is identified from a lifting sensation in the skin. Pricking pain is the main type of brief pain that exists in skin.

However, a pricking pain in the skin becomes a **burning pain** when the stimulus is applied for a long period or over a wider area (Lewis & Hess, 1933; Chery-Croze & Duclaux, 1980). In addition, if a pain continues long after the stimulus has been removed, it continues as a burning pain. Injuries that cause this continuous burning pain in the skin include:

- abrasions, including scratches;
- continued friction;
- freezing;
- heat;
- ultraviolet burns.

To summarise, although skin pain has a very limited repertoire in terms of its fundamental qualitative sensations, the differences that do occur are mainly due to differences in intensity and duration of the pain, and the accompanying sensations which themselves are not painful.

Burning pain sensations have several interesting facets. With mild scratches, there is reddening and whealing in the skin within five minutes, which may be accompanied by slight itching. Then a slight burning is often felt, and by about 12 hours after the injury, the scratched area is red, swollen, tender and produces a more intense burning pain that lasts for a day or more. Pain from freezing the skin has an initial pricking sensation, followed by an itch and tenderness that develops within 20 hours. The lesion is swollen and flushed, eventually producing a burning pain, and it is tender for 4–5 days. In the case of abrasions and thermal burns there is an early pain, whereas with ultraviolet burns the pain develops later and it lasts longer. The pain from a mild burn gradually increases, and it often continues for many minutes or hours after the injury. Once it reaches its peak, it continues at a constant intensity, but there can be episodes of more intense pain superimposed on this background level. Burns that cause blisters can be very tender and are red and swollen.

Cuts and lacerations in tissues below the skin often have a throbbing or beating quality, and the site is tender once it becomes swollen or inflamed. With severe cuts the subject can feel tired. Sprains and fractures have an aching quality, and when there is bruising as well, the pain is also sharp and hot. Amputations have a pounding, jumping, stabbing, tearing, sharp or crushing feel, and leave the subject with a tender wound and a general sense of tiredness. These forms of pain can be divided into two general types: **sharp pains** and **dull pains**. Throbbing and pounding is a dull pain linked to pulse pressure, and jumping or stabbing pains are other names for a sharp pain. A large number of other descriptors are used for pain, and in many cases they do not add much precision or understanding of the suffering (Table 10.2).

Table 10.2 The experience of pain.

Terms used in describing the feeling of pain		
Aching	Burning	Bursting
Throbbing	Shooting	Lightning
Boring	Sharp	Electricity
Drawing	Hot iron	Stinging
Pulling	Soreness	Pricking
Gripping	Knife-like	Needle-like
Cramping	Stabbing	Tingling
Nagging	Toothache	Itching
Sense of pressure	Tearing	
Gnawing	Hot cords	
Beating	Smarting	

Pain can become more intense if venous pressure is raised because of **restricted venous return**. This occurs when tissue swelling above a wound in a limb occludes the veins, the wound region becomes engorged with blood and more painful. There are two components to this: first, pressure from the swelling may directly activate pain receptors; second, the pain will be more protracted and more intense if the pain-provoking substances at the wound cannot be removed through the venous circulation (Lewis & Hess, 1933). Rubbing a bruise can improve venous return.

Pain in one part of the body can reduce or even eliminate pain perception in another region. This is known as **nociceptive inhibitory control** (NIC), and when it occurs throughout the body it is called DNIC (diffuse NIC). NIC is mediated by the *nucleus reticularis dorsalis* in the brainstem. This is useful to know because it means that this form of pain inhibition could be different from the more common forms of inhibition that arise from the periaqueductal grey (PAG) and rostral ventromedial medulla (RVM). DNIC applies to allodynia (pain experienced in response to a stimulus that would not normally provoke pain) as well as nociceptor-mediated pain. In particular, a newly-applied pain will reduce the intensity of allodynia pain, but it does not necessarily change the size of the allodynia field (Witting *et al.*, 1998). DNIC is probably the mechanism that explains why achieving relief from pain due to cancer in one part of the body uncovers pain in another cancerous region. It is a sad fact that clinicians who are trying to provide pain relief sometimes end up chasing pain about the body in patients with well-metastasised cancer.

Distraction can reduce the perception of pain. For example, the competing athlete may not notice a painful injury until the event or game is over. Similarly, if a hungry cat is eating at the time it receives a painful stimulus, it is less likely to respond (Casey & Morrow, 1983). During concentration or mental diversion, a more forceful painful stimulus is required to provoke a behavioural reaction.

In humans, pain can be brought on by **suggestion**. Talking about one's pain 'makes it worse', and distraction helps it subside. For example, phantom-limb pain has been exacerbated when emotionally-laden topics were discussed, and psychiatric patients can develop severe pain when under emotional distress. Some subjects use pain behaviour as a diversion or as a way of recruiting attention or reward. For example, dogs and goats can show foot raising as a form of sympathy lameness (Fox, 1962).

With the possible exception of cats and dogs, animals are given **pain-killing drugs** less often than humans. However, there are four simple procedures, not involving drugs, that can be used to make pain more tolerable. They are:

(1) keep the affected part cool;
(2) maintain the affected part in a horizontal position;
(3) immobilise the affected part;
(4) protect from friction.

In all four procedures, the aim is to control pressure on the wound: keeping the wound cool limits pressure from vasodilatation; keeping the wound raised limits hydrostatic and venous pressures on the wound.

10.3 Ways in Which Animals Express Pain

Pain can be expressed in the following ways:

- escape reactions;
- abnormal posture, gait or speed, guarding behaviour;
- vocalising or aggression during movement or manipulation;
- withdrawal and recoil responses;
- licking, biting, chewing or scratching;
- frequent changes in body position – restlessness, rolling, writhing, kicking, tail-flicking;
- vocalising – groaning, whimpering, crying, squealing, screaming, growling, hissing, barking;
- impaired breathing pattern, shallow breathing, groaning during breathing, increased rate of breathing;
- muscle tension, tremor, twitching, spasm, straining;
- depression, sluggishness, hiding, withdrawal, lying motionless, seeking cover, sleeplessness;
- avoidance behaviour and aversion to the scene of the trauma;

- spontaneous autonomic responses – sweating, tachycardia, hypertension, vaso-constriction and pallor, increased gastro-intestinal secretions, decreased intes-tinal motility, increased intestinal sphincter tone, urinary retention;
- endocrine responses.

One of the difficulties in recognising pain in animals is distinguishing between painful and non-painful behaviours and responses. For example, when an animal is hit by something, it may react physically from the force of the impact, the threat involved in delivery of the blow, the shock or surprise from being hit or from pain itself. Just because the animal recoiled does not mean that it was painful. Some-times we can be convinced that an animal did feel pain, but, since we cannot feel its pain ourselves, we do not appreciate the severity or the type of pain. Instead, we do the best we can to infer the presence and likely severity of pain from the animal's behaviour, and in some instances from its physiological responses. Our appreciation of the likely pain comes from unashamed analogy with comparable cases in humans.

Some examples of **behaviour patterns** that seem to be linked specifically to pain are:

- In guinea pigs and mice, abdominal pain associated with intraperitoneal injec-tion of bradykinin is associated with writhing and tension in the abdominal wall (Collier et al., 1966). In the case of the dog, intra-arterial injections of bradykinin showed that vocalisation was the only consistent behavioural indi-cator of sudden visceral pain (Braun et al., 1961).
- The response to colonic pain from inflating a balloon in the colon of a dog was head-lifting, altered posture, stretching of a hind limb and a change in breath-ing pattern (Houghton et al., 1991).
- When a laboratory rat had its tail pinched it gnawed at an available object. If this was a feed pellet it held the feed pellet in its forepaws, gnawed and ate the pellet in an identical way to normal eating. In the absence of a suitable object to gnaw on, a rat will drink from the water dispenser when its tail is pinched (Rowland & Antelman, 1976).
- Pigs subjected to a remotely-operated laser beam responded by flicking the tail, moving a leg or twitching a muscle (Jarvis et al., 1997).
- In the rat, pain behaviour associated with loose constriction of the sciatic nerve with a ligature is seen as limping, with the toes kept closely together instead of spread out, raising the paw and holding it in a protected position next to the flank while standing or sitting and sleeping or lying on the opposite side (Bennet & Xie, 1988). Rats show paw-lifting, licking and biting when the paw itself is sore, and licking rather than lifting is alleviated by treatment with mor-phine (Bland-Ward & Humphrey, 1997).
- In osteolytic cancer of the femur in the mouse, the pain responses to light pal-pation of the femur are fighting, vocalising and biting (Schwei et al., 1999).

- Ureteric colic is a particularly unpleasant pain in humans. In rats the signs of a painful episode include hump-backed posture, abdomen or flank licking, inward movement of the hind limbs in association with contraction of the flank muscles and squashing of the abdomen against the floor.

One of the most convincing ways of testing whether a particular abnormal behaviour sign is due to pain is to apply a specific analgesic and see whether the abnormality disappears. For example, when chest pain following trauma is treated with an analgesic, one of the most obvious effects is improved ventilation with greater chest expansion. This type of response can be diagnostic as well as aiding therapy. Another example is when muscle pain is relieved by an analgesic, and the animal is able to resume its normal posture or walking speed.

Some species seem to be less expressive about their pain than others. In humans, expressing pain is used as a way of controlling the source of the pain. We cry for help or limp to recruit sympathy and assistance. With the exception of limping, these behaviours are less relevant for animals, and there are fewer benefits from being pain-expressive except in the case of newborn animals. As a result, species such as sheep and deer show limited or very subtle behavioural responses to pain, and this can lead the onlooker to think that they have limited ability to experience pain. Dogs, cats and goats, on the other hand, are more expressive and so they evoke more care and sympathy from care-givers.

The **expression of pain** can be quite different in a newborn compared with an adult animal. In the adult dog, the normal response to a mild electric shock on the leg is withdrawal of that limb, whereas one-to-five-day-old puppies do not show limb withdrawal. Instead, there is generalised flexion of all limbs, as well as raising the head, whining and attempts to crawl away (Fuller et al., 1950).

The same applies in the cases of the human and the rat. In infancy they both show generalised whole-body writhing movements when they experience painful stimulation. As they develop, there is greater inhibition of whole body responses by higher brain centres, leaving the more localised limb response to dominate (Fitzgerald, 1999).

In most neonates, sucking on a teat has a calming and analgesic effect when there has been a painful experience. Both effects appear to be opioid-mediated. Milk has an anti-nociceptive effect, which is naltrexone reversible, as does sucrose but not lactose. The act of sucking plays a large part in producing this analgesia. This was demonstrated by allowing non-nutritive sucking on an anaesthetised dam.

Males are more likely to show reflexive aggression when they experience pain. In rats, this response has been reduced by castration, and so presumably it is linked to testosterone production (Hutchinson et al., 1965). Rats reared in social isolation showed considerably less aggressive behaviour in response to foot shock than rats reared in community conditions. Nevertheless, the fact that it sometimes occurs in socially isolated individuals shows that pain-induced aggression is not a learned reaction.

There may be a genetic component to the expression of pain responses. There is a rat model where two lines have been developed according to differences in the severity of self-mutilation following peripheral nerve denervation (Seltzer, 1995). This trait is transmitted as a single autosomal recessive gene.

10.4 Pain Pathways and Consciousness

A knowledge of pain pathways is helpful in understanding how pain is controlled and modified. It also allows us to predict the limitations of any one drug used for controlling pain. In the past it was thought that pain was modulated within the thalamus of the brain. It is now appreciated that much of the endogenous inhibition occurs within the spinal cord, and that integration with other signals occurs within the reticular formation in the brain.

There are two types of nerve fibre that transmit signals from peripheral receptors to the spinal cord:

(1) Non-noxious sensory signals transmitted by large fast-conducting myelinated Aβ axons.
(2) Noxious and thermal signals conveyed in smaller, slow-conducting, thinly-myelinated Aδ and unmyelinated C-fibres.

The Aδ pain pathway transmits sharp pains and has a faster rate of transmission than the C-fibre pathway which conveys aching pains. C-fibres end exclusively in free nerve endings, whereas Aδ fibres terminate in either a free nerve ending or a specialised receptor.

Pain neurotransmitters associated with free **nerve endings** include substance P, calcitonin gene-related peptide (CGRP), vasoactive intestinal peptide (VIP) and somatostatin. Most neurotransmitters are synthesised in the body of the afferent neurone which is situated in the dorsal root ganglion, and they pass by axonal transport to the peripheral nerve ending or to the central terminal in the spinal cord.

Nerves that convey pain signals enter the **spinal cord** through the dorsal horn. The dorsal horn is arranged in layers, or laminae (Figure 10.1). The Aδ and C-fibres project mainly to laminae I and II which lie nearest the periphery of the dorsal horn, but a smaller number of these fibres project to lamina V. The Aβ fibres that transmit signals from mechanoreceptors terminate in laminae III, IV and V.

There are two major routes that pain signals take between the spinal cord and the medulla of the brain: the **spinothalamic pathway** and the lemniscal pathway. Some signals cross the spinal cord to the anterolateral funiculus on the opposite side, and then ascend to the brain via the spinothalamic tract (Figure 10.2). This tract terminates in the reticular formation of the brainstem and in the thalamus. Damage or surgical severance (cordotomy) of the anterolateral funiculus leads to

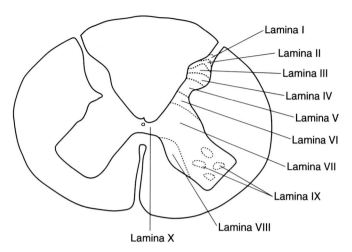

Figure 10.1 Cross section of the monkey spinal cord showing position of the laminae.

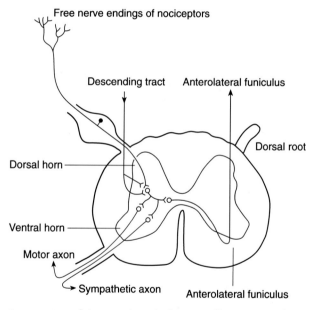

Figure 10.2 Cross section of the spinal cord, showing afferent route of pain pathway to the brain and route of descending inhibition.

loss of pain sensation via this route, and stimulation of the anterolateral funiculus produces a burning pain sensation.

In the **lemniscal pathway**, transmission is via the dorsal column. On entering the brain, the fibres in these tracts synapse at the *medulla oblongata*, cross to the opposite side of the brainstem within the medulla and then project to the thalamus via the medial lemniscus in the reticular formation. From the thalamus, there are projections to the cortex.

Lesioning or damage to the reticular formation produce permanent and irreparable disruption of consciousness, and electrical stimulation of this region causes arousal. During stimulation there is awakening, attentiveness and redirection of that attention. The network from the reticular formation that mediates arousal and helps determine the degree of consciousness is known as the ascending reticular activating system.

Signal modification at the level of the spinal cord has major effects on pain and sensory stimuli that are projected to the brain. **Transmission within the dorsal horn** is modified in three ways:

(1) Transmission can be suppressed by either segmental or descending inhibitory mechanisms. This suppression is mediated by opioid and α-adrenergic receptors, and it leads to reduced pain perception.
(2) Dorsal horn excitability is raised. This sensitisation is initiated by signals projected during peripheral tissue injury, peripheral inflammation and injury to peripheral nerves. It leads to hyperalgesia and allodynia.
(3) The dorsal horn shows persistent hypersensitivity due to structural changes in the pathways. This can occur when there has been injury to a peripheral nerve, or to the spinal cord, and it leads to chronic neuropathic pain.

10.4.1 Suppression of transmission
Transmission in the dorsal horn can be suppressed through three routes:

(1) interneurones which act presynaptically on afferent neurones;
(2) midbrain descending pathways which synapse with the afferent neurone terminal;
(3) segmental projections which synapse with the afferent neurone terminal.

The inhibitory interneurones decrease neurotransmitter release from the afferent neurones by acting on them presynaptically. These inhibitory interneurones are activated from midbrain descending projections in the spinal cord, and by other primary afferent neurones. They help to prevent overstimulation. Some of these interneurones are continuously active.

Pain suppression by descending inhibition can occur for example when emotions, stress, learned behaviours or counterirritation override pain. Segmental inhibition occurs when signals from one part of the body reduce the sense of pain in another body region, both of which project to the same spinal cord segment. For example, licking or rubbing a wound can help reduce pain by segmental inhibition.

Table 10.3 Brain regions that can achieve or mediate inhibitory control of pain.

Brain region	Receptor
Periaqueductal grey (PAG)	μ and κ opioid
Rostral ventromedial medulla (RVM)	μ and δ opioid
Mesencephalic reticular formation	μ opioid
Substantia nigra	μ opioid
Nucleus accumbens and ventral forebrain	μ and ε opioid

Other examples of pain inhibition at the level of the dorsal horn include:

- reduction in pain perception when swimming in cold water – mediated by opioid receptors;
- electric shocks applied to a foot, and raised pain threshold – mediated by opioid, α_2-adrenergic and serotonin receptors;
- reflex reduction in pain associated with cervical probing – mediated by α_2-adrenergic and serotonin receptors.

There are at least six regions in the brain that help to reduce pain perception through **descending inhibition** (Table 10.3). The PAG is one of the main regions. Normally the PAG receives nociceptive input through laminae I and II, and, under the influence of inputs from the amygdala and the *locus coeruleus*, it relays pain-inhibitory signals back down the spinal cord. The types of stimuli that provoke the pain-inhibitory mechanisms include stress and emotional arousal, hence the involvement of the amygdala and *locus coeruleus*. The PAG is also reciprocally innervated with the RVM, which acts as a relay for the pain-inhibitory signals from the PAG, whilst integrating them with signals from the pre-optic area (POA) of the hypothalamus.

10.4.2 Sensitisation

Sensitisation to painful stimuli can occur in three ways:

(1) reduction in threshold of nociceptors;
(2) increase in responsiveness of neurones in the dorsal horn;
(3) recruitment of additional afferent signals and transducing them into pain signals (e.g. allodynia).

Sensitisation is more common in C-fibre pathways than in Aδ pain, and it is mainly mediated through *N*-methyl-D-aspartate (NMDA) receptors. In inflammatory pain there is often up-regulation of Substance P and CGRP in the spinal cord.

Thalamic pain is a form of central sensitisation to pain. It is a disorder in the thalamus causing burning sensations that are projected to regions of the body, which paradoxically have greatly reduced sensitivity in the skin when directly stimulated.

Opioid receptors mediate pain inhibitory mechanisms by decreasing neuronal firing through reduction of the release of excitatory neurotransmitters. In the spinal cord, opioid receptors are present in laminae I and II of the dorsal horn where they inhibit afferent Aδ and C-fibre activity at their synaptic connections. In the midbrain, opioid receptors mediate the signals which bring about descending inhibition in the dorsal horn. Supraspinal opioid systems also decrease nociceptive input to the brain, and these opioid receptors are situated in the brain stem, thalamus, amygdala and hippocampus. The principal opioid receptors are the δ-, μ- and κ-receptors. The δ-receptors respond to enkephalins and β-endorphin. The μ receptors are activated by β-endorphin and mediate the analgesic and euphoric actions of morphine. The endorphins found in bovine and human brain act through μ receptors and are particularly effective against neuropathic pain and allodynia. The κ-receptors are activated by dynorphin.

Opioid peptides drugs can exert effects outside the CNS, and they may play a role in local suppression of inflammatory neuritis. During inflammation, opioid receptors are transported to the periphery along nerve axons. The number of the receptors increases in peripheral nerve terminals, and if inflammation disrupts the perineurium, more opioid receptors are exposed.

10.5 Cortical Regions

Neuroscientists have only recently discovered which cortical sites process pain information and allow the perception of pain. The cortical regions that are most frequently activated during the early stages of pain are the primary somatosensory cortex S1, parietal operculum S2, anterior cingulate cortex, insula, prefrontal cortex and the posterior parietal cortex (Ingvar & Hsieh, 1999).

The primary somatosensory cortex S1 responds to severe painful stimuli and to pain caused by heat or cold. S1 and S2 are both involved in the perception of chronic pain. The posterior parietal cortex is implicated in traumatic and neuropathic pain.

The anterior **cingulate and insula cortical regions** receive input from the thalamus, and so they have a direct link with the spinothalamic tract that carries nociceptive input from the dorsal horn of the spinal cord. These two cortical regions are involved with many forms of pain.

The insula cortex is involved in the mediation of emotional, remembered and autonomic features of a painful experience, and decreased activation of this area is linked to decreased pain intensity. Lesions of the parietoinsula cortex or the underlying internal capsule have been associated with diminished sensibility to pain, an inability to understand pain and insensitivity to heat.

The anterior cingulate cortex integrates the affective components of pain with other inputs that require mental attention (Casey, 1999; Bantick *et al.*, 2002). Activation of the anterior cingulate is associated with the sensation of burning and ice-like pains, headache and the anticipation of a painful experience. Activity in this region increases when the subject is not aware of what is causing the pain, and decreases when the subject recognises the source of the painful experience and the source of an imminent painful experience.

10.6 Applied Neurology of Pain

10.6.1 Headache

Headaches are among the most common types of pain in humans, but they are rarely if ever recognised in animals. This is because little effort has gone into establishing the signs of headache in animals. It is suspected that head-pressing and teeth-grinding indicate a headache, but they could reflect other pains as well. Levine and Wolff (1932) reported increased sweating from the paws of bulbocapnine-immobilised cats when the pial blood vessels were electrically stimulated, and this was thought to be a response to a headache. Similarly, Chorobski and Penfield (1932) observed struggling in lightly anaesthetised monkeys when pial artery dilatation was induced by stimulation of branches of the 5th or 7th cranial nerves. Pial artery dilatation was monitored through a window inserted in the skull over the parietal lobe of the brain, and, as indicated below, it is linked to neuro-vasogenic headaches in humans. More recently, rats have been found to head-groom and head-scratch when meningeal nociceptors were stimulated chemically.

The causes of headaches are inflammation, traction, displacement and distension of pain-sensitive structures in the head (Ray & Wolff, 1940). An individual headache could be due to one of six causes:

(1) traction on the veins and sinuses in the cranium;
(2) traction on the meningeal arteries;
(3) traction on the large arteries at the base of the brain;
(4) distension and dilatation of the intracranial and extracranial arteries;
(5) inflammation near nerve fibres surrounding blood vessels in the head;
(6) pressure on nerves containing pain-afferent fibres.

The pain-sensitive structures in the head were identified during the 1930s by neurosurgeons who operated on the human brain using only a local anaesthetic. Apart from the skull and its overlying tissues, pain could be produced in only the following structures:

• arteries and sinuses associated with the dura;
• the larger basal intracranial arteries;
• choroid plexus.

The brain itself does not possess pain receptors, and invasive injury of the brain parenchyma is not painful except when it stimulates either nerve fibres lining the blood vessels in or on the brain, or a pain afferent pathway entering the brain.

Five types of headache may result from inflammation or mechanical stimulation of cranial neuro-vascular receptors:

(1)   headaches due to chemical agents such as histamine and amyl nitrite;
(2)   migraine headache;
(3)   headache associated with fever or septicaemia;
(4)   headache associated with hypertension;
(5)   postconvulsive headache.

Headaches associated with migraine, raised histamine levels in the circulation, fever and hypertension, are linked to dilatation of the intracranial arteries. The dilatation places pressure on the arterial walls and the perivascular tissues, which triggers trigeminal pathways that provoke further pain. This mechanism has been tested by manipulating blood pressure. Injecting adrenaline to raise the blood pressure at the end of one of these headaches sets it off again, and sudden straining makes a headache worse if it raises blood pressure. Compressing a carotid artery relieves the pain on that side of the head by reducing its blood pressure. A word of caution though for the self-experimenting enthusiast; when the carotid artery is released, the headache returns with a vengeance.

In headaches that are exaggerated by raised pressure in the cerebral arteries, compressing the jugular veins can relieve the headache. Jugular compression will raise cerebrospinal fluid (CSF) pressure, and this can help equilibrate any cerebral oedema as well as the pressure and distension of the intracerebral arteries. The CSF helps to buffer changes in intracranial pressure. When intracranial pressure is high, CSF volume in the cranium declines, and CSF also helps to equilibrate low pressures. If CSF cannot be expelled from the cranium in response to an increase in intracranial pressure, because of a stricture or blockage in the spinal canal, the intracranial pressure is uncorrected and this may exacerbate a headache along with nausea, vomiting and tinnitus.

In some types of headache, compressing the jugular veins will make the headache worse. In those cases, the headache is a referred pain from extracranial arteries. The rise in jugular venous pressure above the occlusion leads to increased tension in the walls of the extracranial arteries, which enhances the pain response. This is probably a mechanism that contributes to some cases of migraine.

Headache during a fever is usually a throbbing pain, which increases gradually to a constant severe pain that is exacerbated with each beat of the heart (Bodley Scott & Warin, 1946). The pain subsides with the fever to regain its throbbing character before disappearing. In most cases there is a referred eye ache which persists after the headache has worn off. Lipopolysaccharide and cytokines such as interferon induce this type of headache, as well as a fever.

Headaches following head injury also have a throbbing quality and can be associated with nausea, sensitivity to light, irritability and drowsiness. Raised intracranial pressure should be suspected, and epidural, subdural and subarachnoid haemorrhages can all produce this type of headache.

Cluster and tension headaches are often repetitive and associated with autonomic signs such as watering of the eyes, nasal congestion and excessive constriction of the pupil (Schoenen & Sándor, 1999). Lacrimation indicates activation of a trigeminal–parasympathetic reflex, and the other autonomic features suggest a stress involvement that is mediated by the hypothalamus.

10.6.2 Spinal cord injury

Spinal cord trauma has occurred in animals when there has been excessive struggling whilst tethered, fighting amongst males, lassoing animals from a moving vehicle, falls in pack-horses and donkeys, road accidents, collapse of buildings and injuries in stockyards. Prognosis and the type of suffering that will occur, depends partly on the extent of the damage to the spinal cord.

People who have had their spinal cord completely severed without loss of consciousness, have reported that it felt like 'a kick in the back', the 'body had been cut in two', an 'electric shock', the 'legs were pulled away' and 'floating, like being in heaven' (Cohen & Rogers, 1942; Bors, 1963). Thereafter, there was paralysis and loss of sensation below the level of the injury.

When the spinal cord is completely severed without loss of consciousness, the victim falls helplessly to the ground, unable to move, except in the case of injury to the lower lumbar cord, when it may be able to move its forequarters. If the spinal cord is partly severed some functions below the injury are retained, but they are not usually normal.

With some spinal injuries, pain is not immediate but instead develops after a few months or, sometimes, after several years. Those pains cannot be described in simple terms, because they change with time. They include root pains, allodynia, central dysaesthesia, hyperalgesia, causalgia and aching at the level of the injury. Fortunately, chronic intractable pain is relatively rare.

---

root pain – severe debilitating pain that arises from damage to the dorsal root ganglia or adjoining nerves

allodynia – condition in which ordinarily non-painful stimuli evoke pain

central dysaesthesia – unpleasant abnormal sensation, usually felt in the skin but is of central origin, and occurs in the absence of direct stimulation. Includes paraesthesias

hyperalgesia – excessive sensibility to pain

causalgia – persistent severe burning pain following damage to a sensory nerve

---

Phantom sensations are common in humans with spinal cord injury. Most of the sensations are unpleasant but bearable. The surface sensations include 'burning', 'tingling', 'pins and needles', 'extremity as though asleep', 'numbness' and 'itching'. Postural phantom sensations include 'gaps' or 'holes' between parts of the phantom which is held together by 'wire' or 'swollen flesh'. Very painful phantoms occur with cauda equina lesions, and in some cases justify cordotomy (Bors, 1963).

Spinal cord injuries can lead to autonomic hyperreflexia. Sympathetic nerve impulses below the lesion are unopposed by descending activity that would normally pass via the intermediolateral column of the spinal cord. This results in episodes of sympathetic nervous outburst which manifest themselves as hypertension, throbbing headache and rhinorrhea. There is often parasympathetic supercompensation (e.g. bradycardia, sweating) above the spinal lesion whilst there is a sympathetic crisis below the lesion. Stimuli which trigger this reflex syndrome include bladder and bowel distension (Landrum *et al.*, 1998).

When presented with an animal that has a spinal cord injury, it is not always possible to make an instant assessment of its prospects. Instead, prognosis is often gauged from the recovery of function over time. This can be important if the animal has experienced **spinal cord concussion** *without* destruction of the cord. In spinal concussion there is temporary loss of reflex activity. Vasomotor reflexes below the level of the lesion are lost, and this will cause a precipitous drop in blood pressure if the impact was in the neck. The concussion may be associated with haemorrhage or oedema within the cord, which will interfere with motor, sensory and visceral function, but can resolve as the swelling subsides. The returning reflexes may be exaggerated, probably from a loss of suprasegmental inhibitory pathways (Simpson, 1963).

Stretching the spinal cord can cause short-term motor and sensory impairment (Chang *et al.*, 1981). Puppies that had their cords stretched by up to 35% of their normal length showed varying degrees of motor dysfunction ranging from inability to walk whilst able to stand, to complete paraplegia. However, motor and sensory function returned within six days. Similarly, stretching peripheral nerves causes transient disturbance of neurotransmission, and it has been used as a way of relieving neuralgia. Sensory nerves are more sensitive to this form of interference than motor nerves, and mammalian nerves are more sensitive than amphibian nerves.

Spinal cord injuries in cats and dogs occur during road accidents, falls or internal trauma (e.g. intervertebral disc extrusion). Complete transection of the spinal cord usually produces a hopeless case for recovery of locomotion, but there is a prospect for return of motor function if the cord is only partly severed (Jeffery & Blakemore, 1999). Humans that have a dislocated vertebral column at the atlanto-occipital axis rarely survive for any length of time. They usually die from shock.

The likelihood of functional regeneration of a damaged spinal cord is greater in fishes and amphibians than in mammals and birds (Kiernan, 1979). The teleost *Sternarchus albifrons* is capable of regenerating a new spinal cord and a new tail, even in adulthood. The fish may be compromised for a long period, as spinal cord regeneration is very slow (about 1 mm per week). Studies with zebrafish have produced good but incomplete recovery of swimming, following sectioning of the spinal cord. One of the reasons for their poorer swimming was that they swam with their fins spread out and this slowed them down. It may be that this was an adaptation which improved their balance.

10.6.3 Causalgia

Causalgia commonly occurs in the first weeks after an injury, following a brief initial period of numbness. It is a neuralgia with a sense of deep burning pain and both primary plus secondary hyperalgesia. It is caused by nerve damage, and in particular by stretching of nerves. It has been suggested that it is due to **ephaptic transmission** in the region of a wound.

Ephaptic transmission occurs when an impulse jumps between two adjacent nerve fibres, one of which is in a primed hyperexcitable state and is triggered by activity in the other. In cases of causalgia, it is thought that the wound leads to hyperexcitability in an afferent nerve, which is then susceptible to receiving this form of nerve cross-talk. The exchange can occur with the sympathetic nervous system. Sympathectomy has arrested causalgia, presumably because efferent impulses in autonomic nerves ephapsed with nociceptive afferent nerves (Keele & Armstrong, 1964). In amputation causalgia, many subjects claim that heat increases and cold eases the pain, and the causalgia may last from three months to over a year.

10.6.4 Phantom pain

Amputation of a limb is almost invariably followed by a feeling that the cut-off part is still there. This feeling is known as phantom-limb sensation. If the phantom-limb feels painful, this is known as phantom-limb pain. If only part of a limb is amputated, and there is pain in the remaining part, this is known as stump pain.

Phantom-limb sensations occur in about 90% of human amputees (Jensen *et al.*, 1983). In some subjects there are constant vivid sensations of the missing limb, whilst in others there are transient tingling sensations in the lost limb. These sensations are common in the distal parts of the limb, and the limb usually feels as if it is an existing part of the body. As time passes, some subjects find that the phantom-limb seems to shorten (telescopes). It is unlikely these non-painful, phantom-limb sensations are a significant source of suffering in animals.

In humans, phantom-limb pain commonly develops within the first four days of amputation. In a survey of 2694 United States military amputees, it was present in 78% of the servicemen (Sherman *et al.*, 1984). It commonly occurred as attacks of pain which usually decreased in duration and frequency with time. At first the pain affected either the whole phantom limb or just the distal part. In about half the affected individuals there was no way of relieving the phantom pain.

In general, phantom pain is more common in subjects who experienced pain in the limb before the amputation. Similarly, studies in laboratory rats have shown that injury of a paw *before* denervation, increased the severity of *subsequent* self-mutilation of the paw (Codere *et al.*, 1986). The pains experienced in humans include knife-like, cramping or sticking pains shortly after the surgery, while squeezing or burning types of phantom pain occur later. A curious feature of phantom-limb pain is that it can be alleviated with either local anaesthetics or transcutaneous electrical nerve stimulation applied to the opposite limb (Gross, 1982). Phantom pains are common after cancer-related amputations.

Phantom pains have been reported for a wide range of body parts. Phantom-eye pain occurs as a headache in eye-cancer patients, and testicular phantoms have been reported following castration. It is not just organs and body parts that are paired and have a counterpart on the other side of the body that can get phantom pain. Unpaired parts in the perineal region have been known to result in phantom pain after removal.

10.6.5 Neuromas

Neuromas contribute towards chronic stump pain in human amputees. Neuromas occur when the severed ends of nerves attempt to regrow. Before this happens the Schwann cells, which are normally responsible for providing energy to the nerve and the insulating myelin sheath, act as guides for the regrowth of the axons. The stump of the severed axon sprouts and these outgrowths spread in all directions. If one of the outgrowths encounters a Schwann cell it receives the nutrients that allow it to grow to the next Schwann cell, thus forming a nerve tract. If the two cut ends of a nerve are situated close enough together, reinnervation can occur. If the outgrowths turn back on themselves and obtain support from a proximal Schwann cell, and if this happens on a relatively large scale, a neuroma is formed.

A neuroma is made up of a large number of small myelinated axons (Holland & Robinson, 1990). They are often embedded with fibroblasts in connective tissue, and can be very sensitive to pain caused by pressure. When present in amputation stumps they may be prone to repeated blows, pressure or irritation because of their unprotected position at the end of the stump. Nevertheless, some neuromas are painless. The reason some are extremely painful and others are painless is not clear, but it could relate to the density of, or pressure bearing on, hypersensitive axon terminals.

Amputation neuromas have been observed in histological sections of the stumps of docked dogs, lambs and pigs (Gross & Carr, 1990; Simonsen *et al.*, 1991; French & Morgan, 1992). They also occur in the beak stump in de-beaked poultry. In the study on dogs, the tail stump neuromas were usually painful, and this caused the dogs to mutilate this region. Human patients suffering from neuroma pain typically complain of a tonic background pain, on top of which they occasionally feel paroxysmal shooting pains.

It is not just cut nerves that form neuromas. Nerves that are damaged by compression or crushing can also develop neuromas (Horch & Lisney, 1981). It seems likely that the rubber rings used for docking could result in neuroma formation.

10.6.6 Neuropathic pain

Neuropathic pain occurs when there has been damage in a nerve either by trauma or disease. Sensitisation starts to develop within hours of the nerve being damaged, and it reaches a peak during the second week. Thereafter, it declines at a variable rate before reaching a plateau of low-grade pain (Seltzer, 1995). Once the region has become sensitised, the pain is provoked by skin stimulation, pressure applied over the nerve or a change in temperature. It is a burning, lancinating, prickling, stinging, shooting or electrical type of pain. With time, it changes to a dull, boring, aching, tingling pain, or discomfort, with sharper pains occurring intermittently. In some subjects the pain gets worse with time, spreads to adjoining regions and is associated with allodynia.

There are about 30 experimental models for neuropathic pain. In one of them, a loosely-constricting ligature is tied around the sciatic nerve in the hind leg of a rat. This causes hyperalgesia and allodynia in the hind paw. The rat walks with a limp and the hind paw is placed clumsily (Bennet & Xie, 1988). The limp is due to reluctance to bear weight on the affected paw. In another model, the sciatic nerve is cut, and after a time the rat mutilates the paw on the affected hind leg (Blumenkopf & Lipman, 1991). In both these models the type of behaviour is due to pain, but the types of pain may be slightly different.

Peripheral neuropathic pain can be initiated by the *nervi nervorum* which are present in the connective-tissue sheath surrounding a nerve. Neuropathic pain may also be due to an adaptive overabundance of sodium channels that control excitability of nociceptor neurones at the site of an injury. In central neuropathies, there is central sensitisation of NMDA glutamatergic receptors in the dorsal horn, and in some cases there is invasion of lamina II by sensory neurones in laminae III and IV, which then activate nociceptive neurones (Attal, 2000). Central perception of neuropathic pain is thought to involve the posterior parietal cortex, but this is not the only function of that cortical region.

In human trigeminal neuralgia there is an intermittent or more persistent, sharp, electric facial pain, which is set off by touch, chewing or cold drafts. In horses, orbital neurectomy can relieve what is thought to be a comparable condition, in which the horse persistently shakes its head and rubs its face on its foreleg (Newton *et al.*, 2000). Neuralgia can be differentiated from some of the other causes of head-shaking by applying local anaesthetic to the apparently affected nerve and looking for relief of the behaviour. The cause of this form of neuropathic pain in horses is not understood.

10.6.7 Nerve compression

Nerve compression can produce action potentials within the axons of the nerve provided the nerve is not damaged. The activation will be painful if the nerve con-

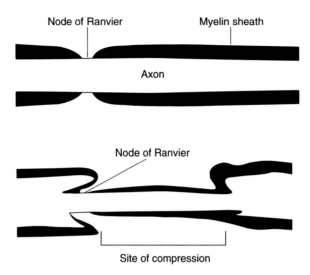

Figure 10.3 Schematic drawing of a nerve before (top) and after (bottom) compression, showing invagination at the node of Ranvier (bottom).

tains fibres that form part of a pain pathway. Often there is a stabbing pain. If the nerve is crushed by the compression, there is a multiple burst of activity in the nerve, leading to multiple, slightly longer-lasting sensations. A chronically trapped nerve often produces a sharp burning pain, accompanied by muscle weakness distal to the entrapment. The pain itself may be situated either at the area of the entrapment or in the distal muscles. Sometimes a trapped nerve gives rise to paraesthesias. In these cases the myelinated nerves become distorted at the node of Ranvier (Figure 10.3). The paraesthesias develop from nervous activity that is transmitted along less severely-distorted myelinated fibres, whereas in entrapment, pain may be mediated by *nervi nervorum*. If the entrapment develops into a neuropathic pain it has a severe burning quality.

The pain from compression of nerves in the spinal cord can be particularly debilitating. Spinal cord compression by a spinal abscess is the commonest cause of posterior paralysis in pigs (Vaughan, 1969). The infection is usually blood-borne from an abscess elsewhere in the body, and, if the abscess bursts, pus may break into the spinal canal. Spinal cord compression by a tumour causes pain, which is often provoked by a particular posture and by coughing.

Nerve compression in a hind limb is quite common in downer cow cases. If the cow is recumbent for prolonged periods a disabling compression of branches of the sciatic and radial nerves can develop. Radial paralysis is obvious from dragging of a hind limb when the cow attempts to rise and knuckling of a hind fetlock. Violent kicking is thought to be a sign of paraesthesias in the limb, and bilateral knuckling of both hind fetlocks is more likely to be associated with back pain. A comparable limb paralysis can occur with peroneal nerve compression in ostriches.

When a subject experiences pain from 'the bends', gas forms in the sheath of myelinated nerves. The pressure on the nerve provokes neuralgia partly from a direct effect of compression, but also from pressure-induced ischaemia (Hornberger, 1950). The pain radiates to other regions.

10.6.8 Anaesthesia dolorosa

When trauma results in a dorsal root being torn away from the spinal cord, severe pain often develops in the denervated region. This phenomenon is similar to the sensitisation occurring in phantom pain, except that the denervated region has not been amputated. It is known as *anaesthesia dolorosa*. The stump in the dorsal root that is still connected with the dorsal horn is hyperexcitable and discharging persistently. In animals, the pain this provokes can lead to self-mutilation of the denervated region. Rats that had the roots at L5 and L6 ligated showed limb guarding, repeated hindpaw lifting, allodynia and hyperalgesia.

10.6.9 Sympathetic nervous system involvement

Normally, sympathetic activity has no direct effect on pain. However, enhanced pain through adrenergic effects has occurred in the following conditions:

- chronic arthritis;
- neuropathic pains, including headache;
- soft-tissue trauma;
- complex regional pain syndromes, such as reflex sympathetic dystrophy and causalgia.

The increased pain is mediated through α-adrenergic receptors which seem to increase or maintain the ongoing low-grade activity of nociceptors, which in turn keep the pain-mediating neurones in a sensitised state. As a result, continuous pain and allodynia can exist in these conditions.

If sympathetic nervous activity leads to poor perfusion of nerves, a dystrophic pain can develop. This is a burning, aching or throbbing pain, that is often accompanied by hyperalgesia, oedema or erythema. It can be triggered by coronary ischaemia, inflammation of a joint capsule, tendonitis and trauma which involves a bruise or sprain.

Within the spinal cord, activation of α-adrenergic receptors can have an analgesic effect, either by endogenous release of noradrenaline by descending pathways from the brain stem or from exogenous spinal administration of agents such as clonidine. The α-adrenergic agonists have a synergistic effect with opioid agonists.

10.6.10 Referred pain

Referred pain occurs when pain is felt at a site which is removed from the site of the lesion. The referred pain is often in the skin surface that is innervated by the same segment of the spinal cord that is receiving signals from the origin of the pain. For example, angina originating in the heart is often referred to the skin on the inside of the arm. This can be due to convergence of signals from the damaged area with other inputs at spinal cord neurones, which summate to produce referral of the pain. Alternatively it may be due to localised axon reflexes within the skin, and summation of inputs from both sites at the thalamic level causing central interpretation of a referred pain (Arendt-Nielsen & Svensson, 2001).

Referred pain is not easily recognised in animals, but gentle palpation of the area to which the pain is referred increases the pain. Local anaesthesia of the zone to which pain is referred sometimes decreases the pain.

10.6.11 Neurotransmitters in pain pathways

There are over 25 naturally-occurring compounds in the body that help to produce pain. Many of them are neurotransmitters, and their role in mediating pain has been demonstrated in the following ways:

- they are present histochemically within pain pathways;
- they provoke or enhance pain responses when administered in conscious subjects;
- they produce pain, hyperalgesia or nociceptor pathway activation that is blocked by analgesic or specific inhibitors of the respective neurotransmitter;
- they are released or accumulate at the site where pain afferent pathways are activated.

With so many pain neurotransmitter substances that have different actions, it is difficult sometimes to know which pain-relieving substance should be given for a particular condition. However, we do know which neurotransmitters are usually involved with the more common types of pain (Table 10.4).

This table does not specify where in the pain pathway the neurotransmitter operates, and this should be taken into account when deciding how to provide pain relief. The following points relate to the individual neurotransmitters:

- Acetylcholine and potassium ions may be responsible for localised early pain that occurs when a site is injured.
- Adenosine triphosphate (ATP) has a particular role in pains that involve leaking of sarcoplasm from unexhausted muscle. Adenosine has a similar role, but it is more likely to leak from metabolically depleted muscle.
- Bradykinin is released from plasma at the site of tissue injury, and can be involved in trauma pain and inflammatory pain.
- Cytokines are released from immune cells such as macrophages, and the pain they provoke accompanies inflammatory pain and cancer pain.
- Glutamate activates NMDA receptors in the dorsal horn of the spinal cord, and is responsible for spinally-mediated hyperalgesia.
- Other neurotransmitters that are present in the spinal cord which may also influence pain signal transmission are the tachykinins (including Substance P), CGRP, bombesin, somatostatin, VIP and nitric oxide.

Table 10.4 Examples of types of pain mediated by some neurotransmitters, receptors or substances.

Neurotransmitter	Type of pain
Acetylcholine	Acute pain in tissue damage
Aspartate	Hyperalgesia
Adenosine/ATP	Hyperalgesia, myonecrosis pain, muscle injury
Bradykinin	Allodynia, cardiac pain, hyperalgesia, inflammatory pain, intestinal pain, oesophageal pain, skin pain
CGRP	Chemical stimuli, joint pain, mechanical stimuli, muscle pain, periosteal pain, sensitisation to inflammatory pain, skin pain, thermal pain, trigeminal headache
Cytokines	Hyperalgesia, inflammatory pain
Glutamate	Hyperalgesia, allodynia, wind-up pain
Histamine	Headache, hyperalgesia, tissue swelling
Hydrochloric acid	Gastric and duodenal ulcer pain
Lactate	Inflammatory pain, ischaemic pain
Leukotriene	Inflammatory pain
Nerve growth factor	Hyperalgesia
Neurokinin	Allodynia, vascular headache
Nitric oxide	Neuritis
Potassium ions	Cardiac pain, ischaemic muscle pain
Prostaglandins	Hyperalgesia, inflammatory pain
Protons	Cardiac pain, inflammatory pain, ischaemic pain, mechanoreceptor sensitisation
Serotonin	Bruises, hyperalgesia, inflammatory pain, migraine, tissue swelling, some forms of gastro-intestinal pain (cancer)
Somatostatin	Thermal pain
Substance P	Arthritic pain, back pain, cardiac pain, hyperalgesia, joint pain, periosteal pain, skin pain, trigeminal headache
Uric acid	Gout
Vasoactive intestinal peptide	Visceral pain

- Histamine is released from mast cells and may be responsible for some forms of trauma pain.
- Nerve growth factor causes proliferation of dendrites, some of which possess nociceptors, and it causes a delayed and relatively long-lasting hyperalgesia. Its production at inflammatory sites, which include the bladder and joints, is stimulated by interleukin-1β. It can also sensitise dorsal root ganglion neurones.
- Protons accumulate in inflamed or ischaemic tissue, and set up a localised response through activation of H^+-gated cation channels in sensory neurones.

- Serotonin is released from platelets, and has a particular role in delayed pain associated with tissue injury.
- Serotonin, bradykinin, prostaglandin and histamine are not responsible for immediate pain during injury, as these substances must first be synthesised or the cells containing these compounds be recruited to the injured site.

The benefits from having multiple pain neurotransmitters are as follows:

- enhanced gating capacity at the level of the spinal cord;
- some neurotransmitters exert a permissive effect for others;
- amplification of stimulus intensity when appropriate;
- allows modification of the receptive field;
- enables specificity in responses according to the type of stimulus in some situations.

10.6.12 Hyperalgesia

Hyperalgesia is a common feature with tissue injury and inflammation. There is enhanced sensitivity to painful stimuli and it takes two forms: in **primary hyperalgesia** there is excessive sensitivity at the site of the injury; in **secondary hyperalgesia** there is increased sensitivity in uninjured tissue surrounding the injury. The zone of secondary hyperalgesia is often present as a halo around the primary zone. The pain in primary hyperalgesia can be provoked by heat, mechanical and chemical stimuli, whereas secondary hyperalgesia only applies to mechanical stimuli.

The primary hyperalgesia that develops, for example, at the site of a burn injury is mediated by sensitisation of nociceptors. The threshold of activation is lowered, and there is enhanced response to stimuli that exceed that threshold. In secondary hyperalgesia, however, there is central sensitisation, often at the level of the spinal cord. The increased sensitivity in secondary hyperalgesia may start the day after the injury, whereas primary hyperalgesia has a quicker onset.

Central sensitisation in the spinal cord occurs when the cord receives repetitive nociceptive signals. This activates improved efficiency in synaptic transmission in the pain-relevant neurones in the dorsal horn. This sensitisation is mediated by NMDA and neurokinin-1 receptors.

Interleukin-1β is an extremely potent hyperalgesic agent when administered systemically at low doses (Ferreira et al., 1988). This effect is mediated by vagal afferents and prostaglandin E_2 (PGE_2) acting on the preoptic area of the hypothalamus and in the neighbouring basal forebrain (Hori et al., 2000). The hyperalgesia is blocked by lesioning either the rostral ventromedial medulla (RVM) or the dorsolateral funiculus which connects the RVM to the dorsal horn in the spinal cord. At high doses, there is analgesia which is mediated by PGE_2 in the ventromedial hypothalamus. This distinction between low and high doses is relevant to the situation where hyperalgesia occurs during the early phase of an acute systemic infection, and is followed by analgesia once a fever sets in. Early clinical signs of hyperalgesia during an acute systemic infection can include myalgia and arthralgia.

If trauma results in disuse of a gland, smooth muscle, skeletal muscle or a nerve, and those parts do not undergo significant atrophy, they can show supersensitivity to a stimulus. In the case of nerves this is known as **denervation supersensitivity,** and if there are pain fibres in the nerve there is enhanced awareness or sensitivity to pain. **Wind-up** is a specific type of hyperalgesia. It occurs when repetitive activation of C-fibres leads to augmented responses to subsequent C-fibre input.

Allodynia is another specific type of hyperalgesia where pain can be provoked using a stimulus that would not normally be painful. For example, receptors normally associated with the sensation of touch acquire the capacity to evoke pain. It can be due to central sensitisation of non-noxious $A\beta$-fibre impulses at the level of the dorsal horn of the spinal cord, or to sensitisation of the peripheral nervous system. Sympathetic efferent activity can contribute to some forms of allodynia through α-adrenergic receptors. Common causes would be inflammation, tissue injury and damage to peripheral nerves. It is often associated with secondary hyperalgesia and neuropathic pain. Simple ways of testing for allodynia in the skin are to stroke, brush or rub the region, or stretch the skin at the affected part, and watch for a pain response.

Erythralgia is redness of the skin which is associated with pain or hyperalgesia. It occurs in inflammatory conditions, chilblains, frostbite and lesions due to defective blood supply.

10.7 Pain in a Given Context

10.7.1 Inflammatory pain

Inflammation is probably the single greatest cause of pain in vertebrate species. The type of pain that is felt varies between different organs. Infection of the cornea produces a persistent dull throbbing pain, osteoarthritis is often a persistent ache interspersed with episodes of stabbing pain and inflammation in the nasal sinuses causes a constant burning pain. Mastitis, which can be a very painful condition for dairy cows, is associated with a feeling of 'hot cords' in women, especially during and after milk let-down.

Acute pancreatitis, cancer of the pancreas and shingles produce some of the severest pains in people. Pancreatitis produces a continuous boring pain, associated with abdominal muscle spasm, reduced diaphragmatic movement and progressive hypoventilation. Part of the pain is attributable to the release of pancreatic enzymes into the abdominal cavity. Peritonitis is almost as bad.

During inflammation, the pain is particularly intense if the swelling is trapped. This occurs for example in inflammation of the laminae in the foot which press against the rigid wall of the hoof in horses and cattle. In dogs, paronychia can be painful for a similar reason. These situations are made worse by the continuous pressure exerted on the foot by weight-bearing and movement.

During inflammation there is hyperalgesia, and, in particular, increased sensitivity to heat. This sensitisation occurs gradually, because the mediators between wound injury and the initiation of inflammation take time to accumulate, and they have to reach an excitation threshold before pain is activated. Sensitisation to mechanical stimuli, such as pain during movement, also takes time to develop, and so movement can be achieved for a short period after an injury or the start of an infection without necessarily incurring pain.

During inflammation, mediators that depolarise terminal nerve endings and produce a sustained excitation of nociceptors and afferent nerves accumulate. The mediators include protons, bradykinin, histamine, serotonin and prostaglandins. The sensitivity of the tissue to these agents is increased by neurotrophic factors, and in particular by nerve growth factor (NGF). The tissue concentration of NGF rises in response to the proinflammatory cytokines interleukin-1β (IL-1β) and tumour necrosis factor-α (TNF-α). Much of the ongoing nociceptor activation can be prevented by neutralising NGF, whereas increasing the concentration of NGF produces hyperalgesia by raising nociceptor activity and responsiveness in the dorsal horn (Koltzenburg, 2000).

Bacterial cell wall components, such as lipopolysaccharide, and cytokines released in response to those components, result in hyperalgesia. In some situations there are specific combinations which provoke inflammatory pain. For example, there are three cytokines which have been implicated in bone pain: granulocyte–macrophage colony stimulating factor (GMCSF); granulocyte colony stimulating factor (GCSF); and interleukin-3 (IL-3). Besides bone pain, they can also mediate the development of headache, myalgia and fever.

The two visible effects of inflammation, vasodilatation and plasma extravasation, are indirect indicators of the likely presence of pain. The vasodilatory response appears as a flare at the site of injury or infection and the extravasation is seen as a wheal or swelling. Both are neurally mediated by vasogenic neuropeptides (e.g. Substance P and CGRP). The vasodilatory response is brought about in three ways:

(1) axon reflex;
(2) spreading depolarisation;
(3) axo-axonal coupling.

The **axon reflex** is a local reflex. When a nociceptor is activated, impulses pass along the afferent nerve towards the spinal cord. Before reaching the dorsal horn, some of the activity is relayed antidromically down other afferent branches that join the nerve (Figure 10.4). The antidromic impulses promote vasodilatation in the skin or mucous membrane neighbouring the nociceptive field. This localised

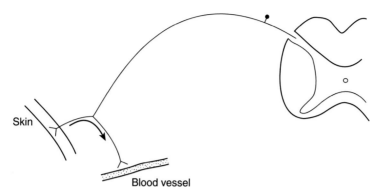

Figure 10.4 Axon reflex from skin to a blood vessel.

reflex is known as axon reflex vasodilation. It can be initiated by histamine through H_1 receptors, and effected by Substance P and CGRP. Localised **sweating** can also occur through the axon reflex (Magerl & Treede, 1996). The vasodilatory response is not necessarily caused by the same concentration of agents that elicits pain. As a result, the redness or flare responses are not precise guides to the pain that is felt, but they are useful indicators of the presence of pain activators in the wound.

10.7.2 Post-operative pain
Some sequels to surgery are:

* pain;
* nausea;
* vomiting;
* intestinal stasis;
* changes in substrate metabolism;
* alterations in electrolyte and water metabolism;
* increased demands placed on the cardiovascular and respiratory systems.

Operations that can lead to long-term pain at or near the surgical site include:

* various operations on the limbs;
* facial surgery;
* mastectomy;
* thoracotomy;
* episiotomy;
* vein-stripping alongside a nerve;
* cholecystectomy.

During recovery following operations on the chest or abdomen there can be the following reflex behavioural responses:

- muscle spasms at the site of the wound;
- muscle contraction on either side of the wound can act as a 'muscle splint', limiting movement and coughing;
- partial closure of the glottis, producing a grunting sound during breathing.

Restrictions on coughing can complicate the clearing of respiratory secretions and lung recovery.

Pain following surgery can result in coronary artery vasospasm through activation of the sympathetic nervous system. When this is associated with raised heart rate and blood pressure, there is potential for myocardial ischaemia and anginal pain.

There are three approaches to controlling post-operative pain:

(1) Allow the animal to recover from anaesthesia, and, when signs of pain such as crying, restlessness, panting, licking or biting the affected area develop, an analgesic is given.
(2) In anticipation of pain on recovery, an analgesic is given after completion of surgery but before recovery.
(3) In anticipation of pain on recovery, an analgesic is given before surgery is started.

Long-term unrelieved pain can lead to self-mutilation. Reducing post-operative pain may help prevent this, and it has been shown to aid recovery. For example, it can reduce pain-provoked reflex vasoconstriction and muscle tension, and so assist perfusion.

10.7.3 Ischaemic and reperfusion pain

When a very tight tourniquet is applied to a limb, there is immediate pain at the site of the tourniquet which subsides within a few minutes as numbness sets in. After about 30 minutes the tingling numbness is gradually replaced by an ache. This ache gets progressively worse, even though the distal part is completely numb, and it is due to ischaemia. If the tourniquet is released, there is immediate relief that is quickly followed by a more severe **reperfusion pain**, which is accompanied by buzzing sensations, tightness, tingling and cramps.

Ischaemic pain occurs in:

- angina;
- some forms of post-operative pain;
- occlusion or injury of major blood vessels;
- 'bends' due to decompression.

It presumably occurs in:

- animals caught in snares and leghold traps;
- castration and tailing with rubber rings;
- prolonged recumbency;
- excessively-tight bandages, harnesses or hobbles.

Tourniquet pain consists of ischaemic pain and pain due to nerve compression. It is often resistant to spinal anaesthesia, and this is because the afferent nerves which are activated by H^+, lactate, adenosine and K^+ at the ligature take the route of the sympathetic chain instead of the spinal cord. Sympathetic afferents are also thought to be the primary mediators of myocardial ischaemic pain (Sutherland *et al.*, 2000).

10.7.4 Electricity
Animals come into contact with electricity in the following ways:

- electric fencing;
- stray currents;
- electric dog collars;
- electric goads;
- electrical stunning;
- electroimmobilisation;
- electrocution units for pest control.

The feeling created by an electric shock is due to two effects: first, there is the direct activation of nerves near the point of contact, and they conduct a barrage of pulses to the brain; second, there is the violent jerk of the muscle contraction.

During electric stunning, if the current is incorrectly applied, the animal can experience an electric shock instead of being immediately stunned (Gregory, 2001). This is common in turkeys, because the wings of the bird hang below its head. The wings make contact with the electrically live water of the water-bath stunner before the head is immersed and the bird is stunned (Plate 4).

The pain that is caused by a shock from an electric dog collar can provoke aggression. This response is not common but has been seen in dominant males which attack a nearby dog on receiving a shock which is part of a training schedule.

If an electric current is sustained for a long period, as in some electroimmobilisation procedures, there is a likely to be delayed-onset muscle pain the next day. This is associated with eccentric contractions, which in general generate a higher force per active fibre. The pain is linked to connective-tissue damage and a non-infected inflammatory response.

10.7.5 Back pain

Back pain and lameness can be due to unusual pressures or injury in the vertebral column and pinching of the spinal cord or spinal nerves. Herniation of an intervertebral disc exerts forces on axons and nerve cell bodies which render the neurones spontaneously active, and hyperexcitable to mechanical and chemical stimuli. Mechanical agitation of the region can be very painful, and chemical mediators of localised inflammation aggravate the pain further. These mediators are released from immune cells recruited to the site, and from the *nucleus pulposus* that is exposed from the ruptured disc (Devor & Seltzer, 1999).

Pain can also arise from direct compression of the cord and its nerves, and from the supra- and interspinous ligaments, facet joints, longitudinal ligaments, outer fibres of the annulus fibrosis and vertebral endplates. The posterior longitudinal ligaments are highly innervated and traction on these ligaments is very painful (Kumer *et al.*, 1996). The spinal *dura* is poorly innervated, and, unlike the *dura* in the cranium, it does not have the capacity to allow the type of neurogenic inflammatory responses that cause headaches.

Debilitating painful back disorders are seen in most species, but especially in dogs, layer hens, broiler chickens, pigs and horses. In dogs, conditions of the lumbar spine that cause back pain include intervertebral disc prolapse, spinal tumours, discospondylitis and osteomyelitis.

Dachshunds and Doberman pinschers are prone to disc herniation (Le Couter & Child, 1995). In the Dachshund the vertebral canal is narrow in relation to the size of the spinal cord, and so any minor extrusion of disc into the epidural space is likely to produce clinical signs. Pain from pinching of the *cauda equina* at the joint between L7 and the sacrum is sometimes seen in German Shepherds, and there is usually ventral displacement of the sacrum relative to the lumbar vertebrae. The region is painful to palpation and during simple hind-leg movements such as standing up and extending the hind leg. Elevation of the tail can also be painful.

In hens, when osteoporosis involves the vertebrae they may fracture, typically at T4 or T5. The spinal cord is compressed causing partial paralysis (Riddell *et al.*, 1968). In broiler chickens, misalignment of vertebrae is known as 'kinky back' or *spondylolisthesis*. In severe cases, it causes posterior paralysis and the birds die from dehydration from not being able to reach the drinkers.

In horses, a painful lameness can occur when pinching of the spinal nerves develops following a violent movement such as jumping.

10.7.6 Bone, joints, tendons and ligaments

Pain can originate in the cortex, marrow or periosteum of bone. During simple accidents and injuries much of the pain is generated from receptors in the periosteum. However, the sensitivity of periosteum varies between sites. For example, in the skull, the periosteum of the occipital and temporal regions has a very low sensitivity to pain, whereas that of the supraorbital ridge is more sensitive (Ray &

Wolff, 1940). In general, bone is less sensitive to pain than joints: for example, when a needle is inserted into the cartilage of the patella, there is a tapping or pressing sensation; when it is pressed against the lining of the joint there is severe pain 'somewhere in the knee' (Gardner, 1950).

The pain-sensitive regions in a joint are the capsule, ligaments, periosteum, perivascular sites and synovial surfaces. The pain receptors respond primarily to pressure. The capsule and ligaments are sensitive to distension from swelling, twisting and stretching. The pain these create has a deep, often sickening quality. It provokes strong autonomic and motor reflexes, including a slowing of the pulse, a fall in blood pressure and nausea. If a joint is swollen, any motion puts pressure on the capsule causing pain. What is ordinarily benign movement is now extremely painful.

The presence of blood in a joint can be painful from two effects: first, if it causes swelling, there will be activation of pressure receptors; in addition, breakdown products from the red blood cells can provoke an inflammatory response which leads to hyperalgesia (Keele & Armstrong, 1964).

Total **rupture of a tendon** is not always painful. It depends on where the rupture has occurred. Most of the nociceptors in tendons are situated close to the muscle attachment and damage in that region is more likely to be painful.

Rupture of a ligament when running or jumping can be very painful and lead to a lasting pain. Rupture of the anterior cruciate ligament is a well-recognised cause of lameness in dogs, and is seen most commonly in the Poodle, Labrador and Retriever breeds (Barnes, 1977). Traumatic disruption of the ligaments in the lower foreleg is a common form of injury and lameness in racehorses (Bowman *et al.*, 1984).

The synovial tissues are innervated by small-diameter fibres that secrete neuropeptides including Substance P and CGRP. Substance P can elicit **arthritic pain**. In osteoarthritis there is sensitisation of afferent nerves to these peptides. Pain arises from the synovial tissues lining the joint, which in turn leads to inactivity and stiffness. In advanced conditions there is destruction of articular cartilage and remodelling of subchondral bone, resulting in deformity and loss of function. There is a persistent ache and stabbing pain during movement or weight-bearing.

Degenerative **osteoarthritis** is seen in elderly animals including old dairy cows, bulls and dogs. It has been a common reason for culling beef breeding bulls (Bellenger, 1971). In cattle, horses and dogs it is a heritable disorder, and in dogs it can develop from hip dysplasia and elbow osteochondrosis. The pain and discomfort are obvious. The animal is lame and finds walking unpleasant. In dogs, often the first sign is a reluctance to climb stairs or jump. There may be episodes of stiffness shortly after the animal stands up, and this progresses eventually to lameness. The dog may be aggressive when interfered with.

Osteochondritis dissecans is a painful condition in humans and animals, where there is erosion of the cartilage in a joint and the underlying bone. In severe cases, the cartilage may peel away from the subchondral bone and lie loose in the synovial space. The pain limits extension of the joint, and there is often intermittent swelling. The joint may lock and sometimes it can be heard to click. In horses it features when there are defects in the blood supply to the joint, and it occurs in metacarpals of trotters because of their unnatural stamping gait. In the past it has been common in breeding pigs, but corrective genetic selection has reduced its prevalence. In deer it has been linked to dietary copper deficiency.

Fast-growing broiler chickens are prone to leg disorders that result in poor walking ability. Most of these disorders are structural growth problems rather than infections, and injecting a non-steroidal anti-inflammatory drug has improved walking ability, suggesting that the structural disorders are painful (McGeown et al., 1999). In addition, when given the opportunity to consume either a normal feed or a feed containing the non-steroidal anti-inflammatory drug carprofen, lame birds selected more of the feed with the pain-relieving drug than the non-lame birds (Danbury et al., 2000).

10.7.7 Muscle pain
Muscle pain occurs with direct trauma, overexertion, inflammation or sustained muscle contraction. It can take a number of forms:

- cramps;
- aches;
- sprains;
- spasms;
- soreness;
- sensitivity to pressure or touch;
- pain that is referred to other parts.

A dull aching pain is more usual than a sharp pain.

Afferent nerve endings are present in the connective tissue and fascia surrounding muscle bundles, between muscle fibres, in blood vessel walls and in tendons. They are particularly dense in the region of tendons and fascia. Some of the nerve endings serve as pain receptors which respond to noxious stimuli. These receptors are responsive to bradykinin, serotonin, histamine and potassium, and they use Substance P, calcitonin gene-related peptide (CGRP) and vasoactive intestinal peptide (VIP) as neurotransmitters. Substance P and CGRP induce oedema and vasodilatation as well as having a direct role in pain-fibre neurotransmission. Oedema favours the accumulation of bradykinin that is derived from blood during inflammatory and ischaemic conditions, and the responses to bradykinin are mediated through specific receptors (Graven-Nielsen & Meuse, 2001).

Deep muscle pain is often diffuse and extends to a large area. The reason is that Substance P and CGRP are released into the muscle from nerve terminals when pain receptors are activated. This occurs as antidromic axon reflexes through the side branches of the neuromuscular network, and these pain agonists can be released into a large volume of muscle.

Muscle can become sensitised to painful stimuli following trauma or unaccustomed exercise. This occurs in two ways: first, pain receptors in muscle can be sensitised to end products of anaerobic metabolism including protons which bind to Na^+ channels in the receptor membrane; second, they can be sensitised by substances from outside the muscle. For example, following injury, bradykinin enters from the bloodstream and increases the pain response to serotonin. The second mechanism involves gradual accumulation of excitatory agents, so it tends to be slower.

Ischaemia alone does not necessarily result in muscle pain, but when combined with exercise it is likely to be painful. It is a continuous pain rather than being synchronised with muscle contraction and relaxation. This suggests that it is not linked to the tension of the muscle acting on nerve endings. Instead it is due to an accumulation of products from muscle contraction. When the circulation is restored the end products can be removed and the pain goes away.

Muscle cramp is an involuntary, very painful contraction which has a highly-active electromyogram (EMG). Spasms are short-lasting and occur, for example, near an injury or an inflamed site. The pain is more likely to be noticed during passive or active movements that cause the muscle to stretch rather than shorten (Macdonald, 1980).

Muscle sprains are a hazard in horses and dogs. They occur mainly when the animal falters, or when there is a sudden change of pace. If opposing muscle groups lose coordination and suddenly act against each other, such as when a horse plunges or slips, they can tear each other at their ligaments or within the belly of a muscle.

Muscle necrosis may occur following exercise if there are macrophage invasion, release of lysosomal enzymes and sufficient hydroxyl radical formation to cause cell injury. The likelihood of free radical accumulation is greatly reduced in animals that are physically fit (Salminen & Vihko, 1983). Muscle necrosis can be associated with pain.

Cystic swellings due to invasion of muscle by warble fly larvae, trichinella and cysticerca can create painful pressure points. Injection of large volumes of drugs intramuscularly causes a deep, dull, diffuse ache. This pain can be controlled by injecting the drug slowly to avoid a rapid localised rise in pressure.

10.7.8 Cardiac and chest pains

Cardiac pain is described as a pressing, constricting or squeezing pain, with periodic bands across the chest. It is often accompanied by nausea and vomiting, and by diffuse sweating and an alarm reaction, sometimes with the feeling of impending death (Procacci *et al.*, 1999). The pain associated with *angina pectoris* is similar, but is not accompanied by nausea, vomiting or the feeling of impending death. There is a deep referred pain with muscle tenderness. The signs of cardiac pain in animals are relatively non-specific, and make this form of pain difficult to diagnose.

The mechanisms evoking cardiac pain are:

- reduced coronary arterial pressure distal to an occlusion, acting on coronary artery pressoreceptors;
- ischaemia, stimulating the myocardial pressoreceptors and chemoreceptors;
- release of pain-producing substances formed by tissue breakdown or platelet disintegration.

Sudden death from coronary occlusion is often reputed to be painless, but some people who survive to relate their experience have complained of severe pain (Saunders & Platt, 1999). The pain caused by longer-term myocardial ischaemia could be due to bradykinin, serotonin, adenosine, histamine, prostaglandins, lactate or potassium activation of chemoreceptors connected to autonomic afferent fibres.

When cardiac-arrest stunning, such as head-to-back stunning, was introduced in abattoirs, there was concern amongst some people that the current that passed through the heart might be painful for the animals. This, however, should not be a problem provided the stunning current is applied correctly and passes through the brain where it induces instantaneous insensibility. Nevertheless, the electrocution system used for the euthanasia of dogs in parts of India could provoke pain because current does not flow through the brain.

It is said that the heart can be pinched and pricked without the conscious subject feeling pain. Bleeding an animal by cardiac puncture is also reputed to be virtually pain and stress free once the operator has perfected the technique (Beckman & Iams, 1979). Cats can even be oblivious of the procedure when it is performed well.

Intracardiac injection of barbiturate is sometimes used as a form of euthanasia, and concerns have been raised that it might be painful. When pentobarbitone is injected percutaneously into a vein and some leaks subcutaneously, there is a rapid physical reaction indicating irritation, if not pain. Whether this irritation occurs in myocardium during an intracardiac injection is not known. However, some animals go limp in about two seconds from starting an intracardiac injection, in which case the pain or discomfort would be brief. In unskilled hands there is a risk of injecting the drug into the lungs without killing the animal, and this will cause signs of respiratory distress.

Pain can occur when there is pericarditis, myocarditis and endocarditis, but it is more frequent in pericarditis. Pain in the oesophagus is sometimes indistinguishable from cardiac pain.

10.7.9 Udder and teats
Udder and teat injuries are very important in dairy farming. Teat soreness causes the cow to object to being milked, and she will kick the cluster off. Teat injuries occur when they get trodden on whilst the cow is sitting, from incorrect vacuum pressures during milking and from accidents with fencing wire.

Teat treading, causing complete loss of a teat, is apt to occur in cows with milk fever, pendulous udders and short stature. Cows with short hind legs place their feet near the udder when rising, and this poses a risk for the lower teats that protrude from a large udder. Teat injury is also more common in cows that are apt to lie down in the dairy yard before milking, but this would not be common except in lame cows. In countries where dairy cows are housed, teat treading is more common where there is no bedding, where the movement of the cow is affected by the design of the cubicles and where slatted floors are used.

Udder oedema is a very painful condition for dairy cows. The udder becomes distended with excessive interstitial fluid from about seven days before calving, and this persists for as many as nine days following calving. A traditional method of treating the condition is to stab the skin on the underside of the udder and allow the fluid to drain. On one occasion when this was done, over five litres of interstitial fluid was collected. This unpleasant condition is due to increased hydrostatic pressure within the blood vessels of the udder, and this develops from raised venous blood pressure (Vestweber & Al-Ani, 1985).

10.7.10 Parturition and dystocia

In women, pain during labour is mainly associated with the early uterine contractions and dilatation of the cervix. Once the cervix is fully dilated the worst of the pain is over. There is, however, some pain from tearing of fascia and from distension of the vaginal canal as the foetus descends down the tract, and from stretching of the perineal region which provokes a sharp localised pain. In some subjects, pain develops in the thighs where it is felt as an aching cramp. Pain is said to be greater in primiparous women.

The pain components are probably similar for the cow. It is also common for the cow to give a roar during the final stages of assisted calving. This coincides with the final pulling of the calf after the head and forelegs have appeared. This additional pain could be due either to the passing of the hips through the pelvis, or to reorientation of the hind legs from a flexed to an extended position within the uterus. The feet of the calf would press against the uterus wall and cause stretching of the uterine ligaments.

The pain threshold during parturition is higher than normal. This is brought about by stretching and stimulation of the cervix and vagina, which provoke reflex opiate-mediated analgesia. In sows, this analgesia does not disappear until the seventh day after farrowing (Jarvis et al., 1997). It is not known whether a cow that is induced to calve, using corticosteroids or prostaglandin, has the same degree of endogenous analgesia as a cow that is at full term and calves naturally, but experience in women suggests that induced labour could be more painful (Paech, 1991). Induction with prostaglandin $F_{2\alpha}$ can have unpleasant side-effects in dogs, including excessive salivation, vomiting, diarrhoea, hyperpnoea, ataxia and anxiety.

Some cases of dystocia are undoubtedly unpleasant for the cow. Problems develop if delivery is protracted and the calf dries out whilst lodged in the uterus and vagina. There is also the risk of damaging the foetus during delivery, and in some situations this could result in subsequent pain for the newborn. For example, assisted parturition can be associated with fractured ribs in the calves and foals (Mee, 1993). The duration of subsequent pain or discomfort in the calf and foal is not easy to predict.

10.7.11 Pain in the neonate

The human infant can experience pain soon after it is born. Circumcision causes pain, and this is seen in short-term alterations in feeding, sleeping and crying behaviours, and in the heart-rate rise at the time of the cutting which can be prevented by applying a local anaesthetic (Anand & Hickey, 1987). In practice, analgesia is rarely given.

In the rat, most of the pain pathways are well-developed by the time of birth in terms of presence of the normal neurotransmitters and the neuroanatomical structures associated with pain-signal transmission. However, it seems unlikely that the full-term foetus, and in particular the foetal lamb, can feel pain before it starts breathing air. This is because the brain is not normally sufficiently oxygenated whilst the foetus is *in utero* to allow perception (Mellor & Gregory, 2003). The foetus can, however, show distinct responses to somatic stimuli which look beguilingly like conscious responses.

Following birth, young infants and animals often show exaggerated responses to pain. This applies to both acute pain and neuropathic pain (Chung *et al.*, 1995). There are still some maturation changes that have yet to occur in the central nervous system, and these modify pain neurotransmission as the infant grows. For example, the expression of c-fos transcription factor in lamina II of the dorsal horn of the rat spinal cord can only be evoked by Aβ-fibre activity in the newborn, whereas it is evoked by Aδ- and C-fibre inputs in the adult (Fitzgerald, 1999).

Painful experiences early in life can sensitise infants to future pain, or make them hyperexcitable when they experience another bout of pain. It has been found that circumcised boys had an increased pain response to vaccination 4–6 months later in comparison with non-circumcised controls (Taddio *et al.*, 1997). This was thought to be due to long-lasting changes in pain behaviour due to central sensitisation, but it is also possible that there was peripheral sensitisation. Tissue damage in the early postnatal period can cause pronounced and lasting sprouting of local nerve terminals, producing an area that is hyperinnervated and hypersensitive. This exaggerated sprouting occurs in A- and C-fibres, but not in sympathetic fibres. C-fibres retain the ability to sprout into adulthood, but A-fibre sprouting only occurs whilst the subject is young.

Trauma

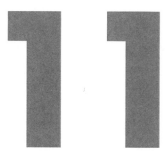

This chapter examines some of the main types of trauma that occur in animals. Where appropriate it explains the pathophysiology following the injury, and draws on information from similar types of trauma in humans.

11.1 Injuries in Selected Body Regions and Tissues

In animals, the legs and feet are the parts of the body that are most frequently injured. These injuries are particularly debilitating for animals that have to find their own feed and water. Some typical examples in farm animals and horses include excessive walking on hard ground causing bruising to the sole, treading on sharp metal objects, becoming entangled in wire, running into obstacles, impact with the ground during a jump or fall, entrapment in a cattle grid or a loading ramp and being kicked by another animal. In general, during the early period following the injury, the deeper the injury the greater the likelihood of pain and lameness, provided a major afferent nerve has not been severed.

Wounds to the neck and upper body are common in cases where animals have run into fencing or been kicked by another animal. Puncture wounds on the body and upper limbs are a common feature of snagging or collision with fixed sharp metal objects (nails, bolts, feeders) or striking a piece of wood that remains embedded in the animal. Injuries to the ventral abdomen can occur when the animal attempts to jump an obstacle.

Mouth and nostril injuries should be given special consideration because in many animals this is the exploratory part of the body and so it is prone to injury, and because of the dramatic effect on subsequent feeding ability and survival. Drenching is one of the most common husbandry treatments given to sheep, and this can present a risk of mouth damage. Injuries can arise from sharp edges forming on the nozzle of the drenching gun through wear and use, incorrect insertion of the nozzle and use of nozzles that are too long. There have been incidents where long nozzles introduced into the mouth too forcefully caused perforation of the back of the mouth. In one report, some sheep died shortly after drenching from ruptured carotid arteries whilst others in the same flock developed a purulent discharge from the nostrils or mouth. Damage as severe as this would not be common, but injury to the inside lining of the cheek and between the tongue and jaw is probably more frequent.

Mouth injuries in horses can occur:

- when worn or badly-fitting bits cut the tongue or lips;
- if a rider is unusually harsh with the reins;
- if the horse has a soft mouth, and rubber, rubber-covered bits or bitless bridles have not been used;
- when a horse rears and pulls away whilst tied by the reins with a bit in its mouth.

Tooth damage is common in cats. In a study in Switzerland it was found that 14% of 200 domestic cats presented at a veterinary clinic had dental fractures. In 95% of cases the canine teeth were involved, and most were crown fractures. The incisors and carnassial teeth are commonly broken in feral cats, and this involves the root as well as the crown (Verstraete et al., 1996). Fighting is a likely cause of canine fractures, and eating bones probably contributes to carnassial tooth damage.

Quite often the speed at impact is important in determining the extent of an injury. This is particularly relevant in the case of abdominal injuries. Slow compression is relatively innocuous, whereas a rapid slam in the viscera can result in liver rupture and death (Lau & Viano, 1981).

11.1.1 Injury to nerves

The painful effects of nerve compression are described in Chapter 10. This section considers the effects on neurotransmission and nerve function. There are three ways in which neurotransmission can be affected:

(1) mild pressure producing ischaemic block;
(2) intermediate pressure disrupting the myelin sheath;
(3) strong pressure disrupting the axon, causing Wallerian degeneration.

Compression of a nerve using 20–30 mm Hg pressure can impair venous flow in the epineurium, but it takes higher pressures (130–150 mm Hg) to cause a block of impulses (Gelberman et al., 1993). When low pressures are applied for brief periods, the effects are rapidly reversible, but higher pressures can cause temporary injury because it takes longer to recover from the structural and functional changes. Both axon conduction and synaptic transmission can be inhibited by pressure effects.

When a nerve is rendered **ischaemic** for sufficient time, it is damaged in two ways:

(1) There is an influx of calcium into the cells via voltage-dependent calcium channels and glutamate-regulated ion channels. Intracellular calcium over-loading leads to cell damage through activation of proteases, lipases and endonucleases.

(2) During reperfusion, at the end of the ischaemic episode, there is release of oxygen radicals, synthesis of nitric oxide and inflammatory reactions, from the sudden availability of oxygen in the presence of enzymes that became activated during the ischaemia. Excessive free-radical formation is cytotoxic.

Injury to peripheral and central nerves results in **Wallerian degeneration** of the nerves. The first stage in this process is shrinking and fragmentation of the axon distal to the injury. The small axonal fragments are enclosed individually in myelin, which digests the dead axon, and then the myelin itself becomes degraded to fat globules by microglia. This pattern of degradation can occur in nerves that are transected, crushed, subjected to toxins or deprived of blood supply, and it is usually completed within a fortnight of the injury (Guth, 1956). It takes two to four days for the nerve distal to a complete transection to lose its ability to conduct an impulse.

If an injury causes localised **demyelination** of a nerve without affecting the axon, that nerve may show ectopic firing. This activity is linked to regrowth of the membrane and it can give rise to pain (Devor & Seltzer, 1999). In other situations, demyelination can disrupt neurotransmission totally.

Damage to a nerve sheath can also render an axon prone to ephaptic transmission. Impulses from one nerve fibre activate impulses in an adjacent fibre or axon. This can be due to failure in insulation and to hyperexcitability in the recipient nerve. Nerves that are severely demyelinated do not show ephapsis, only poorly insulated nerves. The transmission created at ephapses tends to be highly disorganised. It can also be linked to pain, for example in neuromas and in postherpetic neuralgia.

11.2 Some Common Causes of Injury

The cause of an injury has a strong bearing on whether or not it will become infected. Lacerations from sharp objects, such as knives, glass and metal, carry a relatively low risk of infection, whereas shear wounds from nails, barbed wire, bites and sticks carry a high risk. Barbed-wire injuries are particularly serious if there is degloving of a leg, laceration of a joint or injury to the heel. Soft-tissue damage from kicks and collisions are prone to infection if the injury is large. When puncture wounds go unnoticed, they can develop deep-seated infection.

11.2.1 Mustering, fence-line and stockyard injuries

An important principle in mustering livestock is to avoid unnecessary excitement, otherwise the animals are prone to erratic behaviour and may injure themselves or each other in their attempt to escape. The pace that is set should be determined by the slowest animal, whether it be lame or a young animal that is prone to being left behind. Unnecessary excitement can lead to charging the gateways, and some animals may go down or strike a gatepost. The injuries this incurs can lead to abortion in pregnant stock or to implantation losses shortly after mating. In extreme cases, an animal may charge a fence or attempt to clear it by jumping. This usually happens when an animal gets separated from the herd or flock, and it can lead to entanglement in the fence or injuries from the wire.

Maintaining fence-line and stock handling facilities in a serviceable condition is part of good farming practice. One example where this failed was a case in which rains had eroded a gateway at a set of yards, causing a depression in the ground beneath a gate. This encouraged calves to attempt to escape through the gap between the gate and the ground, and two calves ended up with broken backs when they struck the bottom rail of the gate (Edwards et al., 1995). Broken bones in the back can also occur when calves try to turn around in a race or crush. It is usually the processes of the vertebrae that are damaged, rather than the body of the vertebral bones.

Gate-charging can occur when sheep are yarded and an individual becomes separated from its group. It turns back and tries to join another group at the other side of a gate. Gates are often unscreened in forcing pens to encourage a visual draw from groups up ahead, but one of the disadvantages of this is the occasional case of gate charging.

In square holding pens, cattle can bunch up in a corner. They may bury their heads in the corner, and at worst an animal may go down and be trampled. Some corners can be easily eliminated by installing a curved barrier across the inside of the corner. Closing the headbail on a running animal is likely to cause bruising. In addition, catching an animal around the ribs or slamming the gate immediately in front of its head in order to stop it, is liable to cause injuries. Straight neckbars in the headbail are less likely to choke an animal, in comparison with wedge-shaped neckbars, especially if the animal goes down whilst yoked. Curved neckbars give better control of head movement than straight neckbars. In general, cattle are quieter if there is body restraint as well as head restraint. They tend to fight the head restraint when held by the head only. It has been known for animals to lose consciousness when neckbars have compressed the carotid arteries in the neck.

Teat tears used to be common in dairy cows where barbed-wire fencing was used, but now, barbed wire has been replaced by electric fencing on most dairy farms. In its place, one sometimes sees a teat completely severed from the udder when a cow walks though a high-tensile wire fence that is not electrified. When a horse gets entangled in a broken barbed-wire fence, it is apt to plunge and pull backwards repeatedly, making leg wounds worse. Camels can also experience problems because when they are pricked by barbed wire they tend to jump forward, and this can result in them becoming completely ensnared. At one time, barbed wire was used to control flying foxes in orchards. The wires were strung between poles above the orchard to deter these night-time fruit eaters.

Injuries from fence-charging can be fatal. In a report on translocation of wild kangaroos, 14 out of 41 kangaroos were lost as a result of this, and another kangaroo died from drowning (Keep & Fox, 1971). The holding pen should be small (10–15 m²) to control flight speed and reduce the height of jumping. Fences are best made of strong terylene netting instead of wire, timber or steel, and it is not always advisable to muster them at night-time, as they seem then to crash more heavily into obstacles in their path when aroused.

In African wildlife reserves, hartebeest and sable antelope have been known to get entangled in fence wire, to the extent that they had to be destroyed (Lewis & Wilson, 1977). The risk of fence-charging is probably greatest during the panic created by hunting and predation, but it can also occur during chasing by members of the same species. When impala have been mustered into a kraal and then confined in a crush, the mortality rate from injuries has been as high as 30% (Murray et al., 1981). Manual restraint of the animal on its side on the ground, with a blindfold over its eyes, was much less traumatic.

11.2.2 Livestock transport

Livestock inevitably pick up bruising during pre-slaughter handling and transport (Table 11.1). In cattle, bruising is common in the forequarter, but more severe types of bruising occur in the hindquarters (Jarvis et al., 1996). Bruising around the pin bones is common in thin cull dairy cows. Narrow gate openings to trucks, over-vigorous unloading from the truck and forcing the stock too hard in the corridors and raceways are thought to be major causes of bruising (Marshall, 1977).

Cattle normally move cautiously when being introduced to new enclosed surroundings, and forcing them leads to crowding, jostling and striking partitions, corner posts and gateway openings. When crowded they push each other against gateways, and head-butt adjacent animals especially in the flank and lower hindquarters (Blackshaw et al., 1987). Covering dangerous posts with padding

Table 11.1 Prevalence of wounds and bruises in carcasses that required trimming by meat inspection staff in New Zealand meat-processing plants (after Gregory, 1998a).

Species	Wounds and bruises (%)
Cattle	6.0
Deer	4.3
Calves	3.5
Sheep	0.8

could go some way to reducing such bruising. Although it is recommended that horned cattle should not be transported with hornless cattle, one often sees pens of mixed stock (horned and hornless) in the yards at abattoirs. The level of bruising in horned cattle can be double that of hornless cattle (Meischke *et al.*, 1974). Removing the tips of the horns does not necessarily provide any benefit (Wythes *et al.*, 1979).

Bruising from fighting is likely to be worse in pigs that are mixed with unfamiliar animals, and it is a particular problem in boars and bulls. Using sticks instead of electric goads has been associated with more bruising in the skin over the hindquarters (Geverink *et al.*, 1996). Transhipment also increases the prevalence of bruising (Moss & Trimble, 1988).

11.2.3 Road accidents

Vehicle injuries to livestock occur when:

- dry feed is put out in paddocks for stock – cows are prone to being struck, especially if they are hungry and there is competition for the feed;
- vehicles drive over paddocks in the dark, for example driving over a newborn calf when inspecting the calving herd;
- a gate is left open and animals wander onto a roadway.

Kangaroos, white-tailed deer and stray dogs are three uncontrolled mammals that are commonly struck by vehicles on roads. In parts of the Middle East and Central America there is a high incidence of stray-dog road injuries. These dogs are semi-feral, living under or near food factories in the cities during the day, and they come onto the streets at night. Most of the carcasses are seen on the high-speed freeways. In the case of kangaroos and white-tailed deer, most road accidents occur at dawn, dusk and during the first two hours after sunset. In deer there is a seasonal incidence which coincides with the rut. As with stray dogs, the accidents are most common in fast traffic. It has been estimated that 90% of the deer are killed outright when they collide with vehicles, and a further 2% are thought to die shortly afterwards (Allen & McCullough, 1976).

In the past, road accidents have accounted for over half the number of dogs presented at veterinary clinics as trauma cases (Kolata *et al.*, 1974). This number has declined in recent years, but it is still a significant cause of trauma. Pelvic injuries from car accidents are common in medium-sized animals, whilst smaller animals are usually completely crushed. Domestic dogs and cats are usually hit whilst crossing a road, whereas wild animals are more likely to be injured whilst eating road kill, and small birds are prone to being struck in windy conditions, when they are forced to fly closer to the ground.

When a medium- to large-sized animal is hit by a moving vehicle (Plate 5), there are usually two separate impacts: the first is from the direct impact with the vehicle; the second occurs either when the animal is thrown onto the vehicle, or from being thrown against the ground. At the time of impact, the body is often lifted upwards and it may spin or turn onto the bonnet (hood). Catastrophic injuries start to occur when the vehicle is travelling at more than 32 km/h (Weis *et al.*, 1983). If the foot is struck whilst it is weight-bearing there is likely to be more injury in that limb.

Smaller animals are more likely to pass under the car instead of landing on the bonnet. In this situation, they are prone to shearing wounds in the hind leg. This occurs when the leg is scraped along the road as the animal is pushed or towed by the vehicle. The tissues on the medial aspect of the leg are rasped away (Beardsley & Schrader, 1995).

In a study of 200 human road casualties, time to death following an accident was shortest when there was respiratory paralysis and rapidly exsanguinating haemorrhage from a chest injury (McCarroll *et al.*, 1962). Rib ends often punctured the lungs causing a haemothorax. Not infrequently, a transverse fracture or dislocation of a thoracic vertebra was accompanied by fracture of the adjacent ribs, allowing the detached portions of the vertebral column to glide forward, transecting the cord and thoracic aorta. Injuries to the head, pelvis and legs were associated with longer survival, and this gives greater hope when treating these victims.

When death occurred more than 24 hours after injury, the two most common causes of death were pulmonary embolism secondary to a leg fracture and subdural haematoma following head injury. One third of the head injuries were occult injuries, in other words they were hidden or concealed injuries with no overlying fracture or penetrating wound. Most of those cases had a subarachnoid haemorrhage. If the abdomen took the blow, the sudden increase in intravascular pressure sometimes ruptured the aorta. Intra-aortic systolic pressure has to increase ten- to twentyfold to produce this effect.

Laceration or rupture of the liver is a common abdominal injury in road accidents. Typically, a lower rib impacts with the liver, causing crushing, comminution and haemorrhage. Haemorrhage from a lacerated liver is generally faster than from a lacerated spleen. The pelvis protects the major blood vessels in that region, but open pelvic fractures are often associated with severe haemorrhage (Poole *et al.*, 1991). Death is due to irreversible haemorrhagic shock or a coagulopathy.

11.2.4 Floor injuries

The type of floor surface and bedding used in stock housing can influence foot and leg disorders in livestock. In pigs, partially-slatted floors are associated with an increased prevalence of heel erosions, heel flaps, white-line lesions, wall separations and false sand cracks. The danger with slatted floors is uneven distribution of pressure on the surface of the foot. For example, if a toe is pressing on the slat whilst the rest of the foot is over a gap, there is a risk of the toe peeling away from the sole. The width of the slat relative to the width of the gap is critical in avoiding this type of problem. There are advantages in providing slip-resistant floor surfaces, but they must not be too abrasive, otherwise there is a risk of causing too much erosion and in generating uneven pressures which lead to bruising.

Table 11.2 Prevalence of different forms of foot wear and injury in grower pigs.

Foot injury	% of pigs	Comments
Sole erosion	75	Wear of the sole and heel
White-line lesions	55	Damage between the wall and sole of the foot
Toe erosion	33	Absence of horn at the toe
False sand cracks	24	Cracks in the wall of the hoof
Heel flaps	14	Peeling of the horn of the heel
Wall separation	11	Visible gap between the wall and sole

Toe erosion can be common in straw-bedded pigs, but sole erosions, heel erosions and heel flaps are more common in pigs kept on concrete. The risk of injury to the wall of the foot, and the start of white-line disorders, is increased in pigs kept on straw bedding compared with bare concrete, and when pigs slip on wet floors (Mouttotou *et al.*, 1999). The prevalence of different types of foot injury in pigs is shown in Table 11.2.

Overgrowth of the claws from insufficient wear can occur in any animal kept on soft floor surfaces. When this develops, the wall of the claw is prone to tearing away from the sole. In addition, the weight of the foot is thrown back on the heel, and the sole becomes concave rather than flat.

Newborn animals have very soft soles in their feet (Mouttotou & Green, 1999). In piglets, it takes up to four days for the sole and wall to harden. During this period it is helpful to protect the piglets' feet from hard surfaces with litter, otherwise there will be sole bruising and foot tenderness. In many piggeries, farrowing-crate floors are made of round weldmesh or perforated cast iron, but mats can be used to soften the surface during the critical early period.

Soft feet also lead to foot trauma in cattle. When cattle are kept under boggy conditions the horn on their hooves softens and swells and is prone to damage if the animals are made to stand or walk on a hard abrasive surface. This in turn makes the foot more prone to bacterial attack.

11.2.5 Broken bones in layer hens

When a bone is broken, pain arises from distortion and pressure on receptors serving intramedullary nerve fibres, stretching of receptors in periosteum and from pressure on receptors in muscle and soft tissues around the bone. Immediately following the trauma a haematoma develops and the pressure it creates within the compartment triggers further pain from receptors in the fascia and soft tissues. Chemical agents (bradykinin, histamine, potassium and peptide neurotransmitters) accumulate in the damaged tissues, where they sensitise undamaged nociceptors, and the site becomes tender. Those chemical agents also help to initiate an inflammatory response which involves oedema and swelling which provoke further pain through activation of pressor receptors.

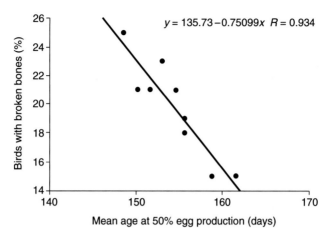

Figure 11.1 Relationship between age at onset of egg-laying and the proportion of hens with broken bones at end of lay.

Bird bones are relatively brittle and prone to fragmenting or shattering on impact. Layer hens develop osteoporosis because of their high turnover of bone in producing eggshells, and, in the case of battery hens, because of their sedentary lifestyle. This makes their bones more likely to break when the birds are taken from their cages at the end of lay. In one study which examined commercial practices in the United Kingdom, 29% of battery hens had broken bones by the time they came to be slaughtered. Birds that reach puberty early are more prone to broken bones when they are caught at the end of lay (Figure 11.1).

Broken bones are not just a problem in battery hens. A quarter of hens from barn units and 12% of hens from free-range units were found to have old breaks by the time they were sent for slaughter. These fractures had occurred during lay and had repaired by the time the birds were culled. Handling the birds causes fresh breaks, and flight accidents contribute to old breaks (Gregory & Wilkins, 1995) (Figure 11.2).

11.2.6 Flight accidents

Birds collide with windows in buildings, motor vehicles, overhead power lines, aeroplanes and fences or walls. Flight accidents are very common amongst some species. In a study of feral rooftop pigeons, 6% of the birds showed evidence of previously broken bones (Gregory & Wilkins, 1991). The fractures were in the furculum, femur, radius and keel, and it was suspected that furculum and keel damage were incurred during collisions or crash landings.

Collision with windows is most common amongst fledglings that have just left the nest. Carter (1967) described an unusual incident in which a flock of starlings flew into a concrete floor. In Scotland, deer fences are a hazard for black grouse

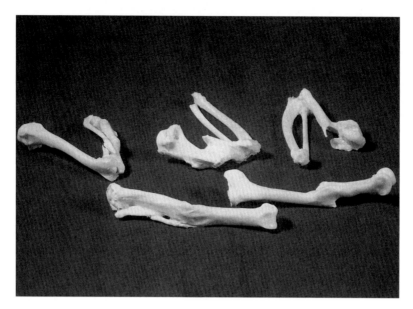

Figure 11.2 Previously broken and mended bones in hens.

and capercaillies where the fences border woodland or a tree belt. Dead birds from a wide range of species are found under electricity power lines. This is more common during migration periods, and most accidents occur with the ground wire. This wire is thinner than the conducting wires and is more difficult to see. Removing the ground wire is not an option, as it leaves the line unprotected against lightning strikes, but making the cables more visible is likely to be effective (Alonso *et al.*, 1994). It has also been recommended that power lines should not be sited in mountain passes along important migration corridors. There are at least three species which have been seriously depleted by wire and cable strikes: these are the barn owl in parts of Europe, the eagle owl in Switzerland, and the Japanese crane, which has now become an endangered species.

Aeroplane strikes by gulls are a hazard at coastal airfields. The number of incidents is highest in the post-breeding season when young gulls are about. Other species commonly involved in aircraft collisions are ducks, starlings and owls. Starlings have been known to disable both engines and cause fatal aircraft crashes.

11.2.7 Fishing
When fish are caught by hook and line, the hope is that the hook will be in the mouth or jaw, but in a minority of fish the hook catches other parts (Table 11.3). Small hooks tend to cause more serious trauma than large hooks (Corbines, 1999). Small hooks tend to lodge in the gut and gills and this causes death from haemorrhages. Similarly, the finer hooks on triple-hook plugs cause higher mortalities than live bait on single large hooks (Nelson, 1998).

Table 11.3 Hooking location in striped bass using different catching methods.

Hooking location	Artificial lures (%)	Live bait (%)
Number of fish	267	124
Jaw	82.4	58.8
Mouth	13.8	24.2
Pharynx	0.4	4.7
Oesophagus	0.7	9.0
Gills and gill arch	1.9	0.5
Head or body	0.7	2.8

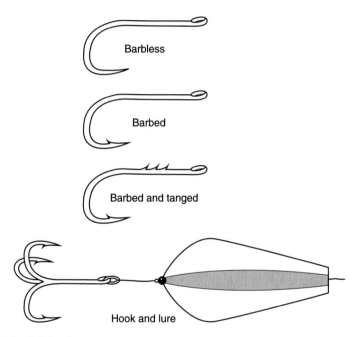

Barbless

Barbed

Barbed and tanged

Hook and lure

Figure 11.3 Fish hooks.

There has been a move away from barbed hooks towards barbless hooks, especially for catch-and-release fishing (Figure 11.3). Barbless hooks are thought to inflict less trauma and so the chances of survival are greater. This has been a controversial topic amongst fishermen, and studies which have compared subsequent mortality in trout caught by the two types of hook have produced conflicting conclusions (Schill & Scarpella, 1997; Taylor & White, 1997).

Commercial fisheries and regulatory authorities are now putting effort into controlling overfishing. Fish which are undersized and catches that exceed specified creel limits are released. One of the problems with this is that fish that are caught from depths greater than 20 m are prone to decompression during rapid ascent. Gas-filled organs such as the gut and swim bladder are overinflated, and so, when they are released, the fish fail to dive and instead float helplessly near the surface. It can take several hours before they manage to adjust the volume of their swim bladders (Bettoli & Osborne, 1998), and the overinflation contributes to mortality amongst released fish. The solution that has been developed is manually to puncture the swim bladder or the abdomen with a hypodermic needle or trochar and cannula. This procedure is only appropriate for certain species (Collins *et al.*, 1999), and the swim bladder is reputed to heal rapidly (Shasteen & Sheehan, 1997).

Boat propellers can cause substantial injury to fish, especially amongst larval and juvenile forms that are unable to escape the turbulence near the boat. Mortality rates of up to 83% have been reported for fish larvae that are in the zone of the propeller. Death is not immediate, taking up to three hours in some cases (Killgore *et al.*, 2001). Propeller-induced trauma is a problem in narrow waterways where the opportunity for escape is reduced.

11.3 Intended or Avoidable Causes of Trauma

This section discusses some of the amputations that are performed on animals without anaesthetics and some of the more common injuries acquired during recreational activities with animals as well as injuries that inevitably occur when animal numbers are controlled by physical methods such as shooting or trapping.

11.3.1 Mulesing

The mulesing procedure was developed in South Australia in 1930 by J.H.W. Mules using Merino lambs. The aim of mulesing is to remove skinfolds surgically to help maintain a clean breech and so reduce the risk of fly strike. Blowflies are attracted to the breech region if it is dirty, sweaty or contaminated or scalded by urine. Mulesing does not eliminate all forms of flystrike, as tail strike, body strike, pizzle strike and head strike can still occur, although these forms of flystrike are less common than breech strike. It is claimed to be a necessary procedure because of the growing resistance of blowfly to insecticides.

In the original method devised by Mules, a fold of skin in the breech region was raised and clamped with a set of Burdizzo emasculators, and then the fold was removed with a sharp knife (Seddon, 1935). This was probably more humane than the present method, where the skin fold is raised and cut off with a set of very sharp shears, without crushing the nerves and blood vessels in the skin with the Burdizzo. Crushing the nerves probably eliminated pain produced by the cutting action and from subsequent stimulation of the edges of the wound. In addition, the clamping effect reduced bleeding, and in some lambs the skin edges that were pressed together by the Burdizzo remained attached to each other. However, Mules' method was not widely adopted because it was slow and cumbersome (Plate 6).

Mulesing is undoubtedly painful for lambs. The animal adopts an abnormal posture and gait, and eats less for two or more days following the operation. Judging from the duration of the plasma cortisol rise, mulesing is a more distressing experience for lambs than either tailing alone or castration plus tailing (Shutt et al., 1987), and the wound usually takes a little over two weeks to heal. However, it is a practice that is strongly defended by many sheep farmers. The suffering associated with flystrike which is not treated is said to be far worse than that experienced following the operation. The blowfly eggs that are laid in the breech region can hatch out within 12–24 hours and it is impossible to inspect stock frequently enough to treat all infested animals.

Poor mulesing technique can increase the suffering. For example, cutting the breech region too close to the midline can cause skin stretching which results in the vulva gaping open. This draws flies to the vulva which irritates the ewe, and it increases the risk of neoplasia if the tail was butted at docking. Careless cutting can take out muscle which causes added pain, and extending the cut too far down the leg results in taut skin above the hock which limits leg flexion during running and walking. Standards and training programmes are in place in Australia to limit these mistakes.

11.3.2 Pizzle dropping

Pizzle dropping is less common than mulesing. It is done to control sheathrot, pizzle strike or urinary calculi. The sheath is severed with a set of hand shears from the underline of the belly to allow the pizzle to droop, and this facilitates drainage of urine (Marchant, 1986). In the case of sheathrot and pizzle strike, the aim is to eliminate fouling of the belly wool with urine. Wool contaminated with urine that has a high nitrogen content is particularly likely to attract blowflies and cause sheathrot, and so the procedure is more common on farms with a high clover content in the sward. In the case of calculi, the aim is to reduce retention of urine in the penis and urethra and the build-up of stones at the flexure. Sheep kept on limestone country are more prone to these calculi, but testosterone implants are now used in wethers as an alternative to pizzle dropping for preventing their formation.

11.3.3 Tail docking and castration

In various countries, **tail docking** is performed on sheep, dairy cows, pigs and dogs. In most cases, the tails are removed without analgesia using either an elastic ring which cuts off the supply of blood, a cautery iron which burns through the tail or a blade.

The types of pain that could be experienced during and following docking include:

- pain associated with cutting the tail;
- inflammatory pain following docking;
- causalgia;
- phantom-limb pain;
- pain associated with neuromas;
- ascending neuritis.

The aim of tailing in sheep is to reduce the prevalence of fly strike. Part of the reason for this is that cutting the tail short, so that it does not press on the vulva, helps reduce the prevalence of urine contamination of the crutch. However, research has shown that when sheep scour butted-tailed sheep are struck more frequently than sheep with long tails (Watts & Marchant, 1977). Nevertheless, tradition has it that removing the whole tail ensures that excessively long tail wool does not get fouled by diarrhoea, and that this helps control tail strike.

In lambs, tail docking with a rubber ring causes similar cortisol responses to those seen with a heated docking iron, whereas tail docking with a knife caused longer-lasting cortisol responses and is not recommended (Stafford & Mellor, 1993).

Tail docking is commonly used in New Zealand in dairy cattle, and to a lesser extent in Victoria, Australia, to avoid swishing dirty tails interfering with milking staff. Petrie (1994) monitored the behaviour of three-to-four-month-old calves when they had a rubber ring placed on the tail as part of the amputation procedure. The signs they showed included tail shaking, vocalisation, running and hind-leg kicking. Calves which received epidural lignocaine before ring attachment did not show these signs until 160 minutes, when the anaesthetic had worn off. The plasma cortisol responses, however, were similar to the control calves which were not docked, and Petrie concluded that over the first eight hours docking was not a major stress for the calves.

Dog breeders justify tail docking on the grounds that it reduces tail injuries. There is some evidence in working gundogs which supports this view. In Sweden, tail docking was banned in 1989. Shortly after introduction of the ban, the Swedish German Pointer Club examined the prevalence of tail damage in 50 litters of undocked working gundogs (Strejffert, 1992). In the autumn of 1990, when the undocked dogs were 1–1.5 years old, 27% of the dogs had experienced tail injuries. By the time the undocked dogs were 2–2.5 years old, 35% of the dogs had experienced tail injuries.

There were four types of tail injury:

(1) bleeding and damaged tips (last 10 cm of the tail);
(2) infected and inflamed tails;

(3) injuries associated with tail lameness;
(4) broken tails.

The injuries were more common or more severe in male dogs, in the more lively dogs and the more the dog was used, especially in thick undergrowth. By the time the survey was nearing completion, tails had to be amputated from 7 out of 92 tail-injured dogs. Other experience has shown that some working gundogs that have had their tails amputated because of tail damage have taken to mutilating their own stumps (Peek, 1995).

Not all breeds of working gundog are prone to tail damage, and so not all of them need to be docked to prevent those injuries. For example, the English Pointer is not docked because it is used in open country rather than thick bush. It has been argued that working spaniels go into undergrowth head first with long hairy ears, and no one chops off their ears (McCreath, 1993).

Overall, the majority of tail injuries are in pups, either from an infection or from bleeding following docking. In those animals it seems that docking has done more harm than good. Nevertheless, when a tail injury does occur, healing can be a slow and difficult process. Mercer (1992) commented that he found some tail injuries the most difficult ones he had to treat, especially when they are at the tip of the tail. There is blood everywhere at every wag and repeated shortening is sometimes needed.

Castration is potentially more painful than tail docking. In young livestock it is performed without analgesia using either an elastrator rubber ring, Burdizzo emasculator or a sharp knife and pulling the testes out. Rubber-ring castration in lambs results in a rapid rise in the plasma cortisol concentration which peaks approximately 40–60 minutes after treatment and returns to baseline levels within approximately 2–3 hours. This response has served as a means of comparing the pain and distress of the different methods, when applied with and without analgesics (Sutherland *et al.*, 1999; Thornton & Waterman-Pearson, 1999). The conclusion is that all the methods are painful.

Castration and tail docking are usually performed at the same time in lambs, and it has been found that when a knife is used for cutting both the tail and the scrotum there is longer-lasting distress (about eight hours) than when two rubber rings are used instead – one ring for the tail and the other placed around the scrotum above the testes. Indeed, when castration and tailing are done together, one of the least painful methods is to use rubber rings (Stafford & Mellor, 1993). The mortality following the different methods of castration and tailing are similar (Fairnie & Cox, 1969).

In lambs, short-scrotum ring placement is used in some flocks where the aim is for male lambs to reach slaughter weight rapidly (Figure 11.4). It caused a plasma cortisol response similar to castration with the ring placed above the testes. In piglets, castration is performed by incising the scrotum with a blade, plucking the testes from the scrotal sac, and cutting or tearing the spermatic cord. All of these

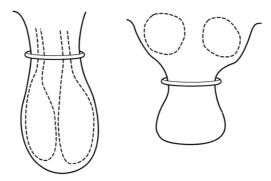

Figure 11.4 Rubber-ring castration above and below (short-scrotum castration) the testes.

acts cause a stronger heart rate when conducted without a local anaesthetic, suggesting that each component is potentially painful (White *et al.*, 1995). Incising the scrotum and severing the spermatic cord were thought to be the most painful components.

Intratesticular injection of phentobarbitone was developed as a method for castrating pigs in the 1950s. There is a reaction at the time of inserting the needle. Substantial pressure is required to inject 10–15 ml of fluid into each testis, but it is claimed that it does not cause appreciable distress in the boar (Dyson, 1964). Nevertheless, the method is not widely used because of concern that it is painful. Phentobarbitone exerts its anaesthetic effect centrally and it is not likely to provide a local anaesthetic effect.

In the past, male birds have been caponised surgically as a routine husbandry procedure. In chickens this practice dates back to the sixteenth century, if not earlier, and it was particularly common in China. It was done to produce a bird with superior eating quality in terms of the succulence of the meat, but when performed by inexperienced hands it carried the risk of rupture of an abdominal vein or peritonitis. In ostriches it was done to reduce feather damage.

11.3.4 Antler removal
In most countries where deer and wapiti are farmed, antlers are harvested for their velvet which is used in the traditional-medicines market in East Asia. The antler is removed using a saw once the animal has been sedated with xylazine and the nerves to the antler have been blocked with lignocaine. This approach has been shown to provide an adequate level of analgesia during the operation. However, xylazine residues have been detected in antler velvet, and there is concern that a carcinogenic metabolite of xylazine (2,6-xylidine), is produced in deer-velvet consumers (Dalefield & Oehme, 1999).

There is growing interest in using drug-free methods of harvesting antler velvet, and, in particular, in applying pressure ligation on the nerves and blood vessels at the base of the antler. This approach is already being used for spiker removal in young stock that are due to be transported for slaughter, and in the future it may be extended to adult animals. It is important to establish whether compression of the antler nerves provokes pain from trapping the nerve, or whether it blocks conduction and induces analgesia.

Whatever method is used for removing the antlers, care needs to be taken to avoid and, if necessary, treat post-operative infections. The wound can become flyblown, and infections have been known to spread through the face, requiring destruction of the animal. This, however, has not been common.

If the antlers are left on the animal, the velvet is shed, and the hard antlers are used as weapons during the rut. The pointed ends of the antlers can cause serious damage to other deer and to stock handlers, and (Plate 7) shows chest puncture wounds in a deer that was transported with other animals that were in hard-antler.

11.3.5 Tooth clipping

Tooth clipping is a normal husbandry practice without analgesia in pigs, llamas and alpacas. It is sometimes performed in laboratory rats without a sedative or analgesic (Quinn et al., 1994).

Tooth clipping in piglets is usually limited to the eye teeth which are liable to cause facial scarring amongst littermates when the piglets compete for a teat. It is thought that facial wounding is associated more with the occasional breakdown of a consistent teat order than with its original development. Reducing the length of these teeth may also save the sow's udder from lacerations. If the teeth are clipped too close to the gum, there is a risk that they will splinter and pulpitis will set in.

In alpacas and llamas, tooth clipping is performed on the wolf or fighting teeth to control damage between sparring males. Typically, the males inflict ear, scrotal and neck skin injuries when fighting. Obstetrical wire or a powered rotary grinder are often used to shorten the teeth every three years. The alternative is to provide the animals with plenty of space so that they can escape from aggressive encounters. A rotary grinder is sometimes used on the incisors in cases of prognathism in show animals. In the words of one alpaca owner, 'they don't like it'.

11.3.6 Declawing

Toe removal or declawing is done in cats that are destructive to furniture, on protruding dew claws in dogs and in turkeys, ducks, cockerels, hens and emus if there is a risk of scratching other birds.

Various techniques are used for declawing cats, but in all procedures it is necessary to remove the dorsal aspect of the ungual crest in order to prevent regrowth (Figure 11.5). The cat is usually sedated or anaesthetised, and the claw removed with nail trimmers, in which case pain will be limited to the post-operative period.

When ducks and turkeys are due to be sent for slaughter they are loaded into transport modules by a team of catchers. If the birds become stressed, they are apt

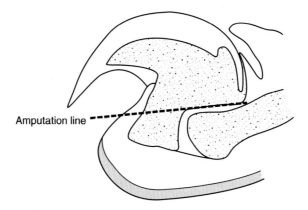

Figure 11.5 Amputation line for use when declawing a cat.

to migrate to one end of the shed where they climb onto each other and inflict back scratching with their claws. This can cause a blemish in the carcass, affecting its marketability. Some companies avoid this problem by amputating the last digit of the toes of the birds when they are chicks. The last digit of the middle toe is sometimes removed in layer hens when problems develop with claw puncture holes in the eggs. Breeder cockerels often have the backward facing toe, or hallux, removed when they are chicks to prevent claw development and damage to the backs of females later on. On some farms emus are declawed with a cautery blade to control damage to other birds and to staff. Either the middle toe or all three toes are declawed.

When declawing has to be performed, the birds should be housed on a soft clean surface rather than on concrete or wire, as this will help to reduce repetitive opening of the wound. Similarly, the birds should be inspected regularly and action taken if birds take to pecking at each other's wounds. There is a risk of claw-bed infections with *Candida* or fungi, especially when declawing is done in older birds. Neuromas in the stump of the chicken's toe are smaller and less complex than those seen in the beak following beak trimming.

11.3.7 Deflighting
Deflighting is done to prevent birds escaping from parks and zoos, and it is used as an alternative to caging birds that are kept in private collections. A range of methods is used, including feather-clipping, wing-wiring, patagiectomy, pinioning and tenonectomy (Figure 11.6). These are usually performed on one wing only to create asymmetry that will unbalance the bird when it attempts to fly. The methods and their complications have been reviewed (Hesterman *et al.*, 2001). The method of choice depends on individual circumstances, but only feather-clipping should be used if a veterinarian is not available to do the other operations using an anaesthetic. Feather-pulling has been performed in the past, particularly in northern

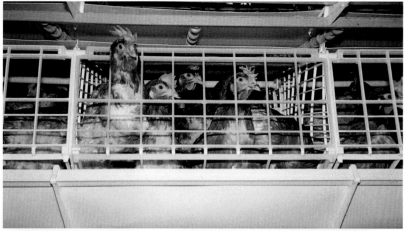

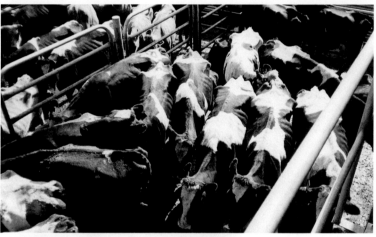

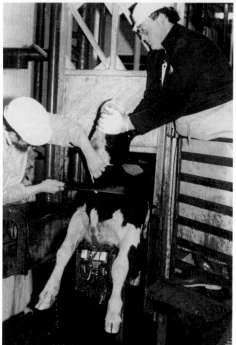

Plate 1 (top) Confinement of hens in a battery cage

Plate 2 (middle) Emaciation in cull dairy cows

Plate 3 (left) Animal about to be slaughtered by shechita

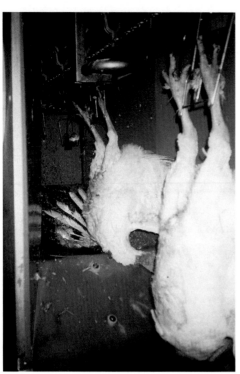

Plate 4 Electrical stunning in turkeys where the left wing dips into the electrically live water before the head

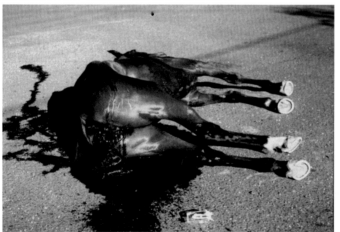

Plate 5 Road accident case (Courtesy of Steve Coleman RSPCA New South Wales)

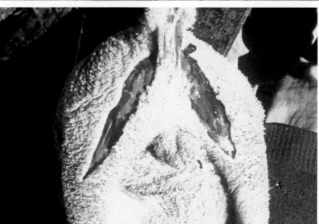

Plate 6 Typical position of the mulesing cuts shown for short-tailed and butted tail ewe lambs

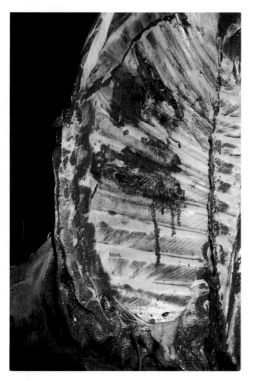

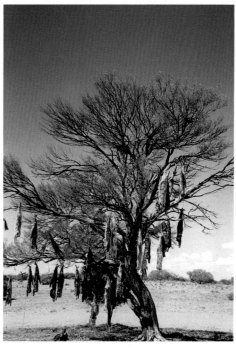

Plate 9 Tree used for displaying trapped feral cat gibbet

Plate 7 Antler puncture wounds in the rib cage of fallow deer

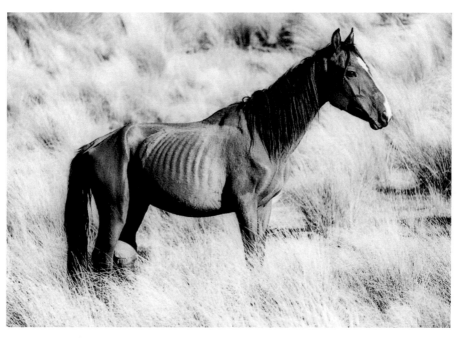

Plate 8 Kaimanawa pony that was shot in the left hind leg during a helicopter cull, 10 months before this photograph was taken (Courtesy of Liz Gillespie and Kate Littin)

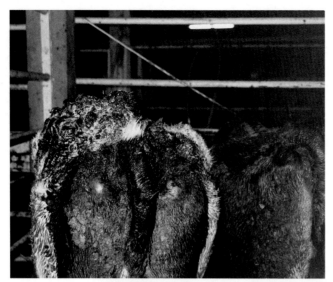

Plate 10 Squamous cell carcinoma in a cow

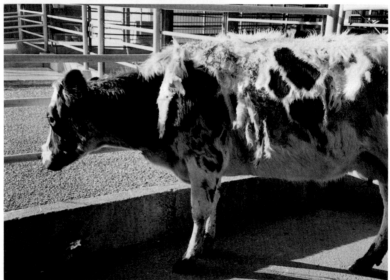

Plate 11
Cow displaying
signs of facial
eczema

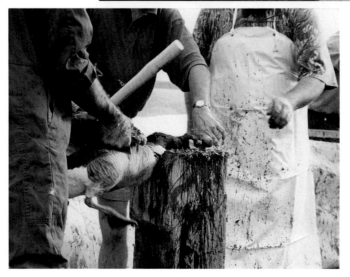

Plate 12 Restraining
and killing method used
during Canada Geese cull

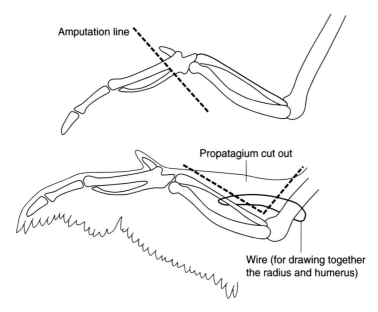

Amputation line

Propatagium cut out

Wire (for drawing together the radius and humerus)

Figure 11.6 Amputation lines used in pinioning and pategiectomy.

Africa, as a way of harvesting feathers from ostriches, but is now regarded as inhumane.

11.3.8 Dubbing

Dubbing is the removal of part of the comb and, sometimes, the wattles from a bird. It is performed in breeder chickens as a way of recognising which genetic line a cockerel came from. When breeder birds are mixed, the birds from the male line have part of their comb removed with a pair of scissors, without anaesthetic, so that any males that crop up because of an error in sexing in the female line can be recognised from their fully grown comb. Combs and wattles are sometimes reduced in game fowl. This helps control physical damage that occurs when two game-fowl cocks get access to each other and have a fight. Breeders also claim that without the comb, the birds are less likely to fight to the death. The alternative is to ensure that male game fowl are never allowed to mix or reach each other between adjacent cages.

11.3.9 Eyestalk and cheliped ablation

Eyestalk ablation is arguably the least commendable practice in modern aquaculture, from an animal welfare perspective. It is practised in breeding stock in farmed crustacea, especially prawns. The animal needs the eyestalks for vision, and they also secrete a number of hormones, one of which inhibits reproduction. Removing the eyestalks takes away that inhibition, and the eyestalks do not regrow. Ablation induces precocious moulting, puberty, mating and reproduction, and it reduces the lifespan of the animal. Although blinded, most species are able to feed, and growth is not suppressed. However, this is not the case in some crab species, which die shortly after ecdysis induced by eyestalk ablation. Instead, ablation of the chelipeds can accelerate moulting without jeopardising their survival.

11.3.10 Beak trimming

Beak trimming is used as a method to reduce the risk of cannibalism in layer hens, broiler breeders, turkeys and breeder ducks. It reduces the weapon that birds use when attacking each other, and it reduces the sensory reward achieved during cannibalism. However, beak trimming is a painful procedure when it involves a large portion of the beak, and it can debilitate the bird making feeding more difficult. The proximal region of the beak is particularly sensitive. If this part is cut and cauterised during beak trimming the bird recoils and tries to shake its head. It is evidently painful. It may also result in a lasting pain when neuromas form in the beak stump.

The chicken's beak is richly innervated and it acts as a sense organ as well as a tool and weapon. It consists of an outer layer of *rhamphotheca* (horn-like material) overlying a relatively thick epidermis. The dermis below the epidermis consists of collagen and elastin fibres, blood vessels, nerve fibres and sensory nerve endings. This is the region from which painful stimuli will be sensed. Sensory reception occurs through free nerve endings and Herbst and Grandry corpuscles within the dermis (Dubbeldam *et al.*, 1994). The free nerve endings are responsive to temperature, mechanical stimulation or to noxious stimuli. Herbst corpuscles act as mechanoreceptors and Grandry corpuscles respond to movement.

The role of the beak as a sensory organ has been explored in greater detail in the duck and pigeon than in the chicken. In the duck, the bill helps to detect and discriminate between prospective food particles. The sensory information is used as directional cues and is especially important in situations where vision is limited (e.g. muddy water). Signals from mechanoreceptors and free nerve endings in the beak project to the brain through branches of the trigeminal nerves (Dubbeldam *et al.*, 1994). Within the brain, mechanosensory information is processed in the *nucleus basalis* in the *telencephalon* (Berkhoudt *et al.*, 1981).

In the pigeon, damage to the nerve tracts that eventually project to the *nucleus basalis* results in impairment of neurosensory control of feeding behaviour. The sense organs in the beak work together with those in the tongue in helping the bird monitor and hence control its feeding actions. When part of the beak is removed, the bird can no longer make use of part of that information. The beak stump does not compensate by having more sensory nerve terminals or sensory corpuscles (Dubbeldam *et al.*, 1994; Gentle *et al.*, 1997). Instead, removal of part of the beak leads to regression of innervation.

Microneuromas develop in the amputation stumps of beak-trimmed chickens when beak trimming is performed at five weeks of age, but they are less likely to form when mild trimming is done at one day old. Severe beak trimming, removing two-thirds of the upper beak, is more likely to result in a persistent neuroma.

11.3.11 Disbudding and horn removal

Horn buds are removed from calves with a cauterising iron, scoop dehorner (Barnes dehorner), saw, guillotine cutters, embryotomy wire, knife or by chemical cauterisation. A local anaesthetic is or is not used, depending on local custom. The plasma cortisol response to disbudding using a scoop dehorner is biphasic. There is an initial response which is prevented by applying a local anaesthetic to the cornual nerves beforehand, and it is followed about two hours later by a more protracted response lasting for at least five hours, which is associated with inflammatory pain. Giving additional local anaesthetic during the second phase merely delays the time at which inflammatory pain sets in (McMeekan *et al.*, 1998).

Disbudding using a hot iron causes an initial cortisol response, which can also be reduced with local anaesthetic, but the second cortisol response due to inflammatory pain is not obvious (Petrie *et al.*, 1996). Instead, the third-degree burns produced by cauterising damage the nerves which mediate the inflammatory pain (Sutherland *et al.*, 2002). In this way, the duration of pain inflicted with the hot-iron method is shorter than that produced by the scoop. This is the case irrespective of whether or not a local anaesthetic is used. However, a local anaesthetic should be used in order to control the pain produced at the time the wound is inflicted.

Horns are usually removed from large cattle with a set of hand-operated guillotine cutters. In Europe it is widely accepted that cattle should be sedated and the horns removed under local anaesthesia, whereas in parts of Australasia this is not the case. Backyard goats would normally be given a local anaesthetic when dehorned by a veterinarian, and a local anaesthetic would usually be recommended for farmed goats as well. It is claimed that elastrator bands cause intense pain when used for dehorning goats. In the United States, range goats are left horned for protection from predators (Bowen, 1977).

When electroimmobilisation has been used in place of a local anaesthetic for dehorning cattle, there was no difference in the plasma cortisol response (Carter *et al.*, 1983). Nor was there any difference between those treatments and the restrained non-dehorned controls, suggesting that in this study the stress of restraint was just as significant as the stress of dehorning.

11.3.12 Blast injuries

Blast injuries are not common in animals, but they have occurred in the following situations:

- intentional underground gas explosions for fox, rabbit, gopher, prairie dog and ground squirrel control;
- control of unwanted animals that live in colonies, such as flying foxes;

- intentional underwater 'fish blasting';
- underwater seismic testing;
- penthrite grenades used in whale hunting;
- bomb and munitions explosions;
- accidental gas explosions.

In underground explosions, animals that are close to the explosion will incur injuries from the blast force, and those at greater distance may experience poisoning from products of the explosion or from oxygen deficiency that develops from the combustion. Kerosene and sulphur, or carbon disulphide, were at one time the preferred explosives for controlling rabbits in warrens, but these have now been replaced by mixtures of propane and oxygen. In the past, the methods used for detonating the explosive were in themselves inhumane. For example, one way of detonating carbon disulphide was to release a rabbit into the burrow with a stick of phosphorus tied to its leg. We do not know much about the effects of underground explosions on rabbits and whether this is a humane method, as few people have gone to the trouble of digging out the warren to see what happened.

During World War II, the biggest hazard to animals from bomb blasts during air raids (see Box 11.1) was injury from collapsing buildings (see below). In an assessment of injuries in 160 traumatised or killed horses kept in stables in London, the most common injury was broken or damaged backs (King & Moller, 1943). When the chest wall was punctured, the horse usually succumbed either to collapse of the lung or to pneumonia. Puncture of the abdomen was often followed by peritonitis, and shrapnel wounds were common and were particularly difficult to treat.

Box 11.1 Injuries to some horses during air raids in World War II

Number of stables damaged	21
Number of horses in the stables	1104
Number of casualties	160
Number of horses killed, destroyed or died	98
Causes of injury	
Bomb blast	26
Shrapnel	49
Fire	17
Building collapse	68

Injuries also developed when horses struggled after being buried in rubble. With animals that are trapped under fallen masonry or timber, there is an inevitable risk of **crush syndrome**. This syndrome develops from crushing of muscle and ischaemic damage to muscle through arrest of blood flow.

When the trapped animal is rescued, reperfusion results in a surge of blood into an anoxaemic capillary bed that has become highly permeable. Plasma pours through the permeable capillary walls into the interstitial spaces causing a prompt swelling. The area becomes red, oedematous and painful, and skin blisters may develop. There is a rapid collapse of blood volume and blood pressure. Myoglobin enters the bloodstream from necrotic muscle, and over the period of a fortnight obstructs the kidney tubules causing 'traumatic anuria'. Myoglobinuria is evident. Reperfusion also allows a sudden surge in oxygen delivery to the injured tissues. The preceding hypoxaemia induces a rise in xanthine oxidase activity which, in the presence of a flush of oxygenated blood, causes localised production of free radicals which, at high concentrations, cause additional tissue damage. When death occurs, it is due to renal failure.

The pressure waves from the explosion cause greatest injury in air-containing organs such as the ears, lungs and intestines. The lungs are particularly susceptible. At one time it was thought that lung injury and haemorrhage were due to the compression wave rupturing the air spaces and surrounding tissue within the lungs. However, it was found, from experimental work in rabbits, that haemorrhages often occurred on the outer surface of the lungs at points corresponding to the position of the ribs (Zuckerman, 1940). This pattern was common in young animals which had compliant rib cages. Evidently, the lungs are bruised by the impact transmitted through the chest wall. Haemorrhages also developed in the mediastinal face of the lungs. The medial lung surface is in fact the part that is most distorted by the pressure wave acting on the rib cage. This situation is analogous to a coin being knocked against a row of other coins, and the end coin flies off (Figure 11.7). The coins in the middle correspond to air-locked alveoli at the centre of the lung that undergo little displacement, whilst the furthest least-constrained coin (mediastinal aspect of the lung) is prone to displacement. In the case of the lung, the displacement results in tearing.

Haemorrhage in the lungs can be linked to pains in the chest and impaired ventilatory function. There is expiratory dyspnoea coupled with grunting, shallow breathing and cyanosis, and the haemorrhagic area may be prone to secondary infection (leading to bronchopneumonia).

Ear injuries can include rupture of the eardrum, middle ossicle displacement and damage to the cochlea. In cochlear damage, the organ of Corti is often dislocated from its attachment to the basilar membrane. There may also be loss of sensory hair cells, which will impair subsequent hearing. In humans, hearing loss following a blast injury is often accompanied by persistent earache (Phillips & Zajtchuk, 1989).

Injury to the intestines is less common than lung and ear injury, except in underwater blasts. Nevertheless, the types of intestinal injury that occur are:

• transmural perforation;
• contusion of the intestines;
• mesenteric laceration.

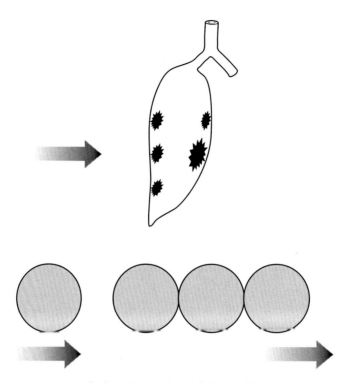

Figure 11.7 Common sites for lung haemorrhages following blast injury. Haemorrhage occurs on the mediastinal aspect of the lung through distortion of the tissue in a manner comparable to the displacement of the furthest coin when a row of coins is struck by a loose one.

Tearing or straining of the mesentery is responsible for stitch-like pain in humans.

In humans, the immediate sensation during a blast wave is severe compression of the chest plus the momentary feeling that 'all the blood was being displaced to my head, making it throb badly' (Anon., 1941). In some cases this is followed by a period of paralysis lasting for half an hour or more, shortly followed by full sensory capacity. In other cases the subjects have been mobile but unable to speak (Gordon, 1918).

The early behavioural responses, after the blast has subsided, are, typically, confusion, depression or dullness, suppression of normal reflexes, deafness, reduced visual function and reduced taste and smell. Memory changes and psychological changes such as fear and anger can occur, or there may be apathy and depression. The behaviour of blast-exposed animals can range from confusion to paralysis. The exact signs depend on the extent and type of damage inflicted on the central nervous system.

Haemorrhages can develop in the brain either from impact when thrown by the blast or from a surge of intravascular pressure to the brain from compression of the thorax and abdomen. At the time of the blast there is a period of apnoea that can last up to a minute and is followed by fast and shallow breathing. Some cases of apparent paralysis may in fact be due to cardiogenic shock. There are hypotension and severe bradycardia, which, in laboratory rats, has been shown to develop within about 15 seconds of the blast. These cardiovascular responses are neurally mediated, as they have been prevented by bilateral vagotomy plus atropine premedication (Irwin *et al.*, 1999).

The medium-term behaviour patterns after a blast can include the following:

- subjects that were disorientated immediately after the blast have been known to develop emotionally-induced convulsive seizures when stressed;
- rabbits have been seen to hop around aimlessly;
- horses showed mild paralysis;
- cows had to be slaughtered because they stopped eating;
- signs of brain injury in dogs include generalised spasms, forced twisting movements of the body, nystagmus, barking whilst in syncope and loss of orientation.

In general, loss of consciousness from the primary blast is rare. The greatest risk of concussion was from being struck by a secondary missile. Concussion can take the form of a **catatonic state** lasting for twelve or more hours after the explosion, during which there is a characteristic physical plasticity and flexibility (Stewart *et al.*, 1941). When the body is manipulated into an unusual posture or orientation, it remains in that position until moved again. Subjects suffering from blast injury often display extreme expiratory dyspnoea. Respiration may be slow and shallow and pain in the chest may modify the breathing pattern, making it short and panting. Tachypnoea may persist for many hours after the blast, and it tends to be more severe in animals that appear to be only moderately injured. In severely-injured mice, monkeys and goats, breathing was instead slow, with expiratory grunting and, in some cases, double expiratory movement (Clemedson, 1956).

Dogs are sometimes trained for land-mine or terrorist explosives detection. During World War II, pointers were the preferred breed for land-mine detection. They were quicker at locating mines than a sapper equipped with conventional detectors (Anon., 1944). By watching the dog, one could tell where mines were not situated. The dogs seemed to move amongst mines without the same risk of setting off a mine as people. The risk of an accident inevitably increased, however, when there were heavy work loads.

High fish mortalities have been observed following seismographic explosions used during oil exploration below the ocean bed (Hubbs & Rechnitzer, 1952). However, this is no longer common because most testing is now done with air guns instead of explosive charges. Blast fishing with dynamite is, however, used to catch fish for the human market on the coral reefs off the Philippines, and was used in recent times off the coast of Tanzania. This practice is widely condemned by conservation groups because of destruction of the coral beds. Fish with swim bladders are particularly susceptible to blast injuries, and explosives such as dynamite, which produce an abrupt shock wave due to a fast burn time, are more damaging than explosives that burn more slowly.

11.3.13 Bullet and shotgun wounds

Shooting an animal in the head at close range is one of the most humane killing methods. The following anecdote from a veterinary practitioner serves as a good example (Rainey, 1933):

> 'The best demonstration ever given to me of how a small bullet will cause instantaneous unconsciousness and certain death to a large animal, was on a coco-nut plantation where a large number of cattle suffering from open tuberculosis had to be killed. The planter, a crack shot, stood beside me in the midst of about 100 cattle in a small paddock and asked me to point out the diseased beasts. Using a 0.22 calibre rifle, fitted with a silencer, he rapidly picked off about a dozen beasts with complete accuracy at ranges up to 25 yards one after another, so that each beast fell dead with one tiny bullet in the brain. The report was so deadened by the silencer, and it was all done so quickly and cleanly, that the other cattle did not take alarm. Every bullet had entered the skull just about where the hair curls on the centre of the forehead.'

Similarly, at close range, a 12-bore shotgun can provide a quick and effective kill. However, on other occasions there have been instances when three 0.22 bullet head shots were needed to fell a steer, and a larger calibre would now be recommended for cattle. Accuracy and a short distance between an animal and marksman are critical when using light firearms and shotguns.

It is very important, for both animal welfare and public perception, to ensure that horses are humanely killed when they are 'put down' with a firearm. This has emerged as a sensitive issue in the case of Kaimanawa pony and brumby culling from helicopters in Australasia. Some ponies and horses have been shot without being immediately killed, and, in one case a pony survived in a disabled state for ten months (Plate 8).

In a helicopter cull conducted in October 2000 by the New South Wales Parks and Wildlife Service, a disabled mare was found with bullet wounds in its shoulder 7–10 days after it had been shot. Aerial culling from helicopters can be haphazard, as both the target and the marksman are moving. Nevertheless it is strongly defended as a more practical option when there are large numbers of animals that have to be culled in extensive or inhospitable terrain. The ideal situation with helicopter culls is to follow any injured but mobile animals to give them a second shot, and to land and off-load operators to despatch any injured fallen animals. These precautions are essential because not every animal will be killed with the first shot.

Most of the information on the effectiveness of shooting during stalking and ground culling, and on the immediacy of the kill, is anecdotal. The accuracy of the shooting has been assessed during kangaroo culls in Australia (Young & Delforce, 1986). The majority of kangaroos (88%) were shot in the head, and a minority in the chest. Dealers pay lower prices for kangaroos shot in the body because of damaged skins and bruising to the carcases, and this has been a strong incentive for performing head shots. Lewis *et al.* (1997) recorded shooting efficiency during night-time impala (*Aepyceros melampus*) culling. Of the animals that were hit, 94% were killed instantaneously, and in the 6% that were wounded the survival time was on average 30 seconds. Bateson (1997) reported that when 44 red deer were shot in the chest, the average distance run before they dropped to the ground was 32 metres, whereas the average distance run by 45 deer shot in the head or neck was 3 metres. There were misadventures, as recorded in the following case:

'On the 25th April 1996 a stag was shot in the left hand side of the head from close range (approximately 5–10 m) after it had lain down in deep bracken, following a chase of approximately 23 km over four hours. The shot broke the upper, vertical section of the lower jaw. The stag immediately leapt to its feet and ran off into nearby woodland. It was killed with a second shot (from a humane killer) about 10–15 minutes later.'

Overall, 11% of red deer that were shot by stalkers were killed with two or more shots, and 7% of the deer took more than two minutes to die. About 2% of the deer escaped wounded (Bateson, 1997).

In a survey of rifle and gunshot wounds in 19 urban dogs and cats in Australia, Keep (1970) reported that 12 animals had been struck by 0.177-calibre air-rifle slugs, two by 0.22-calibre bullets, four by shotgun pellets and one by size 10 shot from a 0.22 long rifle-shot cartridge. An important feature of the study was that many of the owners (16 out of 19) had not suspected that their dog or cat had been shot, and this was only discovered sometime later when a radiograph was taken for an unrelated reason. These types of injury are less common now that there are fewer air rifles in urban communities.

Normally when an air rifle or shotgun pellet lodges in soft tissue without killing an animal it becomes surrounded with fibrin which is non-vascularised. This isolates the pellet and usually arrests the inflammatory response. It also stops the pellet from migrating elsewhere in the body or emerging under the skin. Encapsulation with fibrin does not occur in the case of a shotgun pellet lodged in a joint, and this is a particularly serious injury with lead pellets. The synovial fluid bathing the pellet dissolves some of the lead, causing chronic irritation as well as systemic effects from distribution of the dissolved lead.

Steel shot is now used instead of lead shot in many countries. However, there are disadvantages with steel shot. In the United States there are reports of severe inflammatory reactions from steel shot when it corrodes embedded in non-fatal wounds (Bartels *et al.*, 1991). Tungsten-bismuth-tin, bismuth, tungsten-iron and tungsten-polymer shot are less likely to induce an inflammatory response, in comparison with steel shot.

There are three zones of injury caused by a bullet or shot as it penetrates a tissue (Harvey *et al.*, 1962):

(1) *The temporary cavity*, which is created by radial explosive pressure imparted by a high-velocity bullet as it passes through tissue. This deformation is usually conical or elliptical in shape. It stretches the surrounding tissue, reverberates and leaves behind a tissue pulp. Damage to blood vessels leads to a zone of extravasation, which includes the area of pulped tissue. The temporary cavity can sometimes take the shape of a string of beads, if the bullet has an oscillating yawing motion as it passes through tissue.

(2) *The permanent cavity*, which is the cavity that remains after the temporary cavity has subsided. Its size is governed by the size of the temporary cavity. It is often fusiform in shape and comprises the bullet track and surrounding haemorrhagic area.

(3) *The track* left in the wake of the bullet; part of the permanent cavity.

The size of the temporary cavity can be gauged from the size of the zone of extravasation (Table 11.4). This can be a useful indicator of likely disturbance to surrounding tissue. The size of the entrance and exit holes is a useless indicator of the extent of damage inside.

Low-velocity bullets cause crushing and laceration, whereas a high-velocity missile causes the tissue itself to accelerate, and this gives rise to the larger temporary cavity around the missile tract. The explosive effect produced by the formation and collapse of the temporary cavity results in a zone of bruising and tissue disruption from the stretching, shearing and rupture of vessels, nerves and bone.

When the blast or bullet makes impact with the body there is a massive injury discharge of the nerves that are either damaged or stretched. There is a feeling of general or gross disturbance in the body besides the blow of the impact. The nerves that are damaged may normally serve a wide range of sensory functions, including heat, cold, mechanical sensation, movement and pain perception, and when

Table 11.4 Relative sizes of the different zones of a bullet wound.

Cavity type	Relative cavity volume
Permanent	1
Zone of extravasation	12
Temporary	26

activated in unison there is often an electric shock-like feeling along with the feeling of tissue disturbance ('trauma'). If pain receptors in and around the wound are activated, there is more likely to be an immediate sense of pain, but this may be diluted or overridden by the barrage of impulses from all the other sensory nerves that occurs at the same time. The immediate feelings of trauma are no doubt exaggerated when there is wider tissue disturbance such as that inflicted by high-velocity and **expanding bullets** and close range shotgun blasts.

The construction of a bullet determines whether it penetrates and passes through an animal as a single object, or whether it breaks up on entry. Soft-nosed, hollow-nosed, flat-nosed bullets and bullets with grooves across the tip are more likely to break up ('expanding bullets') and so cause more widespread internal injury. The presence of an entry and an exit wound does not imply that the whole bullet has passed through an animal. High-velocity soft-jacketed bullets tend to leave behind a trail of casing inside the animal.

Military bullets are fully jacketed and are 'non-expanding' when they penetrate a target. They inflict considerably less internal damage than 'expanding' bullets used in hunting, culling and animal euthanasia. For example, in a study on anaesthetised dogs which were shot in the chest at 884 m/s, the internal wound volume with an expanding bullet was 917 cc, compared to 24 cc for a non-expanding bullet with the same velocity (De Muth, 1966). Expanding bullets have been shown to lose 59–77% of their weight in fragments as they break up inside a pig's hind leg (Fackler *et al.*, 1984). This dispersal causes considerable tissue damage, with internal bleeding, and raises the chances of inflicting a lethal wound.

There are five types of bullet motion:

(1) Trajectory motion is the line the bullet takes between the gun and the animal.
(2) Spin or rotation around the long axis of the bullet is caused by the rifling of the gun (Figure 11.8).

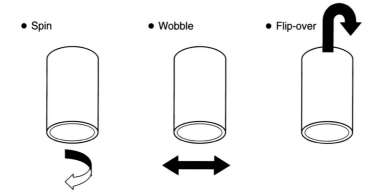

Figure 11.8 Types of bullet motion.

(3) Wobble, in the form of spiralling movement by the tail of the bullet, tends to be greatest at the beginning and end of the flight of a bullet, and is periodic in between.
(4) Flip-over occurs when the nose of the bullet makes impact and the bullet tumbles over itself.
(5) Fragmentation occurs on penetration of the animal, and dispersal in the tissues.

If a bullet yaws as it impacts an animal, or if it enters during a wobble phase in its flight or if it flips over as it enters the body, it tears a bigger hole near the entrance. In these situations, the area of presentation to the skin is larger than the diameter of the bullet, and gyroscopic action reams out a larger internal wound. High-velocity bullets are more likely to flip over and tear out a cavity inside the body. Low-velocity bullets pierce the tissue, creating a hole that corresponds approximately to the diameter of the bullet.

The immense forces generated by high-velocity bullets can cause the following types of damage:

- Muscle can be split along its fascia. Muscle that is ripped from bone does not regain its normal position after collapse of the temporary cavity, and healing can be complicated.
- Hydraulic forces can be set up in blood, which bursts veins at some distance from the wound. Arteries, on the other hand, are more elastic and less prone to this type of damage. Radiographs in the cat have shown the femoral artery can be forced aside by the pressure of the temporary cavity without causing it to rupture, whereas the femur in the same vicinity was broken (Harvey *et al.*, 1962).
- Nerves may show failure in transmission due to compression or stretching, without any outward signs of physical damage. However, when there has been excessive stretching, the nerve may show kinking, and this is a sign that the inner axon has probably broken whilst the neurilemma and myelin sheath are still intact.
- Sometimes it is found that a gas-filled organ, such as the intestine, is ruptured when a bullet passes through the abdomen without directly entering that particular section of gut. It is the negative pressure effect (part B in Figure 11.9) that causes the organ to burst, through expansion of gas inside the intestine, rather than the explosive effect of the temporary cavity (part C).
- Bone fractures can occur at some distance from the track of the bullet, without direct contact between bone and bullet. When a bullet strikes bone, there is usually a comminuted fracture, whereas with high velocity bullets, the bone seems to 'explode' when it receives a direct hit, in a manner similar to the soft tissues around it (Figure 11.10). The bone fragments fly out into the temporary cavity, and, with collapse of the cavity, they are forced back to

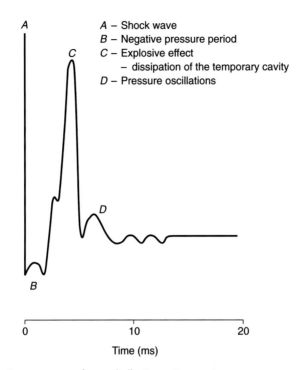

Figure 11.9 Pressure waves from a bullet impacting on tissue.

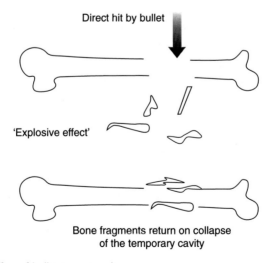

Figure 11.10 Effect of bullet impact on bone.

approximately their former position. The bone fragments act as returning secondary missiles and add to soft-tissue damage.

If a wild animal receives a bullet in the abdomen and the gut is perforated, the risk of death from peritonitis is high, but it is not inevitable. A notable exception, reported in human medicine, was the case of a soldier wounded during the Battle of Loos in World War I, who recovered without surgery. Subsequently, he was wounded again during the Battle of the Somme, and during surgery his earlier wound, which involved several perforations of the small intestine, was discovered. Leakage from the gut had evidently been constrained by loops of the bowel that developed adhesions to the small intestine (Fraser, 1942). An analogous situation has been observed in a dog, and episodic leakage of digesta caused obvious sickness in the animal.

Bullets that pass through layers of wool or dense fur can drag some of the fibre as a cocoon into the wound. This is particularly evident with expanding bullets, whereas round shot and pointed non-expanding bullets tend to split their way through the fleece or coat. Fibre that penetrates in this way inevitably increases the risk of infection.

Tissue will regenerate within the zone of extravasation if it is kept clean. Otherwise, it often harbours pyogenic bacteria and may develop **gas gangrene**. Experience with gunshot wounds in dogs has shown that the risk of osteomyelitis can be quite high, especially in those cases requiring surgical intervention (Doherty & Smith, 1995).

There is also a high risk of gangrene if the wound is untreated and the injury involves damage to the circulation. In its early stages, a gangrenous wound can be painful, partly from the pressure created by gases. During this phase, humans feel anxious and distressed, but as the pain eases the subject starts to feel better. As toxaemia sets in, vomiting and flushes commence, and there is further swelling at the site of the wound which probably helps to disseminate the bacteria. Intoxication with products from autolysis and with bacterial exotoxin make the patient very ill, and the chances of survival are further reduced if the bacteria invade the bloodstream. Overall, the suffering associated with this condition is greatest during the initial stages and during the fulminant phase of the toxaemia. In the later stages the subject is profoundly ill, and seems to submit emotionally to the process.

When a bullet strikes a limb causing haemorrhage which is contained within the limb, there can be a substantial rise in interstitial pressure within the fascia. If the raised pressure reduces capillary perfusion, a condition known as **acute limb compartment syndrome** may develop. This occurs when there is muscle and nerve ischaemia with muscle infarction, nerve damage and swelling. It is a very painful condition, even though there is sensory loss in other respects in the affected area. The pain is out of proportion to the apparent injury, and it is present during passive movement of the limb. Compartment syndrome is not to be confused with crush syndrome. Limb compartment syndrome results from increased pressure while crush syndrome develops from acidosis, hyperkalaemia, myoglobinuria, shock and acute renal failure. An analogous situation to limb compartment syndrome can occur when there is haemorrhage within the abdomen (**abdominal compartment syndrome**).

When an animal is shot but not killed it can suffer from the disabling effects of the injury, from sickness due to infection of the wound and from pain created by the wound. The forms of suffering are itemised in more detail in box 11.2.

Box 11.2

Animal disabled preventing it from:
- escaping or avoiding threatening situations;
- keeping up with the social group;
- feeding and drinking adequately;
- performing particular functions because of damage to a specific body region (e.g. compromised breathing, impaired vision).

Pain and discomfort associated with:
- inflammation at the wound (pain from swelling at the wound, pain from the release of algogenic substances at the wound site, primary and secondary hyperalgesia, allodynia);
- medium-term effects of disruption and damage to tissues (muscle soreness and stiffness);
- chronic effects of injury (causalgia, neuropathic pain, centralised pain, myiasis).

Chronic psychological effects:
- dissociative and/or anxiety disorders.

11.3.14 Hunting

There are three types of hunting:

(1) chase hunting;
(2) trapping;
(3) stalking or shooting at roused animals.

Chase hunting usually depends on out running the hunted animal enabling close enough access to shoot, concuss or stick it, or for the dogs to kill it. Proponents of chase hunting of deer often say that the chase is similar to natural predation, and that hunted species are well-adapted to the chase. It is claimed that if the animal was struck by abject fear or panic, its survival would be compromised. Instead, it must rely on stealth, subtle manoeuvres and outwitting the hunting party, and these must require some control over its own emotions. Others argue that the chase is nothing like natural predation. Prolonged pursuit is unusual during natural predation. Normally, predators such as lions, leopards or wolves depend on catching prey by stalking, ambush or bringing the victim down during a brief pursuit, whereas organised hunting parties use the collective strength of the huntsmen, the pack of dogs or helicopters and open-back trucks to out-compete the animal.

It is inevitable that the opportunities for suffering during chase hunting are considerably greater than during stalking. The stresses and injuries associated with chase hunting can include:

- exertion, fatigue, respiratory distress, exhaustion;
- fear associated with the chase, noise from the hunting party, blocking of escape routes and during close proximity to humans and dogs;
- injuries experienced during the chase;
- biting by the hunting dogs;
- wounding when shot or stuck.

Pig hunting carries some of the highest risks of hunting trauma, for both the pig and for pig-hunting dogs. The usual aim is to chase the pig to exhaustion, and when it has been bailed-up by the dogs, either to shoot or stick it. Some pig-hunters prefer sticking because there is less risk of shooting a dog, but there is a risk of injury to the dogs from the pig with sticking because the dogs have to restrain the pig. This is often done by two dogs, one on each ear, or by one dog holding each leg plus a fifth dog holding an ear. Some dogs develop a knack of biting the scrotum of the pig during the chase and this has been known to stop the pig in its tracks. Pigs have powerful shoulder muscles and when attacking a dog they throw it in the air and then gore it from underneath with their tusks. Eventration in this way can lead to shock and death.

The usual intention when **stalking** deer is to shoot the animal in either the head, neck or chest. When the hunter is within 20 m, a head shot is considered appropriate and at 20–40 m a neck shot is used. At 40–100 m, a chest shot has been recommended (Farm Animal Welfare Council, 1985). With a high-velocity bullet there is a good chance that a head shot will concuss the animal, even when it strikes the jaw instead of the skull. With a neck or chest shot the hope is to sever a major blood vessel and cause a rapid death by haemorrhage. However, as Rainey (1933) pointed out when using a Webley long-barrel revolver firing a 0.450 bullet aimed at the heart, it was unusual to see cattle drop immediately, and there was 'a considerable interval of conscious distress before the animal fell'.

If the spinal cord is struck without incurring much bleeding, the animal may appear, from a distance, to be shot dead, but it could in fact be paralysed and alive. If the spinal cord is damaged above the fifth cervical vertebra, it is likely that the animal will die from being unable to breathe. Damage to the spinal cord below that point without lethal haemorrhage would result in a slow death.

The traditional way of hunting wallaby in Tasmania was to drive the animals from cover with dogs, and then to shoot them with shotguns. On one property as

Table 11.5 Prevalence of shotgun pellets in live ducks in Australia.

Species	Number examined	% with pellets
Mountain duck	400	19.0
Black duck	2544	13.7
Wood duck	696	13.6
Hardhead	351	11.1
Grey teal	38075	9.0
Chestnut teal	3144	6.2
Dusky moorhen	159	0.6
Eastern swamphen	17	0

many as 3000 Rufous and Bennett's wallabies were shot annually. Animals that were not killed outright were either killed by the dogs, re-shot or had their throats cut. Joeys in the pouch were usually concussed. One of the difficulties with re-shooting is in aiming at the head, neck or chest when the main view of the receding target is its hindquarters. **Night shooting** is commonplace for kangaroos, wallabies, foxes and rabbits. The animals are shot from a vehicle whilst frozen by a spotlight.

Non-lethal injuries can occur when a shotgun is fired at a group of birds flying overhead. The birds aligned with the central cluster of pellets will usually be fatally injured. Birds at the perimeter of the volley may be hit by one or two pellets, and they stand a good chance of surviving. The suffering of those survivors is an inevitable welfare problem with shotgun injuries. In a study of shooting wounds in over 45000 live trapped waterfowl in Australia, Norman (1976) found that 14% of ducks had shotgun pellets in their tissues, which were identified radiographically (Table 11.5). The species of larger duck carried more pellets, and one of the Mountain ducks had 13 pellets. In a similar study in the northern hemisphere, 14% of ptarmigans (*Lagopus lagopus*) that were caught with snares were found to be carrying between one and six birdshot pellets, with a mean of 2.7 pellets per bird (Holmstad, 1998).

Catching rattlesnakes (*Crotalus horridus*), and then letting them go is a recreational pastime in the United States. Catching them with a noose is liable to cause more injury to the snake than a hooked stick or snake tongs (Reinert, 1990). In Australia, snakes near homesteads are sometimes shot with a snake gun using 16 gauge shot.

Commercial **whale hunting** is presently practised by Norway and Japan, and it is practised as a subsistence activity around Canada and Greenland. Modern Norwegian and Japanese whaling vessels use a harpoon fitted with a penthrite grenade, but the traditional method is to use a 'cold' harpoon. The cold harpoon is a sharp-pointed barbed iron shaft weighing 12–18 kg. It has a conical piercing head and is used to lance the animal and attach it to the whaling boat with a wire rope.

Table 11.6 Estimated time to death when different parts of a whale's body were struck by a cold harpoon.

Tissue or organ struck by the harpoon	Time to death (seconds)	
	Average	**% of animals**
Central nervous system	69	13
Heart	168	
Blood vessels	364	31
Lungs	467	
Abdomen	725	56
Muscles	1071	

Using the onset of cessation of flipper movement, relaxation of the mandible or sinking without active movement as criteria of death in Minke whales, the time to death on average with the cold harpoon was found to be 11.3 minutes. The longest time to death, in a study of 353 Minke whales, was 62 minutes (Øen, 1995a). The estimated time to death when different parts of the body were struck is shown in Table 11.6. If a whale is struck in the lung and it dives, the water pressure at depth causes the lungs to collapse, and this limits the rate of haemorrhaging and prolongs the time to death. Of the whales shown in Table 11.6, 17% were re-shot with harpoons, and rifle shots were fired into the brain in 56% of the cases. The shooting range was 5–100 m.

With the cold harpoon method, the intention is to hit the animal in the craniothoracic region. This is difficult, however, because this is the region that appears first when a whale surfaces. The gunner has either to anticipate when the whale will surface, or have an extremely fast reaction time, to strike this target. The chances of striking the brain and causing immediate unconsciousness are also low because of the position of and protection around the brain (Figure 11.11). In observations made on a whaling vessel in 1978/9, only 60% of the strikes were in the craniothoracic region (Best, 1996). When an animal is not killed outright, the hunters are careful not to haul it in too fast, otherwise there is a risk that it may free itself and be lost. The larger the whale, the longer this takes, and this delays the time at which the whale can be shot with a rifle. An alternative approach, used by Eskimos, is to tether the harpooned whale to an air-filled bouy. This method entails an even longer delay before the whale is despatched with a rifle or a second harpoon.

When a penthrite-grenade harpoon is used, the time to death is usually quicker (Table 11.7). This harpoon has an explosive head which detonates on penetrating the target (Øen, 1995b). With Norwegian vessels using penthrite-grenade harpoons, about 63% of the whales are thought to be killed immediately by the grenade, whilst with Japanese boats it is thought to be 44% (Kestin, 2001). The

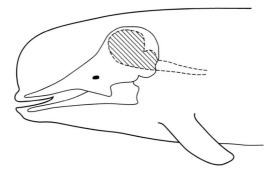

Figure 11.11 Position and size of the pilot whale brain.

Table 11.7 Estimated time to death when different parts of a whale's body were struck by a penthrite-grenade harpoon.

Tissue or organ struck by the harpoon	Time to death (seconds)	
	Average	% of animals
Central nervous system	11	
Heart	27	
Blood vessels	153	52
Lungs	83	
Abdomen	493	48
Muscles	857	

lower rate with Japanese catches is probably due to the delayed fuse used in the Japanese design which can allow the grenade to pass through the whale before detonation. Whales that are not immediately killed are brought to exhaustion whilst towing the boat. They are then hauled alongside and usually shot with a rifle. This is usually completed within 15 minutes of harpooning. In Japanese vessels the whales used to be electrocuted once they had been drawn alongside in an attempt to stop physical activity. This electrocution procedure is no longer commonly used.

11.3.15 Trapping
There are pronounced cultural differences between nations in the acceptability of trapping as a method of pest control. Some countries have strict legislation which prohibits some types of trap, whereas others have a more relaxed, almost 'sporting', attitude towards the control of animals that are regarded as vermin (Plate 9). The classification of animal traps is shown in box 11.3. All traps can cause injuries, but, in general, traps which *contain* an animal cause less damage than *restraining*

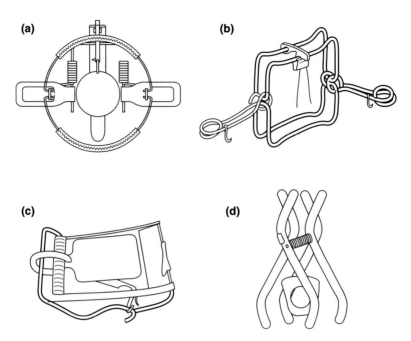

Figure 11.12 Animal traps: (a) leg hold trap (padded); (b) conibear trap; (c) Fenn trap; (d) scissor trap.

traps. Kill traps that kill quickly cause shorter-lasting distress than live traps. Body-catch traps include the scissor-mole trap and the Fenn trap, and in general are not humane (Figure 11.12).

Animals caught in cage and box traps are not likely to experience trauma except when they adopt extreme measures in trying to escape. Normally, foxes either become inactive shortly after capture, or they may pace up and down the box (White *et al.*, 1991). Excitement during transport can be controlled by covering

---

Box 11.3

Live traps	Kill traps
Cage traps	Neck-hold traps
Box traps	Neck snares
Nets	Break-back traps
Pitfall traps	Body-catch trap
Leg snares	Crushing devices
Leg-hold traps	
Glue boards	

the cage with a cloth to exclude light and visual threats. If the caught animal has to be handled or killed at some stage, this is the period when trauma is most likely to occur.

In the past, mist nets were commonly used for catching song birds. Now, they are mainly used for catching birds in research studies. When mist nets have been used for catching forest and heathland birds in Australia, the mortality rate has been 1.3% (Recher *et al.*, 1985). Injuries usually occurred when the birds struggled whilst entangled, and it is important not to provoke struggling when disentangling them.

Net guns are sometimes used for catching feral goats. They are less likely to cause injury when used at waterholes in comparison with firing them from helicopters during a chase (Edge *et al.*, 1989).

Pitfall traps are sometimes used for catching large game for food or for relocation, and wild rodents for research purposes. In Papua New Guinea sharpened stakes are fitted at the bottom of the pit to impale wild pigs, which are used for food.

Research into leg-hold trapping has shown that in red foxes and possums padded traps are less stressful than unpadded traps, and that the longer an animal is held in a leg-hold trap the more stressful it is for the animal (Kreeger *et al.*, 1990; Warburton *et al.*, 1999). The injuries incurred with leg-hold traps in racoons vary from minor soft tissue injury in the case of some animals caught in padded traps, to metacarpal subluxation or phalangeal joint luxation (Proulx *et al.*, 1993). Padded Victor leg-hold traps caused considerably less damage to possums than unpadded versions of the same trap (Warburton, 1992). Lanes-Ace (gin) traps caused substantially more injury than either the padded or unpadded Victor leg-hold traps. Wolves are prone to tooth, lip and gum injuries when they fight leg-hold traps (van Ballenberghe, 1984). They also chew nearby vegetation, and there have been cases where a stick became wedged between the upper molars.

When catching animals with leg-hold traps it is been important to place the traps away from objects that could be used as a purchase that will allow the animal to escape, and not to place them near undergrowth which will allow the chain or wire to get tangled. Foxes and rock wallabies, in particular, can put up an impressive fight against a leg-hold trap, and entanglement increases the chance of a dislocated leg (Meek *et al.*, 1995). Skin lacerations also occur during struggling, and the strength of the trap springs, and the point at which the chain or wire is attached to the jaws of the trap, influences the amount of swivel and potential injury.

The gin trap has been disallowed in many countries. One example of a gin trap is the Lanes-Ace No. 1½ longspring trap. When this trap was compared with a Victor No. 1 padded leg-hold trap for catching possums, the proportion of animals with moderate and severe injuries with the gin trap was 39% whereas for the Victor trap it was only 6%.

Glue boards are used for catching mice and rats in food factories where there is reluctance to use poisons. This method inevitably involves struggling and distress before the animal is found or it dies. It is a relatively inhumane method (Mason & Littin, 2003).

Snares are used in communities where the hunter has time to set and inspect the snares. Wire snares are used widely in Africa, and over the years have often been used for wallaby in Australia. Even though they are potentially inhumane, they are preferred by some trappers because they are cheap, effective and easy to carry around, but they have to be placed on an animal trail and this limits the number of target species. They are usually applied as foot snares, but for some species they act as neck snares. When caught by a foot, 'death is gruesome as the animal fights to free itself, often breaking the captured limb, and dies slowly from shock, blood loss, exhaustion, and starvation' (Noss, 1998). Wire snares tend to be non-selective, and wasteful because of losses to scavengers and decomposition.

The intention with neck snares is to cause a rapid death by strangulation. They may either compress the trachea causing suffocation, or occlude the carotid arteries causing prompt failure in blood supply to the brain. However it does not always work that way. In a study on 65 wild-caught coyote (*Canis latrans*), 59% were caught by the neck, 20% by the flank, 11% the front leg and neck and 10% the foot. Of the total catch, 48% were found alive the morning after the snares were set, but some of these were moribund (Guthery & Beasom, 1978). Clearly they do not always produce a quick kill.

Sometimes the cable snare breaks, and the animal escapes. This could be quite common in some species. For example, in one study 11 out of 45 red duiker (*Cricetomys dorsalis*) were found to have previous wire-snare injuries, the most serious being an individual missing two feet. When a wire is positioned over an artery it can cause long-term arterial spasm (Klenerman, 1962). Theoretically this vascular injury could contribute to the restricted blood supply to a foot or limb in some escapees. In addition, sudden release of a tourniquet can cause shock, through massive loss of fluid from the circulation in the hypoxic limb.

Snares can be made more species- and size-selective with a ferrule which limits the smallest size of the noose. Nevertheless, larger non-target animals can be caught, depending on the lure and how the snare is set.

The majority of kill traps operate in one of two ways. They either clamp the neck or grip the chest. If the neck is clamped, one would hope that this quickly arrests the flow of blood to the brain through the carotid arteries. The aim with a chest clamp should be to inhibit or stop the pumping action of the heart. However, the positioning of the animal in the jaws of the trap cannot be predicted in all cases, and some animals may even be concussed by the jaws striking the head. Sometimes animals are caught by the body in a Conibear trap, where the intention has been to catch them by the neck. The Conibear is the most widely used kill trap for fur-bearing species.

Nutman *et al.* (1998) found that only 22% of brushtail possums (*Trichosurus vulpecula*) that were caught in a Conibear trap had both carotid arteries occluded by the jaws of the trap. There were two reasons for this poor performance. If there was axial rotation of the neck, the carotids were not aligned with the jaws of the trap, and so one or both of them were not clamped. In some cases the carotid arteries were displaced laterally around the sides of the vertebral column. Warburton *et al.* (2000) found that if the jaws of the neck-hold trap are offset from each other, instead of being directly opposed, the neck is stretched into dorso-flexion and this improves the occlusion of the carotid arteries substantially. The time to death was correspondingly reduced. Clearly the way that the jaws of a trap hold the neck is critical, and changes are needed in some designs to improve their humaneness.

11.3.16 Rodeo

The main events in rodeo competitions are bareback riding, saddle-bronc riding, bull riding, steer wrestling, calf roping, steer roping and team roping. The overall prevalence of obvious injuries in the cattle and horses is not high (usually a little under 1%). In the United States, calf roping produces the most injuries, including broken legs and torn ligaments in the stifle joint or shoulder, but bronc injuries have been higher in New Zealand (about 2%).

Most bucking events last for a short time (about 10 seconds) and they rely on the innate bucking drive of the animal, which is reinforced with an electric prod or spurring as they leave the stocks, and with a flank strap secured around the animal which improves the bucking style. Many rodeo associations prohibit the use of sharpened spurs, or spurs with locked rowels, for broncs, and the flank strap has to be lined with soft plastic, felt or sheepskin. This helps to limit the likelihood of cuts on the flank.

The rowels are sometimes locked in the case of bull riding. Steers used for team roping sometimes have their horns wrapped to protect the ears and base of the horns from rope burns. In addition, in some countries a jerk line is used in roping and tying events. This rope feeds from the bridle through a pulley on the saddle, and when the rider dismounts to throw a steer, it jerks as it feeds out. This discourages the horse from moving backwards and dragging the steer. Stock contractors who supply bucking broncs either breed animals from strong bucking lines, or buy in known buckers. It is said that when selecting untried stock a contractor may test 1500 horses to get 30 really good buckers.

Bull running is performed in parts of Spain, Indonesia and India. Bulls are let loose and made to run along the streets of the village. In many cases, it is a hard road surface and injuries to the abdomen and horns occur during falls, but more commonly there are injuries to the limbs.

11.4 Types of Injury

This section examines some general forms of injury that can be either accidental or intentional.

11.4.1 Contact injuries and blisters

Contact injuries include pressure sores, bedsores, saddle and harness sores and other friction sores in the skin. Whenever an animal is haltered, harnessed, tethered, hobbled, caged or stalled, there is a risk of rubbing or pressure sores.

Constant rubbing of the skin produces a burning sensation associated initially with erythema and desquamation. It then leads to **blister** formation, which on bursting directly exposes the pain receptors to any further rubbing motion and to salts that are present on the skin. In long-term low-grade rubbing, calluses may form, and in severe cases there can be ulceration or skin removal exposing tendons, ligaments and muscle. The deeper the injury the greater the risk of infection and septicaemia.

A **callus** is a plaque of keratin resulting from epidermal hyperplasia. The underlying dermis can have increased accumulation of collagen or fibrin around neurovascular bundles, which are tender to pressure. If the callus is situated over a bony prominence it is called a corn, and these can be more painful because of the reduced cushioning. Corns are generally painful when pressed into the skin surface, whereas warts hurt when they are squeezed. Malunion of a bone fracture can produce an exaggerated bony prominence, which if exposed to rubbing injury, will develop a corn.

Examples of **pressure and rubbing sores** are as follows:

- A weanling horse was put out in a paddock with a head halter and left unobserved for a period of more than five months. As the animal grew, the halter became too small. Pressure necrosis set in from the strap over the nasal bones. Enlargement of the nasal bones developed caudal and rostral to the constriction, creating a bulbous appearance in the face.
- Inadequate padding under a saddle giving rise to a saddle sore is mainly seen in endurance rides and in pack horses and camels that are worked for long periods. The skin over bony prominences is most likely to be affected, and so it is animals that are in poor body condition that tend to show skin damage first.
- Chafing from new leather, before it becomes supple, can cause lesions.
- If dirt is trapped between the tack and the animal, because of dirty saddlery, it can cause soreness from rubbing.
- Saddles that are too hard because they are overstuffed with flock can cause soreness.
- Saddles which have become wet, producing lumpy flock with pressure points can cause pressure sores.

- A wrinkle of skin can sometimes get caught under the girth as it is tightened.
- Rug sores can be found, especially on the shoulders, withers and spine.

Pressure sores are a particular hazard when there has been spinal cord injury. Normally, excessive or prolonged pressure on the skin causes discomfort which is relieved by altering body position. In paraplegics, sensation and motor function are absent, and so the subject lacks the incentive and the ability to adjust its position to relieve the contact pressures. In addition, the skin is weakened through atrophy, from reduced collagen synthesis. This probably makes the skin more susceptible to developing sores.

Keeping animals on poorly-managed bedding or litter can lead to bedsores and other skin complaints. For example, hock burn, breast burns and breast blisters are skin conditions that occur in poultry kept on wet or inadequate litter.

Suction can produce skin blisters, erosions and purpura which are sore. When suction from the milking machine has been excessive, a haemorrhage forms at the end of the teat and develops into a black spot. Extreme suction can split the skin resulting in sub-epidermal blisters, in contrast to friction blisters where the split is within the epidermis.

11.4.2 Falls

Examples of injuries or death arising from falls include animals that are thrown from buildings, chicks that drop out of nests and livestock that fall from heights in steep country. Mortality and the types of injury are influenced by the orienta-

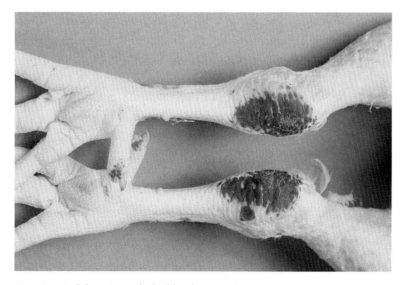

Figure 11.13 Hock burn in a plucked broiler carcass.

tion of the body at impact, the type of surface the animal falls onto and the height of the drop and hence the velocity at impact.

Falls from escarpments have been a significant cause of injury and mortality amongst beef cows, when steep ground has been overstocked. The best pasture becomes limited to poorly accessible ledges and spurs, and accidents happen when stock try to reach this feed.

When cats fall from high rise apartment buildings, they often have a nose bleed, split palate, broken teeth and pneumothorax. Impact on concrete with the feet first is likely to cause injury to the lower legs. If an animal lands on its back, the ribs tend to fracture near the spine, whereas if it lands on its side the ribs tend to fracture near the sternum as well as the spine. Curved ribs in the chest are more likely to fracture than flat ribs. Trunk flexion injuries take the form of broken vertebrae, discs or ligaments, and angulation fractures of the spine may occur if an animal lands on its side. In general, high falls are associated with fractures in the chest, pelvis and thoracic spine, whereas low falls are linked more to limb, head and neck injuries. The most common fall injuries in cats and dogs are in the limbs (Kolata *et al.*, 1974).

The trauma associated with free falls into water include pneumo- and haemo-thoraces with pulmonary contusion and/or lacerations, haemoperitoneum from liver lacerations or pulping and spleen injuries. Free falls onto deep snow are often injury-free up to heights of 12 m, whereas falls from this height onto concrete would often be fatal.

11.4.3 Shock
There are three types of shock following trauma:

(1)   cardiogenic shock;
(2)   haemorrhagic shock;
(3)   shock associated with psychological fright, but without typical cardiogenic shock.

When post-mortems are conducted on trauma cases, it is not always obvious from gross pathology why or how the animal died. Shock may be suspected, and there can be haemorrhage, but it may not be extensive enough to conclude that death arose from haemorrhagic shock. Instead, it may appear that the injury led to a coagulopathy, but this is difficult to prove simply from gross pathology. The chances of death from intravascular coagulation are not great. Most blood clots that form at a wound and enter the bloodstream are trapped by the capillary bed of the lungs. This greatly reduces the risk of a clot blocking a coronary or cerebral artery. However, if the clots form systemically, then it would be possible for a fatal clot to develop in the bloodstream between the left ventricle and either a coronary artery or the brain. An alternative explanation is that there was a fatal cardiogenic or psychological shock.

In **cardiogenic shock** there is profound cardiac inhibition. It has occurred in pithed de-brained animals, and so it is not dependent on intact vagal, spinal cord and brain pathways. For example, in 1831 it was reported that, when a pithed de-brained eel had its stomach violently crushed with a hammer, the heart stopped for a long period, but regained normal function sometime later (Jarcho, 1967). In other studies it has been found that afferent signals that are transmitted from a traumatised region along the spinal cord are essential for the subsequent hypo-tension during the shock phase. Clearly there is more than one physiological explanation.

One of the effects of cardiogenic shock is fluid loss from the capillary bed into the surrounding tissues. This can occur when there is only slight haemorrhage, as demonstrated in a study on anaesthetised dogs (Cleghorn & McKelvey, 1944). The thigh muscles were traumatised by light blows with a mallet without pulping the muscle or inducing haemorrhage. The damaged tissue became engorged with plasma, and blood volume, blood pressure and heart rate collapsed with the onset of shock. Eighty-four per cent of the dogs went into shock, and half of them developed shock in less than five hours. This type of shock is sometimes referred to as secondary shock. From the welfare perspective it is relevant to note that dogs that survived long enough to regain consciousness did not show obvious signs of pain.

When hypotension develops during shock, and if it is sustained for hours, there is an increasing chance of tissue hypoxaemia through capillary stasis. This causes a reflex increase in capillary permeability and progressive loss of fluid and chlo-ride to the intercellular spaces, which loss further compromises venous return and blood pressure. Blood volume is reduced not only by haemorrhage, but also by this increase in capillary permeability. Localised capillary congestion is made worse by localised coagulation of blood (Gando, 2001).

Disseminated intravascular coagulation (DIC) is a common feature in shock, but the mechanisms leading to clotting take time to set in. There are two prerequi-sites for the occurrence of DIC during shock: capillary stagnation and a clotting stimulus. Trauma associated with haemorrhagic shock provides a strong stimulus for blood-clot formation, as does haemolysis (Hardaway et al., 1980). Preventing capillary stagnation can help prevent DIC (Hardaway, 1967).

In **spinal shock** there is loss of vasomotor reflexes below the level of the spinal injury. If the lesion is in the cervical region, there can be a calamitous fall in blood pressure. During recovery, vasomotor reflexes tend to return before somatic reflexes. The returning reflexes may be exaggerated, probably from a loss of suprasegmental inhibitory pathways (Simpson, 1963).

Shock from eventration and **post-operative shock** can occur when there has been severe stimulation of the viscera (Wiggers, 1918). It is a form of secondary shock arising from massive arterial dilatation, and seems to be more common in animals that have some other disease or disorder. It has been induced in dogs by handling the intestines or other viscera roughly during surgery. Blood pressure drops to shock levels, and remains there unless treated (Ivy, 1943). Shock and death from eventration can also occur when large horses are gelded with a blade (Hutchins & Rawlinson, 1972). In about 3% of cases, a section of the small intestine prolapses through the internal inguinal ring and hangs from the open scrotal sac.

Psychological shock is an under-reported response in animals that experience trauma. This is probably because it is not always easy to differentiate it from other causes of shock or lack of movement, and so there is reluctance to use a term that has precise connotations. Psychological traumatic shock can be initiated by a massive injury discharge from nerves at the time of the trauma.

In humans there is a wide range of feelings and behaviours associated with psychological or traumatic shock. They include:

- mental numbing – including reduced involvement, seeking mental escape;
- fatigue;
- anxiety reactions – anxiety, fear of death, sleep disturbance;
- depression – feelings of helplessness, loneliness, isolation;
- psychosomatic reactions – crying, diarrhoea or vomiting, screaming;
- psychotic-like state – disorientation, running amok, fainting, tremors.

In cardiogenic and **haemorrhagic shock** there are profound physical and mental depression, usually accompanied by subnormal body temperature, and lowered blood volume and blood pressure. They are induced and exacerbated by the following conditions:

- fractures;
- wounds;
- visceral perforation;
- surgical intervention;
- eventration;
- burns;
- frostbite;
- crushing injuries;
- prolonged application of a tourniquet;
- exposure to heat;
- exposure to cold;
- exposure to low barometric pressure;
- muscle fatigue with exhaustion;
- acute infections or intoxications.

If an intra-abdominal haemorrhage causes a substantial rise in intra-abdominal pressure (IAP) in combination with a drop in blood volume, there is a syndrome that leads to anuria and reduced cerebral perfusion known as **abdominal compartment syndrome** (Poole et al., 1991). This cascade begins when the raised IAP presses on the mesenteric artery causing impaired perfusion and oxygenation of the gut mucosa; this in turn leads to mucosal acidosis and visceral oedema which raises the IAP even further; the increased IAP also suppresses venous return, raises intrathoracic pressure by displacing the diaphragm, and raises systemic vascular resistance by pressing on the capillary bed, all of which tend to lower the blood supply to the brain. If the raised IAP limits renal blood flow and raises pressure within the renal parenchyma, glomerular filtration rate is reduced and the animal develops anuria.

As a general rule, when blood loss through haemorrhage exceeds 40% of blood volume, the survival time for an animal is inversely related to the additional amount of blood lost. Up to that level, there is no clear relationship between the amount of blood lost and survival time. However, this generalisation may not hold for dogs, and there is remarkable variation between individual dogs. The dog spleen is large and may store up to 15–20% of the total blood volume, and this helps buffer against hypovolaemic shock.

The typical signs during haemorrhagic and hypovolaemic shock are:

- rapid respiratory rate;
- rapid weak pulse;
- physical weakness;
- sluggish depressed senses;
- dehydration and thirst;
- anuria;
- pale mucous membranes;
- slow capillary refill time;
- dark blood;
- variable body temperature (high if agitated and low if comatose) (Jennings 1982). Capillary refill time can be determined by lifting the upper lip and pressing on the gum line. Colour should return to the gum in less than one second. If it takes two to three seconds, peripheral circulation is impaired.

Shock can cause hypothermia, but the hypotension and hypoxaemia will tend to inhibit shivering. These effects could be due in part to reduced oxygen consumption and heat production, and to a central response mediated by the pre-optic area (POA) of the hypothalamus. In some cases, hypothermia may intensify bleeding by prolonging clotting time.

In cases of protracted shock, the subject often succumbs eventually to respiratory failure. This occurs in traumatic, septic and haemorrhagic shock. For example, it occurred in dogs that were bled by about 25% of their total blood volume and developed pulmonary capillary hypoxaemia (Kamada & Smith, 1972). The hypoxaemia produced a secondary increase in capillary permeability which resulted in alveolar oedema, contraction of the alveolar spaces and seepage of serosanguinous fluid into the alveolar spaces.

This form of haemorrhagic pulmonary oedema has been called 'shock lung', 'traumatic wet lung' and 'congestive atelectasis' (lung collapse). The signs include tachypnoea, dyspnoea, cough, cyanosis, respiratory acidosis and physical signs of pulmonary congestion. Not all dogs developed this disorder. However, if the haemorrhage was combined with injury, there was an increased likelihood of pulmonary oedema. This was probably due to the additional lung damage caused by blood clots accumulating in the lung as emboli.

The signs associated with shock can mislead the onlooker into thinking that there is no hope for the animal. There was a case of a dray horse that was housed in a stable that was damaged by a bomb that landed nearby. The animal lay as if dead for over four hours before it was examined. It had a slow weak pulse, and it was decided to fetch a humane killer. Suddenly it shivered all over and got up, but had limited use of its hind quarters. A week later it was able to do light work (Buxton, 1941).

11.4.4 Self-mutilation
Self-mutilation can be due to:

* pain;
* unpleasant dysaesthesias or paraesthesias;
* hyperactivity in the CNS induced by the lesions;
* loss of sensation in the affected part.

When rats have had a sciatic nerve severed, 80% of them mutilated the desensitised region. Pain is thought to have been the main stimulus provoking the self-mutilation (Wall et al., 1979; Blumenkopf & Lipman, 1991), and this response has been used as an experimental model in rats, mice and rabbits for neuropathic pain in humans. In mice, the self-mutilation usually began as a nibbling of the toe nails, and then extended upwards. Local anaesthetics applied to the nerve prior to sectioning prevented self-mutilation, which indicates that injury discharges at the time of the cut were important in initiating the central sensitisation of the dorsal horn of the spinal cord that is often responsible for neuropathic pain.

Self-mutilation also occurs in *anaesthesia dolorosa*, and in other cases of intense nerve irritation such as spinal-nerve compression, and stenosis or attenuation of the *cauda equina*. In the dog, *cauda equina* compression has resulted in self-mutilation of the tail, prepuce, perineal area and limbs (Tavin & Prata, 1980). In laboratory mice there have been outbreaks of self-mutilation of the penis when there was blockage of the urethra (Hong & Ediger, 1978).

Self-mutilation sometimes occurs in animals that are trapped by a leg, for example with a leg-hold trap. This has been seen in racoon and skunk, but it is less common in fox, possum and opossum. There might be two causes for this form of self-mutilation. Firstly, the animal may be desperate to escape, and if the limb is desensitised it mauls its leg to free itself. Secondly, the limb might be attacked if it is a source of pain. Self-mutilation of the digits of the paw has been reported in cats and dogs that experienced peripheral nerve injury following pelvic fractures (Jacobson & Schrader, 1987). Wild raptors will often mutilate themselves when a wing or leg is denervated in a traumatic injury (Holland & Jennings, 1997).

In horses, flank, chest and tail biting can develop as stereotypies (Dodman *et al.*, 1994). The more common expression is flank biting, which responds to opioid antagonists. It is more common in males than females, and in confined horses. It is precipitated by anticipation of feeding, interaction with other horses, inactivity, and states of increased anxiety or arousal. In primates, self-mutilation has occurred in males that have been isolated from counterparts during a socially-formative period of their life.

11.4.5 Autotomy
Autotomy is reflex involuntary shedding of a tail or limb. Tail autotomy occurs in some species of salamander, lizards and rodents, and limb autotomy can occur in Echinoderms and spiders. Many decapod crustaceans shed a limb when threatened or attacked, as a way of avoiding predators. They grasp the attacking predator with a cheliped and then shed the cheliped which remains attached to the predator. Some species of crab, such as *Cyrtograptus angulatus*, are particularly prone to autotomy (Juanes & Smith, 1995). Suffering may develop following autotomy if survival is jeopardised. Some crabs survive autotomy by eating soft invertebrates, algae and grasses instead of their normal diet of hard-shelled bivalves or clams.

Human activities are responsible for substantial limb loss in some crab species, either through intentional harvesting of the claws for human consumption (*Menippe mercenaria*), as a result of incidental damage associated with fishing gear (e.g. trawling) or rejecting sub-legal-sized crabs (e.g. *Ranina ranina*). Sub-legal-sized spanner crabs can lose on average three to four dactyli and seven limbs while being disentangled from commercial tangle nets. Lobsters (*Homarus americanus*) off Prince Edward Island also lose their claws during raking operations used for harvesting Irish moss. Fishermen of southern Spain, the South Atlantic and the gulf states of America intentionally remove the chelipeds of crabs (*Gelasimus tangeri* and *Menippe mercenaria*) in sub-legal-sized catch to stimulate moulting in those that survive and so accelerate the growth of the animal before a subsequent catch (Bennett, 1973). In some parts of the world, young crabs are caught and their legs removed for fishing bait, the torso being thrown back into the sea.

11.4.6 Tail-biting
Tail-biting in pigs can lead to infections, with abscess formation and pyaemia. The precise cause is not always obvious, but predisposing factors include:

- hunger;
- lack of facilities such as bedding, which encourages normal rooting and chewing behaviours;

- early weaning;
- high stocking densities;
- insufficient trough space, leading to frustration at feeding time;
- high temperatures;
- insufficient ventilation;
- very bright light;
- copycat behaviour.

From a postal survey of 46 farms in the United Kingdom, it was reported that farmers recognised it as a problem on farms that had bare concrete floors instead of bedding, had slatted floors, used automatic feeders instead of a manual feeding system and had wet feeding rather than dry feeding (Chambers *et al.*, 1995).

11.4.7 Trauma during pregnancy

The most common cause of foetal death following trauma to the mother is placental abruption. The lining of the uterus is more elastic than the placenta, and so, when the mother's abdomen receives a blunt impact, the uterus deforms while the placenta remains much as it is. This creates a risk that the placenta will separate from the underlying decidua. If there is also an increase in intra-amniotic pressure, the placenta can shear away (Pearlman *et al.*, 1990). When placental abruption occurs in this way, perfusion of the foetus may be compromised. Clinical findings in the mother include abdominal pain, amniotic-fluid leakage and possibly vaginal bleeding. Abortion may not be immediate, but typically occurs within two days, and can be as late as five days after the insult. This involves formation of prostaglandins by decidual lysosomes, which causes uterine contractions.

In humans, stress and psychological trauma have often been thought to be a cause of spontaneous abortion. However, the evidence supporting this is imprecise and there is incomplete agreement about the mechanisms which explain how this occurs.

11.4.8 Beatings and similar forms of abuse

Beatings and whippings are usually suspected from the pattern of the marks on the skin. They are often seen as parallel or criss-cross lines on the animal. On bony parts of the body they tend to be circular bruises. Similarly, kicks tend to produce more or less circular bruises or scars where there is bone close to the skin. Stabbings leave a linear scar, which can be teardrop in shape if the knife had a single cutting edge. Stab wounds in the liver have a characteristic straight edge, whereas splits in the liver have a rougher surface. Sharpened goads leave circular scars which can be similar to cigarette burns.

The internal injuries inflicted by a blunt blow to the abdomen can take a similar form to those described for lung wounds during blast injury. At the site of the blow there is likely to be bruising, and there may be deeper bruising where internal organs have been distorted by the thrust from the blow. The case of a gelding that was kicked by both hind feet of another horse, describes this effect clearly. On being struck, the gelding squealed, backed off, stopped, breathed quickly for a few minutes, staggered and braced himself, then collapsed and died. On post-mortem examination, the abdomen was found to be filled with blood which had arisen entirely from two ruptures on the medial aspect of the spleen. Evidently, the abdomen had been struck in the region of the spleen, which had split on the side *opposite* to the blow where the thrust was least constrained.

Overzealous use of the whip in competitive racing can result in wheals and bruises. In horses these can be on the neck, shoulder or over the ribs, and spur injuries may occur at the flank. Inflammation and swelling with oedema can set in.

Physical abuse may lead to a change in sensitivity to pain. For example, women with a history of physical or sexual abuse had a lower pain threshold in response to finger pressure stimuli than non-abused subjects. It is possible that they more readily labelled stimuli as painful, as distinct from having a physiologically lower pain threshold.

Torture victims often show depression, exhaustion, poor concentration and sleep disturbance (Juhler, 1993). They may also have an abnormal breathing pattern, which, along with other signs is called **chronic hyperventilation syndrome**. The conditions seen in this syndrome are:

- sensation of breathlessness or inability to take a deep enough breath, even though the subject is overbreathing;
- headache;
- weakness and easy fatigue;
- sleep disturbance;
- excessive sweating;
- numbness and tingling;
- giddiness and impaired thinking;
- chest pains;
- aerophagia, resulting in belching;
- dry mouth;
- increased muscle tension and myalgia;
- anxiety, irritability, phobias and panic attacks.

A key physiological response in this syndrome is the reduction in p_aCO_2 from hyperventilation. This produces arterial vasoconstriction and a fall in cerebral oxygenation, which, in turn, is thought to precipitate some of the neurological effects (Turner & Hough, 1993). In some individuals, memory may be impaired. This is due to disturbance of hippocampal function in the brain, which often takes the form of amnesia for the specific traumatic experience, but the associated feelings may keep recurring. Sensitisation (kindling) can occur in repeatedly-traumatised individuals. This involves repeated stimulation of the limbic neuronal circuits which eventually become sensitised and acquire a reduced stimulation threshold. This probably explains their sensitivity to anticipating the return of traumatic events and to their autonomic nervous system imbalance.

Sickness and Disease 12

Disease is one of the most important causes of animal suffering, and yet it is one that is often given the least recognition. To understand the suffering in disease one has to appreciate its pathophysiology and the feelings experienced by humans in comparable situations. Some forms of suffering are peculiar to particular diseases, but there are a number of sensations that are common to a wide range of diseases (Table 12.1).

Ascites is a good example of a specific disorder with fairly precise forms of suffering. This condition is common in broiler chickens, and is associated with congestive heart failure or kidney failure in other species. From experience in humans we know that the raised intraperitoneal pressure from ascitic fluid can cause pain and a sense of dyspnoea, especially during exercise. Pressure on the viscera causes a sense of nausea and suppresses the appetite. Observing the animal's behaviour may tell us whether a particular animal is experiencing these or similar forms of suffering. In people the suffering can be quickly relieved by draining the fluid with a hypodermic needle, and if this procedure improves an animal's behaviour it adds to the evidence that it was indeed suffering.

12.1 Is Suffering an Inevitable Consequence of Being Ill?

There are specific centres in the brain that control general sickness behaviours and some immune responses. This common link makes it difficult to divorce immune responses from sickness behaviour, and presumably sickness perception. This section summarises the evidence behind this dual role for the CNS.

Lesioning the hypothalamus and reticular formation reduces cellular immune system responses in rats, and ablation of the *locus coeruleus* diminishes the ability to mount an antibody response. These three regions also regulate sleep, attentiveness, hunger and body temperature, which are some of the key elements of sickness behaviour. Corticotrophin releasing hormone (CRH) released by these centres

Table 12.1 Some behavioural abnormalities and forms of suffering associated with sickness and disease.

General disturbances	Specific diseases
Loss of appetite	Sore throat
Impaired concentration and memory	Pain in lymph nodes
Fatigue	Fever
Depression	Generalised muscle weakness
Anxiety	Myalgia
Weight loss	Sore sinuses or respiratory tract
Reduced activity	Arthralgia
Anhedonia	Headache
Somnolence	Dyspnoea

activates the hypothalamic-pituitary-adrenal cortex (HPA) axis, and this provides a further link to the metabolic responses that occur in disease states.

Some immune responses can be recruited without involving the brain, but they are associated with sickness behaviours. This peripheral immunity operates through the release of cytokines from infected cells, endothelial cells, fibroblasts, mononuclear phagocytes and lymphocytes in response to toxins produced by the infective micro-organism. The cytokines that are released peripherally act locally, and they can also stimulate the release of cytokines from glial cells within the brain. The CNS response depends on special mechanisms that allow cytokines to bypass the blood–brain barrier, and within the brain they provoke five key sickness behaviours or signs. They are:

(1) fever;
(2) loss of appetite;
(3) impaired memory and learning;
(4) social isolation;
(5) tiredness (Gregory, 1998b).

Cytokines are key agents which recruit both the immune and behavioural responses in sickness.

Feelings of sickness probably depend on activation of the immune system rather than the mere presence of a pathogen or disease condition. Sickness sensation can develop when there is no disease, for example when the immune system is challenged during a vaccination procedure. When people have been vaccinated with attenuated rubella vaccine they have experienced a sickness phase which included depression, social and attention problems and delinquent behaviour (Morag *et al.*, 1998). They did not develop German measles, but their immune system was activated.

12.2 Do the Behaviours Expressed During Sickness Serve a Purpose?

When we develop a **fever** we feel discomfort partly from a knowledge of what is to come but also from the direct effects of the fever. Fever serves some useful purposes. The temperature-raising effect assists body defences by enhancing leucocyte proliferation, promoting antibody production, increasing the rate of neutrophil accumulation at the site of an infection and improving B-lymphocyte responsiveness, all of which help curtail micro-organism growth. In terms of overall outcome, mild to moderate fevers have assisted survival in rabbits that were infected with *Pastuerella multocida* (Kluger & Vaughn, 1978), and allowing a fever to express itself has reduced the severity of influenza infection in ferrets (Husseini *et al.*, 1982).

Infections also induce **sleepiness**, but whether the individual spends more time sleeping depends on circumstances. Sleep is considered beneficial during illness because it may hasten recovery by improving morale and promoting immune function. The evidence that supports this is largely circumstantial. Rabbits that have died following inoculation with live *Staphylococcus aureus* showed reduced neutrophil responses during the infection and spent substantially less time sleeping in comparison with rabbits that overcame the infection (Toth & Kreuger, 1988). In humans, sleep deprivation has been associated with impaired immune function, including natural killer (NK) cell activity, lymphokine-activated killer cell activity, and interleukin-2 (IL-2) production in response to antigen challenge (Irwin *et al.*, 1994, 1996). In rats, fatigue reduced survival after inoculation with bacilli which included anthrax spores, in comparison with animals allowed to rest.

It is often said that one should feed a cold. In other words, do not stop eating when there is a respiratory infection even though **appetite** is suppressed. This axiom may not apply to all disease states. When mice were fasted for varying lengths of time and then injected intravenously with *Listeria monocytogenes* it was found that those that were fasted longest had the lowest subsequent mortality. Similarly, limiting feed intake during the early stages of cancer can help to delay the rate at which it develops (Shields *et al.*, 1991). Evidently, fasting before a disease sets in can afford some protection against the disease. However, other studies have shown that the immune system can be compromised by fasting. For example, feed and water deprivation for two days suppressed the antibody response to inoculation with killed *E. coli* in chickens. We do not have a clear picture of when it is best to stop or start eating, but sickness-induced suppression of eating can be beneficial in some conditions.

In herding species, the urge for **social isolation** during sickness reduces the opportunity for cross-infection. Social isolation may be linked to activity of the *locus coeruleus* in the brain, which is thought to enhance or mediate the sense of nausea, photophobia, phonophobia and headaches during illness.

12.3 Cytokines and Sickness Behaviours

In bacterial infections, cytokine production is induced by cell wall components present in the bacteria, such as lipopolysaccharide (LPS). LPS endotoxin induces a broad range of flu-like sensations, including depression, anhedonia, headache, muscle aches, short-lasting chills and nausea, through the release of cytokines. The psychological effects seem to be correlated with particular cytokines, and they can be reduced by treatment with antidepressants. Part of this effect could be due to suppression of the release of cytokines. For example, antidepressants can suppress the release of IL-1β and IL-6 from monocytes and IL-2 and interferon-γ (IFN-γ) from activated T-cells (Maes *et al.*, 1999).

Cytokines can be either pro-inflammatory or anti-inflammatory. The **pro-inflammatory cytokines** mediate the following:

- fever;
- leukocytosis;
- increased synthesis of acute-phase proteins;
- muscle catabolism;
- stimulation of the HPA;
- activation of leukocytes and endothelial cells.

The precise response depends on the individual cytokines that are present. For example:

- IL-2 produces anhedonia.
- IL-1 and IL-6 promote fever.
- IL-1 and tumour necrosis factor-α (TNF-α) cause an increase in non-REM sleep.
- Interferons cause psychiatric morbidity and flu-like symptoms, including fever, tachycardia, headache, arthralgia, myalgia, and sometimes nausea and vomiting. IL-2 produces similar symptoms, but is more likely to cause peripheral oedema and diarrhoea and less likely to result in myalgia, arthralgia and loss of appetite (Fent & Zbinden, 1987).
- IL-1 can be neurotoxic.

Excessive release of IL-1β, IL-6, TNF-α, IFN-γ and adenosine can promote diffuse intravascular coagulation, and increase the synthesis of nitric oxide in endothelial cells. Nitric oxide promotes vasodilatation, and in extreme situations it exacerbates septic shock reactions.

The pro-inflammatory proliferative cytokines (granulocyte–macrophage colony-stimulating factor (GMCSF), platelet-derived growth factor BB (PDGF-BB) and transforming growth factor β2 (TGF-β2)) also accelerate wound healing.

The **anti-inflammatory cytokines** control inflammatory reactions through autocrine inhibition of pro-inflammatory cytokine production, and some of them promote antibody and allergic responses instead. They include IL-4, IL-10 and TGF-β, and their effects can be beneficial. For example they help to control septic shock.

Several cytokines can activate the HPA, but the pathways vary between the individual cytokines. IL-1α, IL-1β, IL-2, IL-6 and TNF-α stimulate the release of CRH from the hypothalamus. This response is mediated by the induction of nitric oxide, and it leads to activation of the HPA axis through stimulating the release of ACTH.

During fever, the point about which body temperature is regulated is set at a higher level. This readjustment is controlled from the pre-optic area (POA) of the anterior hypothalamus and this centre also mediates sleep. Endogenous agents that reverse the fever include α-melanocyte stimulating hormone (α-MSH), arginine vasopressin, glucocorticoids and IL-10. Although virus infections are often associated with a fever, some small mammals such as mice often show a reduced body temperature. This is probably due to the antipyretic effect of TNF (Conn *et al.*, 1995). The mice try to minimise the fall in their body temperature through behavioural responses.

12.4 Cancer

The most common forms of suffering in subjects dying of cancer are fatigue, pain and dyspnoea. **Fatigue** is often the most distressing symptom. It can be due to the natural progression of the disease and dysfunction of organs, poor feeding, muscle wasting, depression and sleep disorders. In some forms of cancer, the general malaise is made worse by hypercalcaemia and anaemia. Weakness from anaemia can be due to overexpression of IL-1, IL-6 and TNF-α by cancer cells, and suppression of erythropoiesis by these cytokines. Wasting develops from loss of appetite and enhanced hydrolysis of body protein, and TNF, IFN-γ and leukaemia inhibitory factor can mediate this response.

Stress can increase the risk of tumour-cell proliferation. In humans, cancer mortality tends to be high in individuals who have a driving, impatient and sometimes hostile personality. Such people go through states of repeated frustration because of unachieved goals. They alternate between a sense of being able to cope to one of being unable to cope. This pattern is thought to cause repeated episodes of suppression and recovery of the immune system, and to increase the growth of transformed cells (Fox *et al.*, 1987). Some of the ways this occurs are:

- increased β-adrenergic-induced suppression of NK cell activity, and reduced recruitment of spleen cells as anti-tumour cells;

- reduced function of tumour-specific cluster designation 4^+ (CD4$^+$), and inhibition of IL-12 production by adenosine accumulation where large tumours cause localised hypoxic conditions;
- potentiation of capillary growth (angiogenesis) in tumours by glucocorticoids making nutrients more readily available for tumour growth.

In mice infected with mammary tumour virus, handling stress increased the prevalence of mammary tumours from 7% to 92% (Riley, 1975). Stress also reduces the effectiveness of chemotherapy against this form of cancer.

The prevalence of **pain** among patients with newly-diagnosed cancer is about 28%, and this rises as the disease advances and as therapy becomes more aggressive. Unrelieved cancer pain is debilitating, interferes with the ability to eat and sleep and leads to fatigue. Bone metastases are the most common cause of chronic pain in cancer patients. They are often associated with direct invasion of bone marrow with a tumour that has metastasised from soft tissue. The tumour cells adhere to endothelial surfaces within the bone marrow, and the cancer develops through marrow sinusoids to the endosteal bone surface where it causes remodelling of bone. The thoracic vertebrae are a common site where the metastases lodge, and they inflict pain by compressing the spinal cord, stretching the periosteum as the tumour expands, putting pressure on regions where the bone is weakened and collapsing the bone in regions where it has been resorbed (Mercadente, 1997). The pain is often dull, intermittent in nature and occurs as breakthrough pain associated with physical movement or weight bearing. Stabbing pains may be felt when there is nerve compression.

It is well recognised that bone cancer causes pain and discomfort in animals as well as humans (Plate 10). In one of the mouse experimental models for bone cancer, murine osteolytic sarcoma cells are injected into the intramedullary space of the animal's femur (Schwei *et al.*, 1999). Light palpation of the distal femur produces a nocifensive response, including withdrawal of the limb, fighting, vocalising and biting. There is also guarding of the affected limb. This model is being used in designing pain therapies.

12.5 Stress and Immune Function

It is well known that stress can suppress immune function. Stress-induced immune suppression helps to limit and delay inflammatory pain until the immediate danger from the stressor has passed. It also helps prevent abnormal overactivity and exhaustion of the immune system that might otherwise occur during the acute-phase response. In the short term this has benefits, but if the stress-induced suppression persists, there can be unfortunate consequences. In general, chronic stress is immunosuppressive and acute stress is immunoenhancing (Table 12.2). During

Table 12.2 Common effects of acute and chronic stress on immune function.

Acute stress	Chronic stress
↑ leukocyte redeployment	↓ leukocyte proliferation
↑ effector-cell function	↓ effector-cell function
↑ cell-mediated immunity	↓ cell-mediated immunity
↑ humoral immunity	↓ humoral immunity

acute stress, adrenaline and noradrenaline mobilise leukocytes which are distributed through the blood to other organs. Leukocyte uptake during acute stress is usually raised and so there can be a decrease in circulating leukocyte numbers.

The ways in which **chronic stress** suppresses the immune system are highly specific, and only particular types of defence against disease are affected. One of the main inhibitory mechanisms is mediated through T-helper cells (Th). T-helper cells are lymphocytes that enable the destruction of pathogens by interacting with phagocytes.

Stresses that involve the release of glucocorticoids, adrenaline or noradrenaline, and inflammatory responses that provoke histamine or adenosine release, can all result in suppression of IL-12 production. IL-12 is one of the key regulators of the balance between Th1 and Th2 cells. IL-12 encourages a shift away from a Th2 immune response towards a Th1 response. Th1 and Th2 cells have quite distinct cytokine profiles. Th1 cytokines are IFN-γ, TNF-β and IL-2, whilst Th2 cytokines include IL-4, IL-5, IL-6, IL-9, IL-10 and IL-13. The Th2 cytokines are involved in humoral immune responses such as antibody and allergic responses, whereas the Th1 cytokines activate cellular immune responses including cytotoxic, inflammatory and delayed hypersensitivity reactions (Elenkor *et al.*, 2000). Thus, when stress suppresses IL-12 production, the capacity of cellular immune mechanisms is reduced. Th2 responses are still effective, but these are less organ specific than the Th1 responses.

In practical terms, this means that some disorders are more likely to be precipitated by chronic stress than others. These include respiratory disease, toxoplasmosis, *Salmonella* infection and cancer. Infection of an existing gastric ulcer is also likely to be increased, because defence against this happening is largely mediated by Th1 responses. Similarly, traumatic injury, including burns, which provoke intense sympathoadrenomedullary and HPA axis activation, leads to diminished IL-12 and IFN-γ production, and this will promote a Th2 shift which could lead to infection (Molloy *et al.*, 1995). Wound healing is also likely to be delayed. Ischaemia leads to localised build-up of adenosine, which in turn inhibits IL-12 and TNF-α production and potentiation of IL-10, which together produce a Th2 shift and suppression of cellular immune responses.

Another way in which stress can lead to immune suppression is through increasing the release of natural opioids. Endogenous opioids can suppress immune responses by reducing antibody production and NK cell activity through κ-opioid receptors (Rogers *et al.*, 2000). Met-enkephalin, on the other hand, enhances immune reactions.

There is one positive outcome of the immune-suppressing effects of chronic stress. Chronic stress can help to reduce the incidence and severity of autoimmune diseases, and this has been demonstrated in rats using an experimental model for allergic encephalomyelitis.

Some of the stressors that compromise immune function are inevitable aspects of life, whilst others are quite subtle. In humans, psychological stressors such as bereavement, preparing for examinations, marital strife, looking after a spouse with dementia and depressive illness, have been shown to adversely affect immune function. In mice, social disruption, through transferring dominant mice between cages of subordinate mice, increased subsequent mortality to an influenza virus challenge from 11% in unmixed controls to 86% in the mixed dominant mice (Sheridan *et al.*, 2000). In monkeys, low social status has been linked to a greater probability of being infected with an upper respiratory tract infection and gastrointestinal infection with an adenovirus.

Susceptibility to infection is greatest in young, old and immunocompromised individuals. Weaning in very young animals can be a high risk period. During **segregated early weaning** (SEW), piglets are weaned at 5–21 days of age into a low-pathogen environment. The stated purposes with SEW are to eliminate or avoid respiratory diseases in a herd by weaning piglets at a time when immunity to those particular diseases is provided by colostrum-derived immunoglobulins, and to encourage high growth performance. Normally, the piglets' immunity is low at three to four weeks of age. This is because the maternally-derived passive immunity is declining and the piglet's own ability to produce an active immune response has not completely developed. This period of reduced immune protection is known as the **immunity gap**. Weaning during the immunity gap is thought to pose a particular risk for piglet health, and current thinking amongst veterinarians is that this can be avoided by either using SEW or by weaning later, when the piglet can mount its own immune responses.

Early weaning is the least sensible of these two strategies as it is likely to lead to some serious health risks after weaning. It is not always realistic to wean piglets into a pathogen-free environment, and so the weaning ration is usually medicated with antibiotics. These help to control enteric disease and they promote growth rate, but there is growing evidence that such indiscriminate use of antibiotics by the pig industry is leading to antibiotic-resistant strains of bacteria. Weaning at four to five weeks of age would be a more sensible strategy, as it would avoid the immunity gap and it would not require the widespread use of feed antibiotics.

12.6 Corticosteroid Therapy

Corticosteroids are used routinely in veterinary and human medicine to control inflammation, provide relief from pain that is caused by inflammation, induce parturition and, in conjunction with antineoplastic drugs, in treating cancer. Injudicious use of corticosteroids at pharmacological doses can increase the risk of infection through suppression of:

- T-lymphocyte numbers;
- Th cells;
- immunoglobulin levels;
- NK cell activity;
- macrophage antigen expression;
- cytokine production.

These are normal effects of this group of drugs, and one of the implications of inducing calving in dairy cows with long-acting corticosteroids as a routine measure for controlling the calving pattern, is the increased risk of infections. Similarly, hyperactivity of the HPA during depression or chronic stress, leading to high circulating levels of glucocorticoids, causes immune suppression and increased susceptibility to infectious disease (Falaschi *et al.*, 1994). Lower (physiological) concentrations of corticosteroids are more likely to be immunoenhancing.

12.7 Anaemia

Anaemia is associated with a sense of fatigue, dizziness or headaches, and dyspnoea during exertion. In the human being these feelings develop when haemoglobin levels are less than 7 g/100 ml of blood. The heart compensates by increasing stroke volume, and, in severe cases, circulatory congestion similar to that seen in congestive heart failure can develop. In animals, anaemia has been a problem in calves used for white veal production, because of the iron deficient milk diet they receive. Iron deficiency anaemia also occurs in piglets and lambs that are reared indoors without access to iron supplementation.

12.8 Hazards of Improving Disease Control

Some of the tests that are used for genetically-selecting animals for resistance to particular diseases have been criticised because they are very unpleasant for the animals. They involve producing either the clinical or the subclinical condition, and its associated suffering. An example is the facial-eczema test used in sheep in

New Zealand. Facial eczema occurs in cattle, sheep and deer (Plate 11). It is caused by a fungal toxin (sporodesmin) in dead pasture and results in liver damage and photosensitisation when eaten.

The test sheep are dosed with sporodesmin, and liver damage is assessed from the serum gamma glutamyl transferase (sGGT) response. Animals with a high sGGT response are susceptible to the disease. In severely-affected animals there would be photosensitisation, skin soreness and jaundice, but this can be minimised by using subclinical doses of sporodesmin. The adverse welfare consequences with this type of test in susceptible animals are almost inevitable, but the overall saving in suffering through genetic selection helps justify the procedure.

Sometimes the cure is almost as unpleasant as the disease itself. In the past, the gapes in chickens was treated by forcing the birds to breathe in carbolic-acid fumes. Great care was needed to ensure the birds were not overdosed. Nowadays, this parasitic worm is eliminated from the airways of the lungs in a kinder way, with anthelmintic drugs.

12.9 Diseases Used for Controlling Pests

The advantage of using a disease for pest control is that it can be effective against large numbers of the pest species with little expenditure of effort. In some cases it can also be species specific.

Myxomatosis has been used to control rabbits in many countries. The time to death following infection with the myxoma virus varies with the virulence of the strain of virus. It ranges from 10–50 days. With virulent strains, skin swellings appear over the body after four or five days. Conjunctival swellings emerge on the fifth or sixth day and the eyes are completely closed a day or two later (Ross, 1972). Death is often from secondary infection of the respiratory tract. Rabbits that recover from an infection have difficulty seeing, because their eyes are glued together by a tenacious purulent exudate, and their breathing is restricted.

Rabbit calicivirus has been introduced as an alternative to myxomatosis. This virus is thought to cause liver damage which results in the release of clotting factors such as thromboplastin, which causes disseminated intravascular coagulopathy (DIC). This in turn results in a stroke if the clot lodges in the brain, or cardiac irregularities if there is an infarct in the heart, which should be relatively benign ways to die. Unfortunately, this is not always the case. Sometimes there are signs of sickness including anorexia, rapid respiration, cyanosis, ataxia, paddling movements of the limbs and, finally, frenetic behaviour with squealing before death (Chasey, 1997). About 20% of affected rabbits discharge foamy blood from the nostrils. When death is quick, following the stroke or cardiac arrest, it should provide a more humane death than that from myxomatosis.

Digestive System 13

This chapter discusses some of the gut conditions that cause or are linked to suffering. They include nausea, vomiting, dyspepsia, gas distension, constipation, diarrhoea and ulceration.

13.1 Nausea

Nausea, vomiting and diarrhoea are defence mechanisms against the ingestion of toxins and pathogens. Nausea is associated with:

- intoxication;
- gut pathogens;
- motion sickness;
- pregnancy;
- post-operative recovery;
- cancer therapy.

It often precedes vomiting, and it can be conditioned by either the taste, smell or sight of something that previously caused illness. In humans, there is an unpleasant feeling of gastric awareness and imminent vomiting, and there may be cold sweating. This can be more aversive than gut pain. It can be blocked with neurokinin antagonists, which probably act on the *nucleus tractus solitarius* in the brain stem. Nausea is not commonly recognised in animals, but there is no reason to suppose that it does not occur.

13.2 Vomiting and Retching

Some species seem to be more prone to vomiting than others, and it is common amongst sample-feeding species of mammal. Vomiting is a central reflex involving the autonomic nervous system and skeletal muscles. Irritants that initiate nausea and vomiting activate receptors in the gut wall, which include serotonin type 3 and serotonin type 4 receptors. Afferents from the receptors convey signals to the nucleus of the solitary tract and *area prostrema* in the brain. Thereon the nucleus of the solitary tract, lateral tegmental field of the reticular formation and the ventrolateral medulla coordinate the actions in vomiting. Movements of the small intestine, stomach, oesophagus and diaphragm are synchronised to forcibly expel gastric contents through the mouth. In severe episodes, bile from the duodenum may also be ejected. Sectioning the vagus nerves above the level of the heart causes intractable vomiting, and this is partly due to the loss of pulmonary vagal afferents that would otherwise inhibit retching and vomiting. **Retching** occurs when there is a strong involuntary effort to vomit, without expelling gastric contents. **Regurgitation** is the involuntary return of gastric contents, without retching but it may accompany a belch.

The feelings associated with **motion sickness** are drowsiness, cold sweating and salivation, with increased swallowing and nausea. Forms of motion sickness have been observed in horses, dogs, pigs, cows, sheep and chickens. Monkeys, cats, rabbits and guinea-pigs seem to be less susceptible (Tyler & Bard, 1949). In dogs, horizontal motion is more likely than vertical or angular motion to induce motion sickness, but no one component is as effective as a composite of all three (Noble, 1945). Nystagmus is not a common feature of motion sickness, but it can occur in response to rotation. From a teleological perspective, it is doubtful whether motion sickness serves any useful purpose.

Swing sickness is a form of motion sickness that occurs when visual orientation fails to keep up with physical movement. It is more common during motion with the eyes closed or covered, and presumably it would be more common at night-time.

Psychogenic vomiting is an anxiety or frustration-related vomiting which is not usually associated with nausea or retching. Psychological stress can cause this type of vomiting in dogs, for example, during emotional conflicts and separation anxiety.

Airway aspiration of stomach contents is highly irritating. Vomit that settles in the lungs can lead to blood clot formation and obstruction in the pulmonary vessels. This is due to injury of the vessel walls by gastric acid, in combination with raised permeability of the alveolar–capillary membrane, vasospasm and hypoxaemia. In humans the risk of **pulmonary aspiration** of gastric contents is higher during pregnancy, and in animals it can occur when there is a twisted stomach or abomasum.

Dyspepsia is the sensation accompanying indigestion after a meal. It causes discomfort and in some cases can be painful. The forms of discomfort include a sense of fullness, satiety, bloating, rebellious belching, nausea, and retching or vomiting. It is thought that dyspeptic people have a lower vagal tone, which reduces gastric motility allowing greater stomach distension. These people tend to consider themselves as hyper-responsive to stress (Haug *et al.*, 1994). Dyspepsia is not commonly diagnosed in animals, but there is no reason to suppose that it cannot occur in monogastrics.

13.3 Gut Pain

In the healthy stomach, inflammatory injury does not usually give rise to pain. In the past surgeons operated on it using only a sedative and local anaesthetic applied to the abdominal wall (Bonney & Pickering, 1946). Pinching the stomach, inserting a tube through the stomach wall and securing the tube with tension sutures were painless procedures.

Not all the viscera are insensitive to manipulation, however. Stretching the mesenteric attachments to the stomach does cause pain, as well as nausea and tachycardia. Gut pain occurs when there are:

- excessive stretching of the intestine wall;
- spasms or strong contractions within the wall;
- inflammation of the gut wall;
- damage to the mucosa and exposure to irritants, such as hydrochloric acid, that are normally present in the digestive tract.

The first three of these are due to pressure effects. Quite often the pain comes in waves which coincide with contraction phases of the gut. The pain is poorly-localised because there are relatively few pain receptors in the viscera. It may provoke a guarding response as a protective reflex, changes in posture which offset some of the pressure, and autonomic reflexes including sweating, hypotension, nausea and vomiting.

Excessive stretching may be due to build-up of gas, constipation, impaction or abnormal orientation of the gut. When the gut becomes distended with gas, there is initially a bloated feeling, followed by gut pain. Greenwald *et al.* (1969) examined this in finer detail. They found that the normal volume of gas held by the gastrointestinal tract of men is about 110 ml, and the volume produced in a day was about ten times that amount. When the resident volume increased to 500 ml, half the subjects experienced a sense of abdominal fullness. When the gas volume rose to 1090 ml, one in five individuals developed abdominal pain. The distribution of the gas could be important, since as little as 200 ml of gas in the stomach was sufficient to cause pain.

The site at which there is stretching has a strong influence on whether or not the experience is painful. When a balloon catheter is inflated within the rectum, there is a sense of the need to defecate. When the catheter is inserted further, and inflated rapidly within the colon, it causes pain. Similarly, stretching during rapid passage of a large hard bolus in the colon can be quite painful.

There are two types of **constipation**. *Intestinal* constipation occurs when passage through the intestine is delayed whilst defecation is otherwise normal. *Rectal* constipation occurs when there is no delay in the arrival of a stool, but the final expulsion is protracted. In both cases there is stretching of mechanoreceptors, and the consequent pain may be exacerbated by ischaemia within the gut wall. The gut wall has receptors that respond to lactic acid, prostaglandins and free radicals that accumulate during ischaemia.

Dyschezia is the term given to painful defecation. There are two types of pain: a vague dull ache in the proximal part of the rectum which can last for minutes, and a sudden piercing pain usually lasting for a matter of seconds. In humans it has been known for subjects (especially infants) to scream in pain during straining on a stool. In adults this has often been due to a failure to relax the muscles of the pelvic floor, with subsequent loss of coordination in expelling the stool. A short sharp pain can also be due to smooth-muscle spasm that is linked to an anxiety problem.

Difficulty in passing the first stool of meconium is sometimes seen in newborn foals and calves, and in some cases it gives the impression of being a painful experience. Constipation can be a problem in pigs that are confined and take little exercise, and it is not uncommon in dogs. In humans chronic constipation has been associated with mental depression, whereas anxiety is more likely to be associated with a high frequency of bowel movements.

When **diarrhoea** is associated with visceral cramps, there is often a dull diffuse but gripping pain in the abdomen. The spasms that cause the pain are associated with ischaemia and inflammation. Intestinal obstruction and abdominal distension involve a more continuous pain. Pain from peritonitis causes contraction of the abdominal muscles, guarding behaviour and, as a secondary response, gut motility may be reduced. Gas distension causes a diffuse, non-radiating, abdominal pain.

A wide range of abdominal diseases and disorders are associated with visceral pain, including:

- cholecystitis;
- constipation;
- gaseous distension;
- ileitis;
- mesenteric lymphadenitis;
- pancreatitis;
- perforated ulcers;
- peritonitis.

The horse has a very large caecum, and caecal disorders are one of the causes of **colic**. Impaction is the most common caecal disorder, occurring mainly in older horses. It is associated with signs of mild abdominal pain and is caused by impaired outflow of caecal contents whilst fed coarse roughage. The caecum becomes highly stretched by a large, firm, dehydrated mass of digesta (Dart *et al.*, 1997).

Stretching of the mesentery produces a **stitch pain** in humans. Rupture of the mesentery can occur during calving in cows, and this can develop into a problem if a section of the small intestine becomes entrapped in the tear (Garber & Madison, 1991). The cows show obvious signs of abdominal pain, they are depressed, kick at the abdomen, assume a hunch-backed stance, and get up and down frequently. Stitch pain can also be due to ischaemia of the diaphragm. Injury to the liver can cause abdominal pain, as can damage to the spleen. These pains are often aggravated by deep breathing and by movement. Pain arising from the liver may be referred to the right forequarter (Madding & Kennedy, 1971).

Abdominal pain can also be associated with particular forms of poisoning, including poisoning with arsenic, copper, fluoride, lead, mercury, sodium chlorate, thallium rodenticide and zinc phosphide (Humphreys, 1978).

13.4 Diarrhoea

The unpleasant effects of diarrhoea are:

- abdominal pain;
- urge to defecate;
- perianal soreness or discomfort;
- incontinence;
- weakness and lethargy;
- dehydration and thirst.

Diarrhoea may also be associated with fever depending on whether or not there is systemic infection or absorption of toxin.

There are four types of diarrhoea:

(1) osmotic;
(2) malabsorptive;
(3) hypermotile;
(4) secretory.

Each type needs to be treated in a different way when trying to eliminate the underpinning cause. However, in all types it is important to control excessive dehydration otherwise secondary complications set in.

During diarrhoea, the composition of the faeces approaches the composition of the stool that is normally present in the ileum. It contains more water, sodium and bicarbonate than normal faeces. Loss of water in the diarrhoea results in dehydration, but loss of sodium does not usually lead to a sodium deficit, as this is a relatively minor route for sodium excretion relative to sweat and urine. Loss of bicarbonate anions can lead to an *acidosis*, and this could be aggravated by a ketoacidosis if the animal is undernourished or by a lactacidosis if there is poor circulation due to the dehydration. In severe cases of diarrhoea, the dehydration causes a reduction in blood pressure. One of the effects of this is reduced pressure and filtration rate in the kidneys.

Diarrhoea is responsible for a number of farming practices which are themselves stressful. They are dagging, crutching, tail docking and mulesing. In addition, contamination of the skin with diarrhoea can contribute to flystrike and skin sores.

13.5 Gut Injuries

Vomiting is a common feature of stomach or upper-small-intestinal wounds in monogastrics. If this takes the form of persistent retching, there is probably disturbance of vagal activity. If an injury causes the small intestine to burst and contents leak into the abdominal cavity, there is a serious risk of painful peritonitis. The neutral pH, low bacterial count and enzymatic activity of jejunal contents are particularly favourable to bacterial multiplication.

Wild birds are particularly prone to alimentary-tract accidents. These include intussusception, intestinal strangulation, gizzard perforation, phytobezoar and trichobezoar (Reece *et al.*, 1992). Young ratites are prone to proventriculus impaction, especially when reared in isolation from their parents, from whom they can learn appropriate feeding habits.

Injury to the rectum can occur when a veterinarian examines an animal for reproductive purposes or for colic. In general, this form of trauma would be unusual in cattle, but more common in horses. The most common type of rectal tear involves the mucosa and submucosa. Complete perforation of the rectum is unusual, but it can occur when there is contraction around the examiner's hand. Cats show a violent objection to rectal examination.

13.6 Stress and the Gut

Gastrointestinal disorders that can have a psychosomatic origin include:

- nervous anorexia;
- psychogenic vomiting;
- oesophageal and gastric spasms;
- peptic ulcers;
- incontinence;
- chronic diarrhoea;

- spastic colon and mucous colitis;
- chronic constipation.

The effects of acute and chronic stress on gut function are quite different. When animals experience a sudden frightening event, the movement of digesta through the small intestine is reduced, but the rate of movement through the colon increases and this promotes defecation. The fright also inhibits gastric acid secretion and causes mucus release from the colon. All these effects are brought about by corticotrophin releasing hormone (CRH), which is released centrally, acts on the *locus coeruleus*, and is also released from macrophages and leukocytes peripherally. Centrally-released CRH exerts its effects on the gut through vagal efferent pathways, and the effects on colonic motility and rectum evacuation are mediated through serotonin type 3 receptors. Acute stress also increases gastrointestinal permeability through the action of corticosteroids (Meddings & Swain, 2000).

The brain controls colonic activity through routes other than the CRH-vagal axis. Parasympathetic effects are also mediated through pelvic nerves, and sympathetic effects are transmitted along the lumbar colonic, splanchnic and hypogastric nerves. The central regulation of colonic action means that the function of this section of the gut can be a useful indicator of mental disturbances. For example, during post-operative recovery the patient often shows ileus, which is attributable to stress-linked reflexes in the sympathetic nervous pathways.

Chronic stress, such as may be caused by chronic fear, anxiety and anger, increases gastric acid secretion. The acid secretion is thought to be responsible for erosion of the wall of the upper gastrointestinal tract, which can lead to ulcer formation.

13.7 Gastrointestinal Ulcers

In humans, gut ulcer pains are usually described as gnawing or boring pains that come and go. They may be synchronised with hunger pangs, which arise during gastric contractions or from the secretion of acid into the stomach (Carlsson, 1917).

When acid was injected into the stomach of a patient with a stomach ulcer, pain set in after about ten minutes. If the acid was then neutralised with alkali, pain relief came quickly, and was complete by about eight minutes (Bonney & Pickering, 1946). The acid stimulated pain nerve endings in the crater of the ulcer after it had diffused through the layer of mucus. A similar response was evident following a meal. The peak in intragastric acidity and pain awareness is usually reached 1–1.5 hours after food, and duodenal pain usually peaks at two hours after food.

Pain can also occur with non-perforated ulcers. In this situation it may not be the acid which causes the pain. Instead, it is probably due to contractions within the inflamed organ. One sign of this is the link to hunger contractions.

One of the causes of gut ulcers is chronic stress. Three mechanisms have been implicated:

(1)   reduced blood flow to the gut, leading to impaired regeneration once the lesions have developed;
(2)   reduced secretion of mucus, allowing damage to the stomach and duodenal walls by gastric acid;
(3)   inhibition of prostaglandin synthesis by corticosteroids, resulting in impaired repair of gut lesions.

Gut ulcers have been a problem in livestock which received inappropriate feed, or were stressed by restraint, confinement or excessively hard physical training. A survey of 22–24-week-old Dutch veal calves showed that 23% had abomasal ulcers and a further 22% had pyloric scars which were remnants of ulcers (Wiepkema et al., 1987). In pigs, the prevalence of severe gastric ulceration has been as high as 6% (Penny et al., 1972). Gastric ulcers are common in horses undergoing strenuous training, but are usually painless except when they perforate and peritonitis develops. In laboratory rats, gastric ulcers have occurred when there has been stress from a conflict situation or from chronic fear.

Stress-induced gastrointestinal ulceration usually involves the gastroduodenal portion of the tract, but occasionally lesions occur in the distal small intestine and colon. Stress ulcers seem to form where there is localised ischaemia in combination with an irritant which is probably either gastric acid or bile (Gaskill et al., 1984).

Poisoning

14

Suffering associated with poisoning occurs when animals are intentionally poisoned as part of a pest-control programme, or when they inadvertently eat or inhale wartime, environmental or agrochemical toxicants. In some countries poisons are used on a large scale, and the extent of suffering is correspondingly greater. For example, aerial drops of sodium monofluoroacetate (1080) are made in New Zealand native bush as part of the possum and tuberculosis control campaigns, and dichloro-diphenyl-trichloroethane (DDT) poisoning in fish stocks is still a hazard where this insecticide is used to control mosquitoes and malaria. This chapter gives some examples of suffering that can occur with some selected poisons. It does not provide comprehensive coverage of the topic, and the reader is directed to other sources for information on specific toxicants (Radeleff, 1970; Murphy, 1994).

14.1 Wartime Poisons

Agent Orange was used as a chemical defoliant in the Vietnam War between 1962 and 1970. This herbicide contains dioxins as manufacturing impurities, the most important one being 2,3,7,8-tetrachlorodibenzo-p-dioxin (TCDD). The LD_{50} for TCDD in female guinea-pigs is 0.6 µg/kg body weight, and this means it is one of the most toxic synthetic substances that has been made so far. Dioxins are cumulative poisons and their impacts on animals include:

- chloracne and hyperkeratosis;
- suppression of immune responses, especially in young animals;
- teratogenic and foetotoxic effects;
- chick oedema syndrome;
- hepatocellular necrosis and cancer.

When it was realised in the late 1960s that Agent Orange might be teratogenic, it was withdrawn from use by the United States Army. The suffering caused to wildlife in South-east Asia was not evaluated.

During World War II, German scientists synthesised a range of organophosphate compounds that were designed for use as chemical warfare agents. These included **Soman**, which is exceedingly lethal. The signs before death in animals include respiratory distress, tremor, dysmetria, ataxia, excessive salivation and convulsions. Cats that experienced sublethal doses showed visual loss, inability to smell food and motor impairment.

14.2 Environmental Toxicants

DDT was widely used in agriculture during the 1950s, 1960s and 1970s. In addition, in the 1950s the World Health Organisation (WHO) started a global malaria-control programme involving 75 countries where 100 million dwellings were routinely sprayed against mosquitoes, mainly with DDT. By the 1960s it was known that DDT was lethal to fish, that it accumulated in the food chain and damaged the eggs of carnivorous birds such as the peregrine falcon, bald eagle and Californian pelican. Consequently, moves to ban DDT from agricultural use started in the 1970s. Eventually, it was recognised that DDT could be neurotoxic, and it is now suspected that it might be a cause of pancreatic cancer and a form of lymphoma in humans.

From the animal-suffering perspective the main concern is fish. As the concentrations build up in fish there is impaired neural function, which in its early stages appears as irritability or excitability. There is impaired ability to execute learnt responses. It is as if their judgement is affected, because they seem to be prone to making wrong or inappropriate responses. Some species show marked sensitivity to cold and, as intoxication progresses, there are spasms, loss of equilibrium, convulsions and finally death.

Polychlorinated biphenyls (PCBs) are a group of industrial chemicals that have accumulated in the food chain and are thought to be responsible for the immunosuppression that has led to outbreaks of fatal morbillivirus disease in seals and dolphins (Vos *et al.*, 2000). PCBs have also been implicated in immune suppression in young marine birds.

Marine **oil spills** occur in all parts of the industrialised world. In Europe, the Torrey Canyon incident during 1967 was responsible for the death of over 100 000 birds. Cormorants and grebes are especially affected by oil spills. Their feathers become matted with oil and lose their insulating effect. This raises the risk of death from hypothermia in cold environments and hyperthermia in hot conditions. The bird tries to get rid of the oil by preening, and ends up eating some of it. In some respects it is fortunate that oil-contaminated birds lose some of their buoyancy in the water. This forces them to take to the beaches where they can be rescued. When these birds are found, the first step is to flush out their gastrointestinal tracts. Many birds have a ball of feathers, oil and sand in their gizzards from preening, which can cause obstruction. After the gut has been flushed out, the birds can be rehydrated and fed, and then washed and rewarmed.

Shore animals can also be affected by oil spills, especially crabs, shrimps, mussels and barnacles, which succumb to the toxic hydrocarbons they ingest. Naphthalenes accumulate in the liver and brain, and eventually lead to intoxication. There is necrosis of olfactory sensory cells and, in common with most irritants, there is gill hyperplasia. Some petroleum products also coat the gills, preventing gaseous exchange, killing the marine animals by anoxia. Oil spills can also kill algae and plankton on which the fish feed.

Aquatic species are susceptible to poisoning from their own excreta if the water becomes stale. Death is from hypoxaemia or from the direct effects of ammonia in the water. For example, shrimps excrete **ammonia** through their gills as the main end-product of protein metabolism. As ammonia levels in the surrounding water rise, ammonia excretion declines, and re-uptake by the animal occurs. This is measurable from the ammonia concentration in the haemolymph. There is a concomitant decrease in the concentration of respiratory pigment haemocyanin, and this compromises oxygen transport (Chen *et al.*, 1994). During ammonia intoxication, the shrimps switch from carbohydrate to lipid as the main energy source, and this raises the metabolic demand for oxygen (Racotta & Hernández-Herrera, 2000).

There have been occasional reports of mortality in piggeries when the effluent tanks have been emptied. When the effluent was stirred to allow it to be pumped out, there was a large and rapid emission of **hydrogen sulphide** which poisoned the pigs. In humans the usual signs and sensations associated with H_2S inhalation are nausea, sickness, irregular laboured breathing, cold skin, cyanosis and convulsions. Death is from respiratory failure with pulmonary oedema. Exposure to 0.1–0.2% in the atmosphere can be fatal within a few minutes. Chronic exposure to lower concentrations leads to rhinitis, bronchitis, photophobia and headache.

In Japan there is a human disease known as *itai-itai*. The direct translation is 'painful-painful'. It is caused by chronic kidney damage plus painful bone and joint diseases due to eating **cadmium**-contaminated fish taken from rivers near smelting plants. The signs of cadmium poisoning in fish themselves include blindness and bone decalcification.

Ivermectin is a widely used anthelmintic, insecticide and acaricide in livestock. However, it is poisonous to earthworms and dung beetles when it washes onto soil, and to shrimps when used for controlling sea-lice in salmon farms.

14.3 Vertebrate Pesticides

The ideal pesticide is an anaesthetic that puts the animal into an irreversible sleep. However, the use of all anaesthetics is controlled by medical and veterinary practitioners, and none is available for routine use as a pesticide. The nearest compound to an anaesthetic that is used in pest control is the stupefacient **α-chloralose**. It has a bitter taste and so its main use is in birds, which, in general, are less choosy about food flavours. Its weakness is that it sometimes makes a bird drowsy so that it stops eating before it has taken a lethal dose. Death is either from anaesthetic-induced apnoea or from hypothermia, depending on circumstances.

Over the years, **strychnine** has been the most widely-used chemical pesticide. It was discovered in 1817, and at various times it has been the toxicant of choice for crows, moles, wallabies, bandicoots, flying foxes, parrots, rabbits, dingoes, wild dogs, kangaroo rats and rodents, and it is still used for controlling mouse plagues in Australia and gophers and voles in North America. There are anecdotal cases of domestic dogs finding and dying from strychnine-injected eggs or gopher bait.

Strychnine inhibits glycine-mediated neurotransmission in the spinal cord and medulla, and this interferes with post-synaptic inhibition at these sites. The signs of strychnine poisoning are as follows: within ten minutes to two hours of eating the poison, the animal becomes apprehensive, nervous, tense and stiff. Seizures occur, often in response to noise, light or touch, and they terminate with extensor rigidity in a 'sawhorse' posture (Murphy, 1994). Death is from respiratory failure.

One of the most potent pesticides in use today is **1080** (sodium monofluoroacetate). It has been used for controlling kangaroos, wallabies, dingoes, feral pigs and rabbits. It is now widely used in New Zealand for controlling the Australian brushtail possum (*Trichosurus vulpecula*) and in Australia against red fox. In other countries it is considered too toxic to be used except under confined conditions, for example against ship rats. 1080 is a tricarboxylic acid (TCA) cycle blocker, affecting brain and heart function. The signs of poisoning in humans include nausea and apprehension, muscle twitching, tremors, cardiac irregularities, convulsions, coma and then death. In Australia, wild pigs (*Sus scrofa*) often have easy access to 1080 fox baits, and death follows within two hours to five days. In the intervening period there is frequent vomiting (O'Brien, 1988).

Anticoagulants are the most widely used poisons for controlling rodents. The favoured anticoagulant presently is brodifacoum, which was originally developed to combat warfarin-resistant rodents, but has subsequently been used against many agricultural and forest pests throughout the world. It competitively inhibits recycling of vitamin K, leading to depletion of vitamin K-dependent clotting factors. The impaired clotting is accompanied by weakening of blood-vessel walls. Death is from spontaneous haemorrhaging or bleeding. Sites that are prone to bleeding are those that normally move a lot, such as the lungs, heart, intestines and joints.

There are two ways in which anticoagulants cause suffering: first, they cause a slow death with a relatively long sickness period. In possums, the signs of illness last for 6–13 days before death at about 21 days (Littin *et al.*, 2002). These signs include abnormal breathing, diarrhoea, shivering and trembling, external bleeding and spasms. Second, some haemorrhages can be painful, causing swelling within confined spaces in tissues (compartment syndrome effect). If haemorrhaging is chronic but not lethal, jaundice may set in due to absorption and breakdown of blood pigments.

Cholecalciferol causes sickness and death from hypercalcaemia. Hypercalcaemia is associated with nausea, occasional vomiting, anorexia, depression, thirst, constipation, weakness, dehydration, mental disturbances and confusion. It is a particularly unpleasant form of protracted malaise. The animals fail to groom themselves, and the abdominal wall is tense, possibly in association with gastric ulcers. Death may follow seizures and is often due to kidney failure through calcium accumulation. In the words of a medical endocrinologist who induced hypercalcaemia in himself as part of a research study 'I have never felt so ill in all my life'.

Phosphorus is used as a pesticide for controlling cockroaches, rats and possums, and it is one of the more common agents used for suicide amongst young women in the Middle East (Fahim *et al.*, 1990). It has been used for bird species, such as ravens at lambing time. Affected animals usually show restlessness before a period of subdued activity, disorientation and coma prior to death. Animals that fail to eat a lethal dose, and animals that lose part of a dose from vomiting, can die at a later stage from liver failure. Normally, when a lethal dose is consumed, death is from myocardial infarction (Pietras *et al.*, 1968), and in possums the time to death is about 25 hours. When the stomach is opened post-mortem, phosphoric acid fumes are liberated as the contents are exposed to air.

One of the newer rodenticides is **bromethalin**. It is an oxidative phosphorylation uncoupler and starts to have effects within ten hours. There are ataxia, vomiting, tremors, hyperexcitability, vocalisation and seizures before death occurs after a period of coma that can last for days.

Various approaches have been used to inflict death by constipation. In former times plaster of Paris was mixed with flour and sugar in a formulation that was used for controlling sparrows. More recently, a cellulose derivative was marketed as a compound for blocking up the intestines of rats.

Chloropicrin is used as a fumigant with diesel fumes in rabbit and fox holes. It is an intensely irritating vapour and is an inhumane control method. **Carbon monoxide** is used against foxes in their dens and is to be preferred. The pesticides which probably cause the least suffering in terms of sickness and distress before death are α-chloralose, potassium cyanide and carbon monoxide (Mason & Littin, 2003).

Rotenone (derris powder) is used for poisoning unwanted fish. Between 1988 and 2000, 110 tonnes were used in North America for this purpose, and for quantifying fish populations. Its species-specificity in fish has allowed the retention of game species, whilst unwanted species, such as catfish, have been controlled. It is recognised as an environmental carcinogen for mammals, causing mammary tumours at high concentrations, and has become a controversial pesticide because of the ways in which it has been used. In animals that survive rotenone poisoning, there can be signs similar to Parkinson's disease due to destruction of dopaminergic neurones in the *substantia nigra* of the brain. This is also a potential risk with using cyanide as a pesticide.

Respiratory System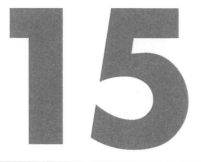

This chapter considers the forms of suffering connected with the respiratory system. The situations that cause suffering include:

- asphyxiation and choking;
- breathlessness;
- drowning;
- carbon dioxide inhalation;
- irritation of the respiratory tract.

The physical mechanisms that cause respiratory distress are linked either to an inability to breathe, or to irritation of the respiratory tract. The chemical mechanisms that cause respiratory distress are exposure either to excessive amounts of carbon dioxide or to chemical irritants. Normally animals protect themselves from inhaling physical and chemical contaminants through the following:

- closure of the glottis followed by swallowing;
- adhesion of inhaled particles to the mucus layer in the respiratory tract and coughing them up;
- bronchosecretion and ciliary propulsion of the mucus layer to the mouth;
- breath-holding and bronchoconstriction, which help limit the intake and absorption of smoke or gases.

These mechanisms sometimes lose coordination, and they can be compromised by injury or infection.

This chapter also considers the signs of discomfort or suffering that are expressed in an animal's breathing behaviour. In humans the breathing pattern is a way of expressing one's emotions. It can be voluntary or involuntary. For example, a person can display:

- a gasp of surprise;
- a sigh of sadness;

- exhalation from frustration;
- altered breathing during laughing and crying;
- hyperventilation during anxiety, panic or fear.

Over-breathing and chronic hyperventilation during anxiety can lower the blood CO_2 tension. A low p_aCO_2 produces arterial vasoconstriction and cerebral hypoxaemia, which can lead to headaches. This syndrome is sometimes associated with aerophagia resulting in belching air, dry mouth and sleep disturbances.

Animals also express emotions through their breathing pattern, but not necessarily in the same manner as humans. For example, dogs can show anticipatory hypoventilation (Anderson, 1994). Grunting can be a sign of abdominal pain in cattle, and panting is an obvious sign of either heat stress or exertion. They may not be purposeful expressions in communication, but they can be useful signs of an animal's predicament.

15.1 Asphyxia

During asphyxia the subject is unable to breathe. This occurs during:

- exposure to muscle relaxants;
- bloat;
- respiratory disease;
- smothering;
- chest compression;
- strangulation;
- atmospheric decompression.

Breathing movements are controlled voluntarily by the cortex of the brain, and involuntarily by the pons and medulla. The main motor nerves that activate inspiratory movement are in the phrenic nerve, which emerges from the spinal cord at C3–C5 in the neck. Injury to the spinal cord above these segments leads to death from asphyxiation (inability to breathe). The main motor nerves which control expiratory movements are in the external intercostal nerves which join the spinal cord in the thoracic region. When cattle are slaughtered without stunning by the puntilla method, the spinal cord is severed at C1. If they are not bled immediately, the animals die from asphyxia (Gregory, 1998a).

The activity of the respiratory centre in the medulla, which controls involuntary breathing is modified by neurones projecting from the pons and the vagus nerves. When the pons is damaged, respiration becomes slower and tidal volume greater. The vagus nerves relay signals from mechanoreceptors in the lungs which inhibit respiration. Damage to the vagus nerves results in prolonged inspiration.

Succinylcholine is used in some parts of the world as a way of immobilising and euthanasing free-ranging animals. It is used in northern Russia for killing seals, in Africa for capturing wild game for translocation, veterinary care or other purposes and in various countries for restraining crocodiles and alligators. This drug is principally a smooth-muscle relaxant, but at high doses it is a neuromuscular blocker, and it is the paralysing effect that is used when darting an animal. Measurement of the plasma catecholamine and cortisol responses to succinylcholine in Cape buffalo (*Syncerus caffer*) has shown that it is a highly stressful restraining method, and respiratory compromise could be contributing to the distress. For this reason, its use is disallowed in some countries.

Bloat is another cause of asphyxia which can be very unpleasant for the animal. When a cow develops bloat there is a rise in pressure inside its abdomen. This has two effects: first, the diaphragm is displaced towards the thorax. This reduces the intrathoracic space, the lungs are compressed and inspiratory volume is reduced. The animal becomes breathless because physical breathing movements are impaired, and because it develops hypercapnia. Second, if intra-abdominal pressure rises out of control, the vena cava is compressed and the flow of blood back to the heart is reduced. In severe cases this reduces cardiac output and the animal faints because of an inadequate supply of blood to the brain. The behavioural signs during bloat indicate severe discomfort and distress (Boda *et al.*, 1956). Similarly, ascites in broilers can limit breathing and cause a sense of breathlessness especially when the birds take exercise through wing flapping.

Death by strangulation is not common in either humans or animals, but it does occur. In humans, **strangulation** is often accompanied by petechiae, cyanosis, congestion and oedema above the level of neck compression. Petechiae are not proof of death from asphyxiation. They are also seen in many non-asphyxial deaths, and they indicate death from any cause where there has been increased venous pressure from terminal right heart failure. If there is strenuous unsuccessful effort to inhale, the barrier between the alveoli and capillaries in the lungs can be ruptured and there will be frothy blood in the airways.

If asphyxia lasts for longer than ten minutes before a subject dies, there is usually irreversible damage to the brain. This applies to subjects with a normal body temperature, but people have survived without breathing for over an hour if the temperature is reduced (Gooden, 1992). Young animals are less susceptible to brain damage from asphyxia and anoxia than adults. In addition, the respiratory centre in the medulla continues to function for longer in neonates following arrest of blood flow to the brain (Kabat, 1940).

15.2 Breathlessness

Breathlessness can be caused by asphyxia or hypercapnia. It is a particularly unpleasant form of suffering. It is incapacitating and breathing requires continuous effort. The subject comes to a standstill and struggles for breath from a sense of 'air hunger'. In extreme situations in humans there can be a sense of imminent death or a fear of death, and panic may set in.

Breathlessness during **breath-holding** and **smothering** is thought to be due to muscle spasms and contractions in the chest and abdomen. This explanation developed from work in conscious volunteers who were paralysed with curare and ventilated artificially by machine. When ventilation was stopped it was found that they could tolerate apnoea for four or more minutes with none of the discomfort that normally accompanies breath-holding (Campbell *et al.*, 1967). In non-curarised subjects, breath-holding was associated with spasms in the abdominal muscles, and it was tolerated for a minute or less before the sense of breathlessness became so strong that they were obliged to breathe normally.

The contractions during breath-holding or smothering occur as waves of negative pressure, or attempts to inhale. The drive for these contractions is greatly reduced if the subject can perform the physical motions of breathing, even when there is no effect on oxygen or carbon dioxide tensions in the bloodstream. In other words, it is the physical contractions that help relieve the sense of breathlessness. The involuntary inspiratory contractions can also be inhibited if cold air is blown through the nose and pharynx during breath-holding (McBride & Whitelaw, 1981).

To summarise, the sense of breathlessness from breath-holding or being unable to breathe is highly dependent on muscle contractions in the chest, and the urge to breathe can be dulled either by complete muscle paralysis, by performing the physical actions of breathing or by stimulation of airway receptors in the upper respiratory tract.

Fibrosis of the lungs from disease can cause breathlessness. Fibrosis occurs during the healing process following an infection (e.g. pneumonia), and, in extreme situations, the lung is converted into a more-or-less solid mass of fibrous tissue. Providing better ventilation for a housed animal that has dyspnoea due to lung disease will help it cope with any shortage of oxygen, and it will flush away exhaled pathogens, but it may not completely relieve the sense of breathlessness if breathing movements are constrained.

We have little understanding of what causes the corresponding sense of breathlessness and suffocation in a fish, if in fact these sensations do exist. Do fish experience something similar when they are out of water and unable to irrigate their gills? Does compression of the operculum and gills during trawl fishing cause a sense of suffocation? Some species of reptile can hold their breath for very long periods and presumably they are less prone to developing breathlessness. The iguana (*Iguana iguana*) can breath-hold for up to $4\frac{1}{2}$ hours, and turtles (*Pseudemys* species) have survived up to 27 hours without breathing.

In humans, the initial response to immersion in cold water is a reflex inspiratory gasp. It seems to 'take the breath away'. This is not the same thing as breathlessness.

Breathing is not inhibited and hypercapnia does not develop. The reflex is quickly followed by hyperventilation, tachycardia, peripheral vasoconstriction and a rise in blood pressure.

15.3 Carbon Dioxide Inhalation

Carbon dioxide is the other potent stimulus of breathlessness. A small rise in blood CO_2 tension leads to an increase in involuntary ventilation. Chemoreceptors in the medulla and in the carotid and aortic bodies, are activated by CO_2, and receptors in the carotid and aortic bodies are activated if there is at the same time a reduction in p_aO_2. Hypercapnia can occur either from breathing in carbon dioxide, from excessive metabolism in tissues which liberate CO_2 into the bloodstream or from failure to extract CO_2 from the blood and exhale it. Normally, hypercapnia will stimulate ventilation. If, however, the blood pCO_2 rises too high, CO_2 intoxication occurs, the nervous system is suppressed (including the medulla) and unconsciousness sets in. Exposure to CO_2 has been shown to be aversive (Leach et al., 2002).

Carbon dioxide is used for killing animals in the following situations:

- stunning pigs;
- stunning chickens;
- killing farmed salmon;
- killing farmed fur-bearing species;
- euthanasia of unwanted day-old chicks;
- euthanasia of unwanted cats and puppies;
- killing small laboratory animals such as mice and rats.

The time to loss of consciousness depends on how the carbon dioxide is administered. If the animal is lowered into a chamber that is pre-filled with CO_2, loss of consciousness is quicker than placing the animal in the chamber before the gas (Glen & Scott, 1973).

Some animals show hyperactivity before they collapse. In cats this takes the form of hyperventilation, licking, sneezing, moving about the cage and trying to reach its highest point. There may also be some yowling. When there is no excitement, the cats sway from side to side for about 20 seconds before falling onto their sides.

When pigs inhale an atmosphere containing more than 30% CO_2 they experience respiratory distress (Raj & Gregory, 1996). However, at high concentrations (90% CO_2 or more), the onset of unconsciousness is rapid, and the duration of breathlessness is correspondingly short. In practice, high concentrations are used in abattoirs, to allow a fast line speed.

15.4 Drowning

The way that an animal or human drowns has a strong bearing on whether or not there is suffering. People who have been rescued from death by drowning often say that before losing consciousness they experienced no suffering. When there was no inhalation of water, one person said that he saw 'panoramic views of part of my life' before losing consciousness, and others report that they had pleasant dreams during recovery. Whereas, when water has been inhaled, the tales are of fear and pain in the middle of the chest. It should be noted that, as with any form of hypoxia, there will be some retrograde amnesia, in which case the recollections may be incomplete.

During drowning, there is an initial resistance to inhaling water, and a sense of breathlessness and suffocation. If water is inhaled, the irritation of the upper respiratory tract provokes reflex coughing during which more water is inhaled. Shortage of oxygen leads to loss of neural function, and the glottis muscles relax allowing more water to enter the lungs. In some instances, the subject either resists inhaling water, or, with the first gasp of water there is a laryngospasm and death results from asphyxia without appreciable intake of water into the lungs.

If water is inhaled, it can irritate the alveoli, and this sets up a localised vaso-constriction and hypoxia. This in turn results in accumulation of fluid in the inter-stitial space (pulmonary oedema), and some fluid may leak into the alveolar air spaces adding to the burden. The irritating effect of the inhaled water is a key component in the reactions, and the degree of irritation is influenced by the fluid's tonicity, temperature and the presence of contaminants (Yagil et al., 1983). Chlorinated fresh water has a stronger irritant action than fresh water alone, and this is no doubt relevant when nocturnal animals fall into outdoor swimming pools. Fresh water is more likely than sea water to lead to loss of surfactant lining the alveoli, and when this happens there will be areas of collapse in the lungs.

Drowning occurs during:

- misadventure;
- destruction of unwanted animals;
- submersion trapping of beaver and muskrat;
- inhalation of specific poisonous gases which cause secretion of fluid by the lungs;
- inhalation of blood following injury;
- inhalation of vomit.

Drowning from misadventure is a common problem during the wet season in buffalo calves in east and south-east Asia. Broiler chicks may drown if their drinking water is provided in an open trough, especially if there is competition at the trough because the water is available only intermittently (Abdelsamie & Yadiwilo, 1981). Regurgitation and inhalation of stomach contents can be a problem in non-ruminants, and inhalation of rumen contents sometimes occurs in cows with milk fever, especially when the cow is lying with its head downhill. It does not normally lead to drowning, but can lead to pneumonia, as can inhaling drenching fluid.

Water traps have been, and still are, used for catching mice, and they are occasionally used for rats. **Submersion traps** are used for catching beaver in Canada and muskrat in the Netherlands. With submersion traps, the intention is to kill the animals by drowning. A weighted leg-hold trap is set alongside a waterway. When an animal is caught in the trap it usually dives with the trap into the water, and the weight prevents the animal from rising to the surface to breathe. The trap has to be set alongside deep water to produce death by drowning, otherwise the tethered animal stays alive by swimming at the surface.

Beaver show a forced diving response during submersion, in which heart rate drops and blood is directed to the brain. This allows them to withstand submersion for up to five minutes (Clausen & Ersland, 1970/71). When held under water by a submersible trap the time to an isoelectric EEG is about nine minutes. They usually die without water entering their lungs. Instead they succumb to submersion asphyxia plus self-intoxication with CO_2 (Gilbert & Gofton, 1982). About 50% of muskrats are thought to die from wet drowning. In other words, their lungs contain water. The time to an isoelectric EEG in muskrats is about four minutes. In both species, physical struggling ceases about one minute before electrocerebral silence.

The length of survival during submersion depends on whether the subject manages to maintain an effective diving response. The purpose of the diving response is to conserve oxygen for the brain and heart during the dive. The **dive reflex** consists of bradycardia with simultaneous breath-holding, and is stimulated by sensory receptors that supply signals to the trigeminal nerves. It occurs during forced submersion in water, and is less pronounced during voluntary immersion.

Animals that have a short breath-hold duration are likely to be more prone to death from drowning. Excitement and physical exertion will reduce survival, and sudden immersion in cold water, as distinct from warm water, reduces breath-holding duration. If the animal is hypothermic it has a reduced metabolic rate, and this can provide some protection from hypoxia and a longer survival.

In about 25% of human cases of near-drowning, the subject dies within the following four days (Rivers *et al.*, 1970). There are two common causes of these delayed deaths: in some subjects there is an encephalopathy secondary to brain hypoxia and oedema; in others, water that was in the lungs leaves behind particulate matter, such as diatoms, which set up an inflammatory response. There is exudation of serous fluid into the alveoli which causes obstruction to breathing and death occurs from **secondary drowning** if a significant proportion of the alveolar air space is lost. This is an unpleasant way to die. There is rapid shallow breathing due to the inability to inflate the lungs, burning sensations in the chest, pleuritic pain, production of a frothy pink sputum and a hoarse rasping cough.

The inflammatory response may be associated with pyrexia, and body temperature should be closely monitored for early signs of this condition.

Drowning in fresh water is different physiologically from drowning in sea water. Fresh water is hypotonic so it is absorbed by the lungs and dilutes the plasma causing intravascular haemolysis. Sea water is hypertonic and draws fluid from the lungs and circulation resulting in internal dehydration. Diarrhoea from irritation of the alimentary tract can develop during recovery and this may amplify the dehydration.

15.5 Pulmonary Oedema

Pulmonary oedema is a common terminal stage in many animal diseases. In severe cases there is dyspnoea which is obvious from heaving breathing through the mouth. The animal may stand with its front legs spread apart, head hung low and nostrils flared. In humans, there is restlessness, weakness, a dry non-productive cough and there may be chest pain. Respiration becomes difficult, laboured and it is usually faster. Gurgling sounds may be heard and there may be a frothy sputum.

Pulmonary oedema is usually caused by raised permeability of the lung capillaries leading to leakage of fluid into the interstitial tissue. It can be due to increased calibre of the pulmonary capillaries because of high capillary pressure, hypoxia, opening of channels between endothelial cells in the capillary wall (e.g. through the action of histamine, serotonin or corticosteroids), rupture of the capillary wall, direct effects of nerve stimulation or changes in the mucoprotein layer lining the alveoli.

Pulmonary oedema can occur in cases of:

- head injury or cerebral disease;
- arterial hypertension;
- mitral stenosis;
- coronary heart disease;
- pulmonary heart disease;
- myocarditis;
- high altitude;
- shock;
- allergy or infections;
- inhalation of toxic gases;
- drowning.

Two mechanisms contribute to pulmonary oedema following head or spinal injury: first, there is massive sympathetic stimulation which causes peripheral vasoconstriction and elevation of blood pressure throughout the pulmonary circulation. In other words, there is a prompt shifting of blood from the systemic to the pulmonary circulation. Second, the resulting vascular congestion in the lungs causes overloading of the left ventricle. When peripheral vasoconstriction and left ventricle overloading occur together, there is back pressure acting against the pulmonary capillary bed, and this forces fluid into the interstitial space of the lungs (Luisada, 1967). This type of oedema is known as **neurogenic pulmonary oedema**.

In other forms of pulmonary oedema there can be collapse of the peripheral circulation instead of an active vasoconstriction. This happens when sudden trauma causes shock through the so-called **pulmonary defensive reflex** (Irwin *et al.*, 1999). The mechanical injury results in fluid leaking from lung capillaries into the interstitial space, where it exerts pressure on C-fibre nerve endings, which activate vagal pathways that ascend to the solitary tract nucleus and forebrain. This provokes reflex reductions in α- and β-adrenergic activity in the sympathetic nervous system innervating capillaries in muscle and skin, and increased cholinergic activity to the heart. The bradycardia, in combination with suppressed sympathetic responses, results in cardiogenic shock, which can set in immediately after the injury. The initial leakiness of the capillary bed is due to disruption and separation of adjacent endothelial cells within the capillary walls. When large amounts of fluid leak from the capillaries, some fluid invades the air spaces in the alveoli. This limits breathing, and in advanced states results in breathlessness followed by drowning in one's own serum.

Oversecretion of adrenaline can exacerbate pulmonary oedema (Cheng, 1975). At high levels, adrenaline causes pulmonary hypertension with impaired clearance of blood by the venous drainage. As with most cases of pulmonary congestion, where there is overstretching of capillaries, there is a risk of fluid escaping into the interstitial space and compromising normal lung movement. Animals that experience this problem sometimes develop a pinkish froth in their lungs. This could be due either to capillary damage or to elevated hydrostatic pressure which forces red blood cells through gaps in the capillary wall.

The inhalation of toxic gases, such as phosgene, and severe burns to the lung, also cause prompt endothelial cell separation and oedema. In former times, α-naphthylthiourea (ANTU) was used as a rat poison, and its intended action was to increase the permeability of lung venules and capillaries causing death by drowning. Normally, the animal protects itself from this type of drowning by a combination of coughing up the fluid, forced evaporation during breathing and reabsorption of the fluid. In the case of ANTU poisoning, the rate of removal cannot compete with the continuous outpouring from the capillaries.

15.6 Hypoxia

Oxygen deficiency is not a painful experience, except in rare angina states. Low O_2 is less potent than high CO_2 as a respiratory stimulant, and the likelihood of breathlessness during hypoxia is relatively low. Instead, the symptoms of progressive hypoxia in humans are usually a dulling of intellect and judgement without the subject being aware of what is happening. In addition, the power of memory is affected, so the subject may not recall anything afterwards. In some individuals, there are uncontrolled emotional outbursts (ranging from laughter to tears), and the subject becomes irrational, in a manner similar to excessive alcohol consumption (Ernsting, 1965). This has two implications: first, hypoxia is a potentially humane method of euthanasia if it induces comparable effects in animals; second, in unintended exposure to hypoxia, there is a serious danger that the subject will fail to notice the problem before it is too late to react. Failing consciousness may be the first indication that the oxygen supply is inadequate.

Hypoxia can occur during the inhalation of nitrogen or other inert gases. It can also occur during underwater diving, high-altitude oxygen deficit and sudden decompression. If the hypoxia is gradual there is likely to be a longer warning period prior to the loss of consciousness, and so the subject will be able to do something about it. In that situation the sensations are broader, and some people experience dyspnoea and apprehension (Table 15.1).

When consciousness is lost, anoxic convulsions set in. These seizures are violent, and they occur because cortical activity in the brain is suppressed before that in the brainstem. Activity in the reticular formation would normally cause involuntary rigidity and convulsive activity in the body, if it were not for the fact that it is suppressed by signals descending from the cortex. Removal of activity in the cortex of the brain by hypoxia allows the convulsive signals to predominate, and

Table 15.1 Prevalence of different sensations during hypoxia in humans.

Sensation	% of subjects
Visual disturbance	64
Dizziness	57
Light headaches	49
Inability to think clearly	42
Tingling	37
Muscle incoordination	37
Numbness	21
Unsteadiness	20
Apprehension	19
Euphoria	19
Fatigue	15
Sweating	15
Dyspnoea	14
Sleepiness	13

the body starts convulsing. This occurs at a time when cortical activity has disappeared, and so the convulsions are not associated with consciousness. Owing to their severity, the convulsions are ugly to watch.

Oxygen depletion is a problem for fish living in freshwater streams and lakes which have been polluted with organic effluents. A fish can only assess the oxygen content of water *after* its body has become hypoxic (Erichsen Jones, 1952). Once this happens, it will show one of two responses. It may rise to the surface to breathe air, which can be recognised from a gulping or coughing-like action. This can be a useful sign of hypoxia, but needs to be distinguished from air breaths taken to improve buoyancy. Alternatively, it will increase the amplitude and frequency of its respiratory movements and, if this does not suffice, it will make random movements which develop into violent struggling. If the fish manages to escape to well-oxygenated water, the hyperactivity stops abruptly. The onset of this escape behaviour is very rapid if water temperature is high.

The air-breathing vertebrate with the highest known tolerance for hypoxia is the painted turtle, *Chrysemys picta*. It can survive hypoxia at 3°C for up to five months. It has two adaptations: first, it can decrease energy metabolism to about 10% of normal rate when it becomes hypoxic. However, in doing this it switches to anaerobic glycolysis generating lactic acid instead of carbon dioxide, and this poses a threat from systemic acidosis. The second adaptation is protection against that acidosis by the buffering action of its shell. Carbonates are released from bone and shell to buffer systemic lactic acid, and lactate moves into shell and bone where it is buffered and stored (Jackson, 2000).

15.7 Altitude Sickness

In humans, the feelings experienced during altitude sickness are headache, nausea, irritability, fatigue, insomnia, breathlessness and vomiting. These signs develop 8–24 hours after being exposed to high altitude, and last four to eight days. The hypoxia causes dilatation of blood capillaries and this can lead to an increase in pressure within the brain. Fluid migrates from the capillaries into brain tissue causing cerebral oedema, which results in feelings of sickness.

Angiotensin converting enzyme (ACE) serves an important role in adaptation to high altitude. This enzyme is present in lung capillary endothelial cells and acts on two components present in the bloodstream: it converts angiotensin I to angiotensin II and it degrades bradykinin. Angiotensin II is a vasopressor peptide, and bradykinin increases capillary permeability and so provokes oedema. When an animal is introduced to a high altitude or is subjected to some other hypoxic situation, such as chronic exercise, ACE is inhibited by the oxygen deficit. This allows systemic vascular resistance to fall, through the reduction in angiotensin II, and, along with changes in activity of the sympathetic nervous system, blood flow is redistributed away from the viscera towards the brain, heart and muscles. This response is beneficial, but, if bradykinin increases out of control, it can precipitate pulmonary oedema. The risk of this is especially high if there is respiratory acidosis superimposed on the hypoxia, and the animal is then in extreme danger of respiratory failure (O'Brodovich *et al.*, 1981).

Altitude sickness is not common in animals. There is a **congestive heart failure** condition called 'high mountain disease' or 'brisket disease' which occurs in a small proportion of cattle ranging above 2200 metres. The animals appear depressed and develop subcutaneous oedema, especially in the brisket region, which progresses to ascites. There are signs of dyspnoea, cyanosis and reluctance to move, and they may die if there is forced exertion (Alexander & Jensen, 1959).

15.8 Decompression

Decompression has been tested for use as a method of euthanasia, but it is not in general use. It is not possible to condone or castigate this method without considering the time–pressure profiles for the respective species (Latner, 1942). Some authorities who have used it in primates, claimed that it appeared to be relatively humane, whereas some of the side-effects that will be described here suggest otherwise.

Depending on the circumstances, death can be from anoxia, atelectasis or congestion of the air spaces with fluid, and the exact cause of death is important from the humanitarian perspective. The easiest way to induce decompression is to puncture a diaphragm between an evacuated chamber and another chamber holding the animal. The potential disadvantages with this method are:

- inner ear damage, which can be painful: the inner ear system has fluid-filled cavities within rigid bone and the sudden negative pressure causes bubble formation within this fluid, capillary rupture and haemorrhage;
- reflex emesis;
- pain can occur in animals with blocked sinuses from an earlier infection;
- gas expansion in the intestinal tract is liable to cause voiding and abdominal pain at pressures with an altitude equivalent of 12 200 m;
- breathlessness in animals that are not rendered immediately unconscious – animals that die promptly from explosive decompression may have collapsed lungs and ruptured alveoli with flooding of the air spaces with blood.

Depending on the extent of the pressure drop, body water loses its gases and it may vaporise. In amphibians the body can swell considerably due to expansion effects of water vaporisation, and the water vapour may be vented through the mouth and cloaca (Hornberger, 1950). When explosive decompression has been tested in rats, they were killed within 40 seconds of reducing the pressure to 21 mm Hg (altitude equivalent of 24 300 m) (Hall & Corey, 1950). It is worth noting that retrospective reports in humans included sensations of a painful blow in the chest, difficulty in inhaling and soreness in the trachea and large bronchi. Recovery was associated with a sense of being drunk, nausea and cold sweating followed by chest pains.

15.9 Collapse of the Lung and Pneumothorax

In the normal lung the alveolar tissue is coated with a surfactant, which prevents the alveolar walls from collapsing into the air spaces. In some lung diseases there is increased permeability of the alveolar–capillary barrier and proteins leak from the circulation into the alveolar air space where they inhibit surfactant function. Inflammatory mediators can also inhibit surfactants. When loss of the surfactant permits collapse of a lung region, acute respiratory distress syndrome may develop.

Lung collapse (atelectasis) in terrestrial animals also occurs when there is failure of lung inflation after birth and as a sequel to pneumothorax. Failure of lung inflation in the newborn is not likely to be associated with much, if any, suffering, as it is thought that the animal has to breathe in order to initiate consciousness following birth (Mellor & Gregory, 2003). In other situations, pneumothorax and atelectasis are associated with breathlessness and chest pains. The chest pains are sharp at onset, and develop into a steady ache.

Fish have their own form of respiratory system collapse. Normally the gills are perfused with oxygenated water, but, when a fish is removed from water, its lamellae collapse and adjacent filaments adhere to one another. This reduces the surface area for gas exchange and the fish goes into oxygen deficit. This situation occurs in catch-and-release angling, and the aim should be to minimise the period that the fish is held out of water.

15.10 Asthma and Allergies

Asthmatic attacks can be frightening to the point of causing panic. In severe attacks there is an intense urge to escape, along with feelings of chest pain, dyspnoea, choking or smothering, rapid heartbeat, sweating, trembling or shaking, nausea and numbness (Carr, 1999). Milder forms of asthma include wheezing, shortness of breath, chest tightness, recurrent cough, congestion and hyperventilation.

In asthma, exposure to a specific allergen causes histamine release from mast cells lining the respiratory tract. The histamine stimulates reflex bronchoconstriction through activation of the irritant-receptor–vagus nerve pathway. When an acute inflammatory response develops, other histamine-containing cells, such as polymorphonuclear eosinophils, are recruited, more histamine is released and the responses can get out of control.

A number of species have been used in experimental models of asthma, including mice, rats, guinea-pigs, ferrets, hamsters, rabbits, dogs, sheep, pigs, horses and primates. For example, in dogs, asthmatic attacks have been produced experimentally using aerosols of the nematodes *Toxocara canis, Ascaris suis* or grass pollen. One of the naturally-occurring asthmatic conditions is fog fever in cattle. This can occur when they gorge on lush pasture that is rich in nitrogen. Tryptophan in the grass is converted to 3-methyl indole in the rumen, which is then absorbed and transported to the lungs where it causes an allergic response. There is respiratory distress and the animals have particular trouble in exhaling.

15.11 Ammonia

Ammonia production is a problem in poorly-ventilated sheds where animals are kept on damp litter. The amount of ammonia that is produced in livestock buildings is substantial. Of the nitrogen eaten by sows, 20–23% is emitted as ammonia (Groenestein *et al.*, 2001). There has been a lot of discussion about the acceptable upper limit for the atmospheric ammonia concentration in livestock buildings. The threshold limit value (TLV) is the concentration which a man can tolerate for eight hours per day for five days a week without detrimental effects. The recognised TLV for ammonia in the United States is 25 ppm. The lower limit which is unpleasant for animals has not been clearly established, but is often set at 20 or 25 ppm. Jones *et al.* (1996) established that the concentration which is aversive to growing pigs is somewhere between 10 and 20 ppm. At concentrations higher than this, ammonia causes hyperplasia of tracheal epithelium, the cilia lining the tract progressively disappear, a mucilaginous exudate is formed and ultimately there is an inflammatory response. The respiratory tract may be sensitive to concentrations lower than this – 3 ppm can cause ciliostasis in rat trachea.

15.12 Signs of Respiratory Distress

The signs or symptoms of respiratory distress include:

- coughing;
- sneezing;
- wheezing;
- laboured breathing;
- chest pain.

When considering the physical agents that cause respiratory distress, it is best to start with the receptors that are present along the walls of the airways. The main receptors in the respiratory system are:

- stretch receptors in airway smooth muscle;
- irritant stretch receptors, which respond to chemical irritants and inhaled dust;
- C-fibre receptors which respond to lung oedema, congestion and pneumonia. They act as mechanoreceptors, are activated during exertion and mediate the sense of breathlessness that can occur during pulmonary oedema. Some of the C-fibres contain Substance P, neurokinins and CGRP and are involved in bronchoconstriction.

There are two types of irritant receptor in the lining of the respiratory tract, namely those of the upper and lower respiratory tracts. The large airways of the upper respiratory tract have cough receptors which are sensitive to dust, inflammation, mucus and foreign bodies. When irritated, these receptors initiate coughing through a vagal–medullary pathway. The lower respiratory tract has few cough receptors, and so coughing is a sign of upper, rather than lower, respiratory tract infection or irritation. As a result, pneumonia is not usually associated with coughing. The lower respiratory tract has irritant receptors which are activated by dust, histamine, anaphylaxis, pulmonary embolism and pneumothorax, but they stimulate reflex hyperpnoea instead of coughing. These receptors become sensitised during chronic suppurative lung infection or inhalation of ammonia.

The involvement of the central nervous system in coughing has two implications:

(1) coughing can be psychogenic – e.g. caused by anxiety or a habit disorder;
(2) centrally-acting drugs (antitussives) can be used to control coughing.

There are different types of coughing, and these can be helpful in understanding the cause of the irritation:

- persistent coughing during the day that disappears during sleep or following distraction suggests psychogenic origin;
- coughing associated with eating could suggest a swallowing problem, gastro-oesophageal reflux, obstruction of the pharynx;
- seasonal coughing suggests an allergy;
- coughing with dyspnoea indicates airway obstruction, restrictive lung disease or congestive heart failure;
- coughing and wheezing can be a sign of asthma or a foreign body blocking the respiratory tract;
- cough producing sputum indicates an infection.

Different types of sputum indicate different problems:

- clear mucus – dust or allergy;
- purulent – infection;

- brown – altered blood (e.g. pneumonia);
- blood-stained – fresh damage in the tract (e.g. tuberculosis).

Wheezing is associated with narrowing of the large airways either from oedema, mucus or a smooth-muscle contraction. Sounds that can be detected with a stethoscope are crackles, 'creaking-shoe' noises and clicks. Creaking-shoe sounds occur with pleural friction during rubbing. When a lung collapses or consolidates during disease it conducts sound more readily than if it were full of air, and the sound spreads less.

'Roaring' in horses occurs when one or both vocal cords hangs across the glottis. It can develop from demyelination of the laryngeal nerve and paralysis of the muscles that should hold the cords in position. The cords obstruct breathing and cause dyspnoea.

Dyspnoea (laboured breathing) is a sign of respiratory distress. It can be due to acute respiratory obstruction, emphysema, adhesive pleurisy, congestive heart failure, pulmonary embolism, acute paralysis, anaemia, acidosis, hypercapnia and pulmonary fibrosis. It is usually associated with exercise intolerance.

Coughing in fish helps to remove small irritating particles from the surface of the gill lamellae (Ballintijn & Jüch, 1984). Larger particles are removed by spitting. In some species, coughing occurs at regular intervals and is not a sign of irritation of the gills. It is provoked by an involuntary pattern generator in the medulla.

15.13 Agonal Gasping

When an animal is killed by concussion, it sometimes happens that there is a protracted period of inspiratory spasms called agonal gasps before the animal dies. These are low-frequency inhalations that are quite distinct from normal breathing. They occur whilst the animal is lying unconscious on its side. They have a guttural sound and the neck usually flexes during the gasp. They are due to residual medullary activity in the brainstem. The gasps cause pulsatile oxygenation of the blood, which allows strengthening of the pulse. As the pulse gradually loses its strength during a gasp interval, the brainstem becomes hypercapnic and this provokes another gasp, which in turn causes another resurgence in the strength of the pulse.

This cycle can allow an unconscious animal to survive for a long time, and it can be disturbing for onlookers. Death can be hastened either by concussing the animal again, or, in the case of small stock, compressing the chest to suppress cardiac action. The chest compression needs to stop the action of the heart with a sustained pressure, as mild or repeated chest compression during hypotension would have an opposite effect and improve circulation within the brain (Wolff & Forbes, 1928).

Dying

16

Many of us will realise when we are dying. In fact, during the final weeks, about 75% of bedridden subjects are aware that they are about to die, even though they prefer not to admit it. For some the prospect is distressing. For others it is a release and viewed as inevitable and desirable.

The anxious patient is often afraid to be left alone, and fear or anxiety stem from feelings of:

- separation;
- unfulfilled responsibilities;
- the unknown;
- loss and failure.

It would be fanciful to suppose that animals are equally aware of their situation as death draws closer. In fact, research indicates that watching other animals being killed is not necessarily stressful for the observing animal (Anil *et al.*, 1997). However, two lessons come from considering the suffering associated with dying in humans. First, some forms of terminal suffering can be treated and controlled. The second point is that dying can be a lonely experience. For pack, herd or flock animals, forced separation during the final days may add to the misery.

In modern medical practice, efforts are made to relieve suffering when people are about to die. Pain, nausea and vomiting are controlled with drugs, but quite often there is dyspnoea, which is more difficult to manage (Rees, 1972). Other common causes of suffering are anxiety, depression, incontinence and bedsores.

The main reasons for emotional and physical distress in patients dying of cancer are **fatigue**, anorexia and pain (Ross & Alexander, 2001). Fatigue is a sense of tiredness, a general lack of energy not relieved by rest, diminished mental capacity and subjective weakness associated with difficulty in performing activities of daily living. It is debilitating and destroys the quality of life.

Experienced nurses are skilled at recognising the signs of approaching death, and often make more reliable predictions than other professionals. The signs they note are:

- a greater depth of weakness;
- increasing apprehension, restlessness and irritability, partly because of less self-control;
- greater sensitivity to 'minor' discomforts;
- a need for continual contact and reassurance.

This experience has been invaluable to the sufferer and relations in preparing for departure and loss.

16.1 Euthanasia

We usually feel obliged to terminate suffering in animals that are dying, by killing them humanely. Humane animal euthanasia:

- is painless;
- does not involve fear or distress before, during or following administering of the killing agent;
- does not provoke fear or distress in other animals that witness the killing or are close at hand.

This definition is helpful in setting standards for euthanasia or destruction of animals. The death does not have to be immediate provided it is stress free.

Not all killing methods fulfil all the above criteria. Those that do not are not necessarily unacceptable, as there may be no alternatives for a particular situation. For example, there are few alternatives to catching a river trout other than with a hook and line, and this method is inevitably distressing once the animal is hooked and when it is taken out of water. Some methods involve a low level of distress, or the distress is sufficiently short-lasting, to be considered acceptable. This is usually assumed to be the case with carbon dioxide stunning in pigs, but the animals inevitably experience breathlessness before they collapse unconscious.

The euthanasia method itself should not add to any suffering, but additional suffering can occur in the following ways:

- stress of capture and restraint;
- stress associated with administration of the euthanasing agents;
- misapplication or misadventure when administering the euthanasing agent.

The **stress of capture and restraint** is a real problem when a fractious dog has to be euthanased using a lethal injection. A dog-catcher noose and pole is often

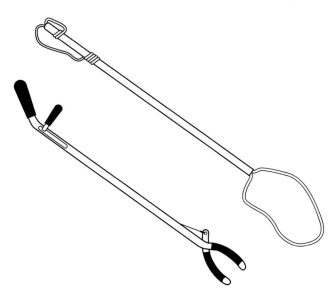

Figure 16.1 Dog catcher and fox grabber

used, and the animal is pinned to the ground at its neck (Figure 16.1). The dog is then either muzzled or, if it is safe, injected without a muzzle. In some situations it would be less stressful and safer to shoot the animal, or to shut it in a carbon monoxide euthanasia cabinet. The method of choice depends on human safety, available equipment and expertise, and minimising stress for the dog.

Carbon monoxide is used in dogs and, less commonly, in mink, and there are mixed views about its suitability. This gas combines with haemoglobin and gradually displaces the available oxygen from the bloodstream, causing the animal to die from hypoxia. The gas is toxic at low concentrations and produces few adverse signs. Respiration is normal and there is no obvious salivation or tears. It does not induce loss of consciousness quickly, typically taking about five minutes. Some dogs give a howl just before collapsing unconscious, and this has been upsetting for staff who are in charge of the procedure. When unconsciousness does not occur quickly, the sensations associated with carbon monoxide poisoning in humans include dizziness, weakness, nausea, vomiting, headache, excessive sweating, pyrexia, mental dullness and confusion.

In most countries, the administration of an anaesthetic for euthanasia purposes can only be given by a veterinarian. This has raised the question of whether or not an intravenous **injection of air** could be used instead by non-veterinarians. Normally, when air is inadvertently administered intravenously it is trapped by the lungs where it is gradually absorbed at a rate of about 2 ml per minute from the bloodstream (Ohkuda *et al.*, 1981). Animals can tolerate relatively large volumes of intravenous air before the lungs are overloaded and lethal air emboli collect in

Table 16.1 Foetal survival rate following onset of failure in the blood supply through the umbilical cord in cattle.

Clamping time (min)	Survival rate (%)
0	100
4	75
6	33
8	0

the brain or coronary vessels. This makes the method unpredictable, and so it is not recommended.

Sometimes there is concern about how foetuses should be managed when pregnant animals are being killed. This is relevant to the **harvesting of foetal tissue** in slaughterhouses for oriental medicine. The risks are that the hypoxaemia during slaughter will stimulate the advanced foetus to breathe and act independently. If those attempts coincided with evisceration on the slaughterline and the foetus was able to breathe air, it could initiate consciousness. The likelihood of this happening depends on how soon after slaughter the foetus is removed. In cattle foetuses, failure of the blood supply has to last for more than six minutes to ensure death of the foetus (Table 16.1). In practice, evisceration does not normally occur within six minutes of slaughter.

Microwaves are used for laboratory rodent euthanasia especially in research involving post-mortem neurochemistry. They cause heating of tissues and in the brain this induces petit mal or grand mal epileptiform activity plus physical convulsions (Guy & Chou, 1982). The method is humane provided appropriate wavelengths and energies are used. At low energies, microwave irradiation causes hyperactivity before collapse. Low frequencies have a greater depth of penetration and high frequencies (e.g. 2450 MHz) cause rapid surface heating with a risk of skin burns.

Advice on specific euthanasia methods for animals can be found in AVMA (2001).

16.2 Decapitation

Decapitation, neck dislocation or severing the spinal cord are sometimes used as killing methods for poultry, laboratory rodents and fish. Neck stabbing, or puntilla, was a common method for killing cattle, but its use is now limited to parts of Africa and Spanish bullfighting.

When decapitation and neck dislocation are not associated with concussion to the head, it is unlikely that there is instantaneous unconsciousness. When chickens have had their necks dislocated or they have been decapitated, the evoked responses in the visual region of the brain in the isolated head have been identical to the evoked responses before dislocation or decapitation (Gregory & Wotton, 1990), whereas, following concussion the visual evoked responses were lost immediately. The implication is that neither neck dislocation nor decapitation caused immediate disturbance of neurotransmission in the brain.

Various attempts have been made to revive the isolated head after decapitation. In humans, these attempts have been unsuccessful, and in the dog and rabbit it has been possible to revive only the respiratory, cardioregulatory and vasomotor centres in the brain after circulation had been arrested for about 30 minutes.

16.3 Religious Slaughter

The risks of suffering during religious slaughter are greater than for conventional slaughter methods that use stunning in three respects. First, cutting the neck of a conscious animal requires a robust restraining method, which in some situations is stressful for the animal. Second, the injury discharge when nerves in the neck are severed, and subsequent activity in nerves adjacent to the wound, would cause a sense of trauma and in some instances there could be pain. Third, subsequent bleeding from the neck wound could be distressing.

When an animal is stunned properly before the cut is made, the third risk is removed. The first risk still exists with conventional stunning and slaughter but to a lesser degree, because vigorous forms of restraint are not necessary. The second risk is replaced with the risk of pain or discomfort during the application of the stunning device. With stunning methods that cause instantaneous unconsciousness, this is not relevant. Overall, the theoretical risks of discomfort and pain are greater with religious slaughter, but whether this is the case in practice depends on how it is done, and on the stunning and slaughter methods that are used for comparison.

16.4 Death from Brain Injury

There are nine types of brain injury or insult that can result in death:

(1) ischaemia;
(2) anoxia;
(3) trauma;
(4) haemorrhage;
(5) metabolic abnormalities;
(6) toxins;
(7) inflammation;
(8) tumours;
(9) rise in temperature.

What concerns us is the perceptions that intervene before unconsciousness and death set in. By implication, which types of brain injury are likely to be associated with apprehension, or even suffering ?

When an animal is euthanased with an anaesthetic overdose, the various mental faculties disappear in quick succession. Vision is the first conscious faculty to be affected, and blurring of vision is the first untoward effect that is felt. The rapid disappearance of overall consciousness means that the potential for suffering is brief.

During death from a cardiac arrest or arrest of breathing, there can be a sudden sense of impending death which could be distressing for a short period. When conscious volunteers have had the blood flow to the brain in the carotid and vertebral arteries clamped off with an inflatable cuff they lost consciousness in, on average, 6–7 seconds. The eyelids drooped, the head dropped down and they slumped in the chair (Rossen *et al.*, 1943). Afterwards, the subjects recalled that there was narrowing of the field of vision, blurring of vision whilst being able to hear, flashes of light, paraesthesias and then loss of consciousness. In a limited number of people there was a shooting pain down an arm or leg, and in others anoxic convulsions on release of pressure in the cuff. Taken together, this indicates that loss of consciousness during cerebral ischaemia is not inevitably an unpleasant experience.

Victims experiencing a dislocated neck at the base of the skull rarely survive any length of time. They die from acute neurogenic shock and in some cases there could be a sense of breathlessness from being unable to breathe. Hypoglycaemia and haemorrhage are associated with a sense of weakness and fatigue before the loss of consciousness.

When the brain is poorly perfused, certain regions are more prone to ischaemic injury than others. The hippocampus is vulnerable in the adult and newborn, and so amnesia is a common repercussion following non-fatal hypoxaemic episodes. In the foetal lamb, the rank order of damage is parasagittal cortex > hippocampal CA1, CA2 and CA3 regions > lateral cortex, hippocampal CA4, striatum > amygdala, dentate gyrus, thalamus and cerebellum. The resilience of the thalamus and cerebellum allows rudimentary functions, including motor coordination, to persist in cases of brain injury.

Trauma is the main cause of death in people who are under 45, and head injury accounts for 40% of these deaths. Head injuries in animals occur during collisions with gates and partitions, motor vehicle accidents, falls, kicks and during euthanasia. There are two mechanisms involved in death from head injury, and they differ in the types of suffering they produce. Primary injuries occur in the brain as a direct result of the physical impact, and include abrasion, shearing, coup, contre coup and compression injuries.

Secondary brain injuries arise when there is reduced energy or oxygen supply because of oedema or haemorrhage. Oedema and haemorrhage cause a rise in intracerebral pressure, which in turn can compress the main arteries that supply blood within the brain, and this results in unconsciousness, but may be preceded by headaches if the process is drawn out. The headaches are due to activation of specific tissues in the brain rather than a generalised increase in intracranial pressure.

Not all penetrating head injuries cause immediate unconsciousness. There was a case of a German mechanic who was struck by a spinning propeller at an airfield. He did not lose consciousness, and stated that he could not see any more. When taken to the hospital he gave an exact description of the accident, and he showed no symptoms of concussion other than loss of vision. He died shortly afterwards from an unarrestable brain haemorrhage. At autopsy it was found that the occipital bone and the visual cortex had been severed completely (Spatz, 1950).

Experience from other post-mortem examinations has shown that when there is a haemorrhage in the brain stem, the head injury is likely to be instantly fatal. In the case of crushed skulls it is common to find that either the falx or the tentorium slice deeply into the brain, tearing the large blood vessels as well.

The most common cause of death following head injury is subdural haemorrhage. The haemorrhage arises from one of three sources:

(1)   direct injury of cortical arteries and veins by a penetrating object;
(2)   contusion and pulping of the cerebrum;
(3)   tearing of the veins that bridge the subdural space between the surface of the brain and the dural sinuses (Figure 16.2) (Gennarelli & Thibault, 1982).

16.5 Recognising Insensibility and Brain Death

Diagnosing **consciousness** can be a confusing procedure. During dying there can be gradations and episodes of conscious-like behaviour interspersed with periods of coma, and the same applies during recovery from serious injuries. For example, there was a case where a soldier took weeks to recover from a head injury. First, he showed some crude forms of arousal, later there was a return of speech but at an emotionally facile level and then he regained peripheral sensory function with intelligent speech (Gregory & Shaw, 2000). Clearly, recovery in such cases is protracted and there is no distinct interface between consciousness and unconsciousness. We have no exact words to describe these gradations in consciousness or unconsciousness, and the same applies to fading consciousness during dying.

The **reticular formation** in the brainstem is an important relay point which coordinates consciousness. It receives incoming signals from the anterolateral funiculus, trigeminal nucleus and cranial nerves, as well as inputs from the cerebral

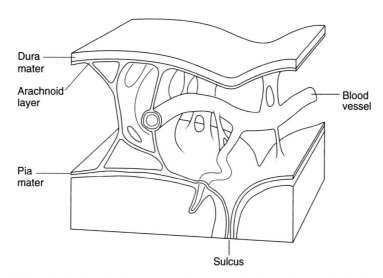

Figure 16.2 Section through the meninges showing a blood vessel in the subdural space.

cortex, thalamus and hypothalamus. It also sends signals back to these regions, and is a major relay point for signals that descend the spinal cord. It is not surprising, therefore, that damage to this region has catastrophic effects on consciousness. Mild insults can influence affective responses and emotional behaviour, through disturbance of signals that normally come from the limbic system, whilst involuntary behaviours are normal. At the other extreme, electrical stimulation of the reticular formation in a normal subject causes arousal. There is awakening and attentiveness. Instantaneous disruption of the reticular formation, along with other parts of the brainstem, will cause immediate unconsciousness progressing to death.

Brain death is usually identified by testing brainstem reflexes. Brainstem reflexes are preferred to spinal reflexes because the latter can occur independently of brain function, as in animals that have a severed spinal cord.

There are 12 pairs of cranial nerves that connect with the ventral surface of the brain, and most of them have sensory as well as motor functions. For example, stimulation of the back of the mouth activates sensory receptors which convey signals along the ninth (glossopharyngeal) cranial nerve, and, if the brainstem is functioning, there will be reflex gagging which is activated by efferent fibres in the same nerve.

There are four other cranial-nerve reflexes which are used routinely in assessing brainstem death (Pallis, 1982). They are: (1) absence of a pupillary response to a beam of light shone in the eye; (2) absence of blinking in response to irritation of the cornea; (3) absence of eye movement in response to an infusion of ice cold water into an ear; (4) absence of grimacing in response to compression of a supraorbital ridge.

These tests have to be modified to suit particular species. For example, in poultry the absence of a nictating membrane response to irritation of the cornea is used instead of absence of an eyelid blink. Often the brainstem is the last region in the brain to die, but there are exceptions (Roine *et al.*, 1988).

Dying can be an ugly process, and some deaths are worse than others (Plate 12). Only the leaves on the trees die beautifully.

References

Abdelsamie, R. E. & Yadiwilo, F. (1981) Water consumption and the effects of water restriction on performance of broilers in the tropics. *British Poultry Science* **22**, 423–9.

Abramson, L. Y. & Seligman, M. E. P. (1977) Modeling psychopathology in the laboratory: history and rationale. In: *Psychopathology: experimental models* (eds J. D. Maser & M. E. P. Seligman), pp. 1–26. W. H. Freeman and Co., San Francisco.

Agar, W. E. (1925) Trial and error and intelligence in the behaviour of certain arthropods. *Australian Journal of Experimental Biology and Medical Science* **2**, 151–5.

Alexander, A. F. & Jensen, R. (1959) Gross cardiac changes in cattle with high mountain (brisket) disease and in experimental cattle maintained at high altitudes. *American Journal of Veterinary Research* **20**, 68–9.

Allen, R. E. & McCullough, D. R. (1976) Deer–car accidents in southern Michigan. *Journal of Wildlife Management* **40**, 317–25.

Alonso, J. C., Alonso, J. A. & Muñoz-Pulido, R. (1994) Mitigation of bird collisions with transmission lines through ground wire marking. *Biological Conservation* **67**, 129–34.

Anand, K. J. S. & Hickey, P. R. (1987) Pain and its effects in the human neonate and fetus. *New England Journal of Medicine* **317**, 1321–9.

Andersen, H. S., Sestoft, D. & Lillebæk, T. (2000) A longitudinal study of prisoners on remand: psychiatric prevalence, incidence and psychopathology in solitary vs. non-solitary confinement. *Acta Psychiatrica Scandinavica* **102**, 19–25.

Anderson, D. E. (1994) Behavior analysis and the search for the origins of hypertension. *Journal of the Experimental Analysis of Behavior* **61**, 255–61.

Anil, M. H., McKinstry, J. L., Field, M. & Rodway, R. G. (1997) Lack of evidence for stress being caused to pigs by witnessing the slaughter of conspecifics. *Animal Welfare* **6**, 3–8.

Anisman, H., Kokkinidis, L., Borowski, T. & Merali, Z. (1998) Differential effects of interleukin (IL) -1β, IL-2 and IL-6 on responding for rewarding lateral hypothalamic stimulation. *Brain Research* **779**, 177–87.

Anon. (1941) Experiences of blast. *Lancet* i, 586.

Anon. (1943) Psychiatric battle casualties. *Journal of the American Medical Association* **123**, 499.

Anon. (1944) Dogs as mine 'pointers'. *Veterinary Record* **56**, 363.

Apter, R. C. & Householder, D. D. (1996) Weaning and weaning management of foals: a review and some recommendations. *Journal of Equine Veterinary Science* 16, 428–35.

Arbit, J. (1957) Diurnal cycles and learning in earthworms. *Science* 126, 654–5.

Arendt-Nielsen, L. & Svensson, P. (2001) Referred muscle pain: basic and clinical findings. *Clinical Journal of Pain* 17, 11–19.

Armus, H. L. (1970) Conditioning of the sensitive plant, *Mimosa pudica*. In: *Comparative Psychology. Research in Animal Behavior* (eds M. R. Denny & S. C. Ratner), pp. 597–600. Dorsey Press, Illinois.

Attal, N. (2000) Chronic neuropathic pain: mechanisms and treatment. *Clinical Journal of Pain* 16, S118–30.

AVMA (2001) 2000 report of the AVMA panel on euthanasia. *Journal of the American Veterinary Medical Association* 218, 669–96.

Bailey, C. J., Reid, S. W. J., Hodgson, D. R., Bourke, J. M. & Rose, R. J. (1998) Flat, hurdle and steeple racing: risk factors for musculoskeletal injury. *Equine Veterinary Journal* 30, 498–503.

Ballintijn, C. M. & Jüch, P. J. W. (1984) Interaction of respiration with coughing, feeding, vision and occulomotor control in fish. *Brain, Behavior and Evolution* 25, 99–108.

Bantick, S. J., Wise, R. G., Ploghaus, A., Clare, S., Smith, S. M. & Tracey, I. (2002) Imaging how attention modulates pain in humans using functional MRI. *Brain* 125, 310–19.

Barker Jørgensen, C. B. (1994) Water economy in a terrestrial toad (*Bufo bufo*), with special reference to cutaneous drinking and urinary bladder function. *Comparative Biochemistry and Physiology* 109A, 311–24.

Barlow, C. G. & Bock, K. (1984) Predation of fish in farm dams by cormorants, *Phalacrocorax* spp. *Australian Wildlife Research* 11, 559–66.

Barnes, A. J. (1977) Rupture of the anterior cruciate ligament of the dog: a survey from practices in the Kent region BSAVA. *Journal of Small Animal Practice* 18, 55–9.

Bartels, K. E., Stair, E. L. & Cohen, R. E. (1991) Corrosion potential of steel bird shot in dogs. *Journal of the American Veterinary Medicine Association* 199, 856–63.

Bateson, P. (1997) The behavioural and physiological effects of culling red deer. *Report to the Council of the National Trust.* United Kingdom.

Beardsley, S. L. & Schrader, S. C. (1995) Treatment of dogs with wounds of the limbs caused by shearing forces: 98 cases (1975–1993). *Journal of the American Veterinary Medical Association* 207, 1071–4.

Beckman, D. L. & Iams, S. G. (1979) Circulating catecholamines in cats before and after lethal head injury. *Proceedings of the Society for Experimental Biology and Medicine* 160, 200–202.

Beise, R. D., Carstens, E. & Kohlloffel, L. U. (1998) Psychophysical study of stinging pain evoked by brief freezing of superficial skin and ensuing short-lasting changes in sensations of cool and cold pain. *Pain* 74, 275–86.

Bell, F. R. & Itabisashi, T. (1973) The electroencephalogram of sheep and goats with special reference to rumination. *Physiology and Behavior* 11, 503–14.

Bellenger, C. R. (1971) Bull wastage in beef cattle. *Australian Veterinary Journal* 47, 83–90.

Ben-Nathan, D. & Fenerstein, G. (1990) The influence of cold or isolation stress on resistance of mice to West Nile virus encephalitis. *Experientia* 46, 285–90.

Bennet, G. J. & Xie, Y.-K. (1988) A peripheral mononeuropathy in rats that produces disorders of pain sensation like those seen in man. *Pain* 33, 87–107.

Bennett, D. B. (1973) The effect of limb loss and regeneration on the growth of the edible crab, *Cancer pagurus*, L. *Journal of Experimental Marine Biology and Ecology* 13, 45–53.

Berkhoudt, H., Dubbeldam, J. L. & Zielstra, S. (1981) Studies on the somatotopy of the trigeminal system in the mallard. *Journal of Comparative Neurology* 196, 407–20.

Berner, G. E., Garrett, C. C., Jones, D. C. & Noer, R. J. (1926) The effect of external temperature on second wind. *American Journal of Physiology* 76, 586–92.

Berryman, J. C. (1986) Parental behaviour in rodents. In: *Parental Behaviour.* (eds W. Sluckin & M. Herbert). Basil Blackwell Ltd, Oxford.

Bertrand, E., Smedja, C., Mauborgne, A., Roques, B. P. & Daugé, V. (1997) Social interaction increases the extracellular levels of [met] enkephalin in the nucleus accumbens of control but not of chronic mild stressed rats. *Neuroscience* 80, 17–20.

Best, J. B. (1964) Behaviour of *Planaria* in instrumental learning paradigms. *Animal Behaviour Supplement* 1, 69–75.

Best, P. B. (1996) The external locations of harpoon wounds on Minke whales taken in Antarctic commercial whaling operations, 1978/79 season. *Animal Welfare* 5, 57–62.

Bettoli, P. W. & Osborne, R. S. (1998) Hooking mortality and behavior of striped bass following catch and release angling. *North American Journal of Fisheries Management* 18, 609–15.

Bianca, W. & Hales, J. R. S. (1970) Sweating, panting and body temperature of newborn and one-year-old calves at high environmental temperatures. *British Veterinary Journal* 126, 45–53.

Blackshaw, J. K., Blackshaw, A. W. & Kusano, T. (1987) Cattle behaviour in a saleyard and its potential to cause bruising. *Australian Journal of Experimental Agriculture* 27, 753–7.

Bland-Ward, P. A. & Humphrey, P. P. A. (1997) Acute nociception mediated by hindpaw P2X receptor activation in the rat. *British Journal of Pharmacology* 122, 365–71.

Blenk, K.-H., Janig, W., Michaelis, M. & Vogel, C. (1996) Prolonged injury discharge in unmyelinated nerve fibres following transection of the sural nerve in rats. *Neuroscience Letters* 215, 185–8.

Blount, W. P. (1944) Chemical warfare and farm animals. *Veterinary Journal* 100, 249–57.

Blumenkopf, B. & Lipman, J. J. (1991) Studies in autotomy; its pathophysiology and usefulness as a model of chronic pain. *Pain* 45, 203–209.

Boda, J. M., Cupps, P. T., Covin, H. & Cole, H. H. (1956) The sequence of events preceding death of a cow in acute experimental bloat on fresh alfalfa tops. *Journal of the American Veterinary Medical Association* 128, 532–5.

Bodley Scott, R. & Warin, R. P. (1946) Observations of the headache accompanying fever. *Clinical Science* 6, 51–61.

Bolhuis, J. J. (1991) Mechanisms of avian imprinting: a review. *Biological Reviews* **66**, 303–45.

Bonney, G. L. W. & Pickering, G. W. (1946) Observations on the mechanism of pain in ulcer of the stomach and duodenum. Part II – the location of the pain nerve endings. *Clinical Science* **6**, 91–111.

Bors, E. (1963) Phantom limbs in patients with spinal cord injury. In: *Spinal Injuries. Proceedings of a Symposium Held in the Royal College of Surgeons of Edinburgh*, pp. 15–32. Morrison and Gibb Ltd, London.

Bouzeghrane, F., Fagette, S., Somody, L., Allevade, A.-M., Gharib, C. & Ganquelin, G. (1996) Restraint vs. hindlimb suspension on fluid and electrolyte balance in rats. *Journal of Applied Physiology* **80**, 1993–2001.

Bowen, J. S. (1977) Dehorning the mature goat. *Journal of the American Veterinary Medical Association* **171**, 1249–50.

Bowman, K. F., Leitch, M., Nunamaker, D. M. *et al.* (1984) Complications during treatment of traumatic disruption of the suspensory apparatus in thoroughbred horses. *Journal of the American Veterinary Medical Association* **184**, 706–15.

Boycott, B. B. (1960) The functioning of the statocysts of *Octopus vulgaris*. *Proceedings of the Royal Society of London, B* **152**, 78–87.

Braun, C., Guzman, F., Horton, E. W., Lim, R. K. S. & Potter, G. D. (1961) Visceral receptors, pain, bradykinin, and analgesic agents. *Journal of Physiology* **155**, 13.

Busnel, M. C. & Molin, D. (1978) Preliminary results of the effects of noise on gestating mice and their pups. In: *Effects of Noise on Wildlife* (eds J. L. Fletch & R. G. Busnel). Academic Press, New York.

Buxton, H. F. (1941) A blasted horse – and others. *Lancet* i, 261.

Campbell, E. J. M., Freedman, S., Clark, T. J. H., Robson, J. G. & Norman, J. (1967) The effect of muscular paralysis induced by tubocurarine on the duration and sensation of breath-holding. *Clinical Science* **32**, 425–32.

Carlson, A. J. (1918) Contributions to the physiology of the stomach. XLV. Hunger, appetite and gastric juice secretion in man during prolonged fasting (fifteen days). *American Journal of Physiology* **45**, 120–46.

Carlsson, A. J. (1917) Contributions to the physiology of the stomach. XLIV. The origin of the epigastric pains in cases of gastric and duodenal ulcer. *American Journal of Physiology* **45**, 81–91.

Carr, R. E. (1999) Panic disorder and asthma. *Journal of Asthma* **36**, 143–52.

Carter, H. E. J. (1967) Flock of starlings hitting ground. *British Birds* **60**, 304–305.

Carter, P. D., Johnston, N. E., Corner, L. A. & Jarrett, R. G. (1983) Observations on the effect of electro-immobilisation on the dehorning of cattle. *Australian Veterinary Journal* **60**, 17–19.

Casey, K. L. (1999) Forebrain mechanisms of nociception and pain: analysis through imaging. *Proceedings of the National Academy of Science* **96**, 7668–74.

Casey, K. L. & Morrow, T. J. (1983) Nocifensive responses to cutaneous thermal stimuli in the cat: stimulus-response profiles, latencies, and afferent activity. *Journal of Neurophysiology* **50**, 1497–515.

Chambers, C., Powell, L., Wilson, E. & Green, L. E. (1995) A postal survey of tail biting in pigs in south west England. *Veterinary Record* **136**, 147–8.

Chang, G.-L., Hung, T.-K., Bleyaert, A. & Janetta, P. J. (1981) Stress–strain measurement of the spinal cord of puppies and their neurological evaluation. *Journal of Trauma* **21**, 807–10.

Chang, S.-S. & Rasmussen, A. F. (1965) Stress-induced suppression of interferon production in virus-infected mice. *Nature* **205**, 623–4.

Chapman, R. E., Bennett, J. W. & Carter, N. B. (1984) Erythemal response of biologically denuded sheep to sunlight and the effect on skin structure and wool growth. *Australian Journal of Biological Sciences* **37**, 217–35.

Chapman, R. E., Fell, L. R. & Shutt, D. A. (1994) A comparison of stress in surgically and non-surgically mulesed sheep. *Australian Veterinary Journal* **71**, 243–7.

Chasey, D. (1997) Rabbit haemorrhagic disease: the new scourge of *Orctolagus cuniculus*. *Laboratory Animals* **31**, 33–44.

Chen, J.-C., Cheng, S.-Y. & Chen, C.-T. (1994) Changes of haemocyanin, protein and free amino acid levels in the haemolymph of *Penaeus japonicus* exposed to ambient ammonia. *Comparative Biochemistry and Physiology* **109A**, 339–47.

Cheng, C. P. K. (1975) Haemodynamic changes in adrenaline-induced acute massive lung oedema. *Cardiovascular Research* **9**, 105–11.

Chery-Croze, S. & Duclaux, R. (1980) Discrimination of painful stimuli in human beings: influence of stimulation area. *Journal of Neurophysiology* **44**, 1–10.

Chew, R. M. (1961) Water metabolism of desert-inhabiting vertebrates. *Biological Reviews* **36**, 1–31.

Chiueh, C. C. & Kopin, I. J. (1978) Hyperresponsivity of spontaneously hypertensive rat to indirect measurement of blood pressure. *American Journal of Physiology* **234**, H690–5.

Chorobski, J. & Penfield, W. (1932) Cerebral vasodilator nerves and their pathway from the medulla oblongata. *Archives of Neurology and Psychiatry* **28**, 1257–89.

Chu, C. S. (1981) New concepts of pulmonary burn injury. *Journal of Trauma* **21**, 958–61.

Chung, J. M., Choi, Y., Yoon, Y. W. & Na, H. S. (1995) Effects of age on behavioral signs of neuropathic pain in an experimental rat model. *Neuroscience Letters* **183**, 54–7.

Clausen, G. & Ersland, A. (1970/71) Blood O_2 and acid-base changes in the beaver during submersion. *Respiration Physiology* **11**, 104–12.

Cleghorn, R. A. & McKelvey, A. D. (1944) Studies of shock produced by muscle trauma. I. Methods; mortality; cardiovascular, blood concentration, and sugar changes. *Canadian Journal of Research* **E22**, 12–25.

Clemedson, C.-J. (1956) Blast injury. *Physiological Reviews* **36**, 336–54.

Codere, T. J., Grimes, R. W. & Melzack, R. (1986) Autotomy after nerve sections in the rat is influenced by tonic descending inhibition from locus coeruleus. *Neuroscience Letters* **67**, 82–6.

Cohen, H. & Rogers, L. (1942) War injuries of the spine and cord. In: *Surgery of Modern Warfare*, Vol. 1 (ed. H. Bailey), pp. 333–46. E&S Livingstone, Edinburgh.

Cohen, N. D., Peloso, J. G., Mundy, G. D. *et al.* (1997) Racing-related factors and results of prerace physical inspection and their association with musculoskeletal injuries incurred in Thoroughbreds during races. *Journal of the American Veterinary Medical Association* **211**, 454–63.

Collier, H. O. J., James, G. W. L. & Schneider, C. (1966) Antagonism by aspirin and fenamates of bronchoconstriction and nociception induced by adenosine-5'-triphosphate. *Nature* **212**, 411–12.

Collins, M. R., McGovern, J. C., Sedberry, G. R., Meister, H. S. & Pardieck, R. (1999) Swim bladder deflation in blacksea bass and vermilion snapper: potential for increasing postrelease survival. *North American Journal of Fisheries Management* **19**, 828–32.

Conn, C. A., McClellan, J. L., Maassab, H. F., Smitka, C. W., Majde, J. A. & Kluger, M. J. (1995) Cytokines and the acute phase response to influenza virus in mice. *American Journal of Physiology* **268**, R78–84.

Corbines, G. D. (1999) Large hooks reduce catch-and-release mortality of blue cod *Parapercis colias* in the Marlborough Sounds of New Zealand. *North American Journal of Fisheries Management* **19**, 992–8.

Dalefield, R. R. & Oehme, F. W. (1999) Deer velvet antler: some unanswered questions on toxicology. *Veterinary and Human Toxicology* **41**, 39–41.

Dalton, R. G. (1964) Water diuresis in cattle. *British Veterinary Journal* **120**, 69–77.

Dalton, R. G. (1967) The effect of starvation on the fluid and electrolyte metabolism of neonatal calves. *British Veterinary Journal* **123**, 237–46.

Danbury, T. C., Weeks, C. A., Chambers, J. P., Waterman-Pearson, A. E. & Kestin, S. C. (2000) Self-selection of the analgesic drug carprofen by lame broiler chickens. *Veterinary Record* **146**, 307–11.

Dart, A. J., Hodgson, D. R. & Snyder, J. R. (1997) Caecal disease in equids. *Australian Veterinary Journal* **75**, 552–7.

Davidson, R. J., Marshall, J. R., Tomarken, A. J. & Henriques, J. B. (2000) While a phobic waits: regional brain electrical and autonomic activity in social phobics during anticipation of public speaking. *Biological Psychiatry* **47**, 85–95.

Davis, P. E. (1967) The diagnosis and treatment of muscle injuries in the racing greyhound. *Australian Veterinary Journal* **43**, 519–23.

Davis, P. E., Bellenger, C. R. & Turner, D. M. (1969) Fractures of the sesamoid bones in the greyhound. *Australian Veterinary Journal* **45**, 15–19.

De Muth, W. E. (1966) Bullet velocity and design as determinants of wounding capability: an experimental study. *Journal of Trauma* **6**, 222–32.

Dennis, S. M. (1969) Predators and perinatal mortality of lambs in Western Australia. *Australian Veterinary Journal* **45**, 6–9.

Denton, D., Shade, R., Zamarippa, F. *et al.* (1999) Neuroimaging of genesis and satiation of thirst and an interoceptor-driven theory of origins of primary consciousness. *Proceedings of the National Academy of Sciences* **96**, 6304–309.

Devor, M. & Seltzer, Z. (1999) Pathophysiology of damaged nerves in relation to chronic pain. In: *Textbook of Pain* (eds P. D. Wall & R. Melzack), 4th edn. Churchill Livingstone, Edinburgh.

Dielenberg, R. A. & McGregor, I. S. (1999) Habituation of the hiding response to cat odor in rats (*Rattus norvegicus*). *Journal of Comparative Psychology* **113**, 376–87.

Dodman, N. H., Normile, J. A., Shuster, L. & Rand, W. (1994) Equine self-mutilation syndrome (57 cases). *Journal of the American Veterinary Medical Association* **204**, 1219–23.

Doherty, M. A. & Smith, M. H. (1995) Contamination and infection of fractures resulting from gunshot trauma in dogs: 20 cases (1987–1992). *Journal of the American Veterinary Medical Association* **206**, 203–205.

Dubbeldam, J. L., de Bakker, M. A. G. & Bout, R. G. (1994) The composition of trigeminal nerve branches in normal adult chicken and after debeaking at different ages. *Journal of Anatomy* **186**, 619–27.

Duncan, I. J. H. & Wood-Gush, D. G. M. (1971) Frustration and aggression in the domestic fowl. *Animal Behaviour* **19**, 500–504.

Duncan, I. J. H. & Wood-Gush, D. G. M. (1972) Thwarting of feeding behaviour in the domestic fowl. *Animal Behaviour* **20**, 444–51.

Dyson, J. A. (1964) Castration of the mature boar with reference to general anaesthesia induced by intratesticular injection of pentobarbitone sodium. *Veterinary Record* **76**, 28–9.

Edge, W. D., Olson-Edge, S. L. & O'Gara, B. W. (1989) Capturing wild goats and urial with a remotely fired net-gun. *Australian Wildlife Research* **16**, 313–15.

Edwards, J. F., Wikse, S. E., Loy, J. K. & Field, R. W. (1995) Vertebral fracture associated with trauma during movement and restraint of cattle. *Journal of the American Veterinary Medical Association* **207**, 934–5.

Elenkor, I. J., Chrousos, G. P. & Wilder, R. L. (2000) Neuroendocrine regulation of IL-12 and TNF-α/IL-10 balance. *Annals of the New York Academy of Sciences* **917**, 94–105.

Erichsen Jones, J. R. (1952) The reactions of fish to water of low oxygen concentration. *Journal of Experimental Biology* **29**, 403–15.

Ernsting, J. (1965) The effects of anoxia on the central nervous system. In: *A Textbook of Aviation Physiology* (ed. J. A. Gillies). Pergamon Press, Oxford.

Erwin, W. J. & Stasiak, R. H. (1979) Vertebrate mortality during the burning of reestablished prairie in Nebraska. *American Midland Naturalist* **101**, 247–9.

Evans, C. L. (1966) Physiological mechanisms that underlie sweating in the horse. *British Veterinary Journal* **122**, 117–23.

Fackler, M. L., Surinchak, J. S., Malinowski, J. A. & Bowen, R. E. (1984) Bullet fragmentation: a major cause of tissue disruption. *Journal of Trauma* **24**, 35–9.

Fahim, F. A., El-Sabbagh, M., Saleh, N. A. & Sallam, U. S. (1990) Biochemical changes associated with acute phosphorus poisoning. *General Pharmacology* **21**, 899–904.

Fairnie, I. J. & Cox, K. J. (1969) Deaths in lambs after emasculation and tail docking. *Australian Veterinary Journal* **45**, 39.

Falaschi, P., Martocchia, A., Proietti, A., Pastore, R. & D'Urso, R. (1994) Immune system and the hypothalamus–pituitary–adrenal axis. *Annals of the New York Academy of Sciences* **741**, 223–33.

Farm Animal Welfare Council (1985) *Report on the Welfare of Farmed Deer.* Farm Animal Welfare Council, UK.

Fent, K. & Zbinden, G. (1987) Toxicity of interferon and interleukin. *Trends in Pharmacological Sciences* 8, 100–105.

Fernandez de Molina, A. & Hunsperger, R. W. (1962) Organisation of the subcortical system governing defence and flight reactions in the cat. *Journal of Physiology* 160, 200–13.

Ferreira, S. H., Lorenzetti, B. B., Bristow, A. F. & Poole, S. (1988) Interleukin-1β as a potent hyperalgesic agent antagonized by a tripeptide analogue. *Nature* 334, 698–700.

Fitzgerald, M. (1999) Development and neurobiology of pain. In: *Textbook of Pain* (eds P. D. Wall & R. Melzack), 4th edn, pp. 235–51. Churchill Livingstone, Edinburgh.

Flynn, J. P. (1967) The neural basis of aggression in cats. In: *Neurophysiology of Emotion* (ed. D. C. Glass), pp. 40–60. The Rockefeller University Press and Russell Sage Foundation, New York.

Fox, B. H., Ragland, D. R., Brand, R. J. & Rosenman, R. H. (1987) Type A behavior and cancer mortality. *Annals of the New York Academy of Sciences* 496, 620–27.

Fox, M. W. (1962) Observations on paw raising and sympathy lameness in dogs. *Veterinary Record* 74, 895–6.

Fraser, J. (1942) Intra-abdominal procedures, including wounds of the small intestine and mesentery. In: *Surgery of Modern Warfare*, Vol. 1 (ed. H. Bailey), pp. 403–11. E&S Livingstone, Edinburgh.

French, N. P. & Morgan, K. L. (1992) Neuromata in docked lambs' tails. *Research in Veterinary Science* 52, 389–90.

Fuller, J. L. & Clark, L. D. (1966) Effects of rearing with specific stimuli upon postisolation behavior in dogs. *Journal of Comparative and Physiological Psychology* 61, 258–67.

Fuller, J. L., Easler, C. A. & Banks, E. M. (1950) Formation of conditioned avoidance responses in young puppies. *American Journal of Physiology* 160, 462–6.

Gagge, A. P. & Herrington, L. P. (1947) Physiological effects of heat and cold. *Annual Review of Physiology* 9, 409–28.

Gando, S. (2001) Disseminated intravascular coagulation in trauma patients. *Seminars in Thrombosis and Haemostasis* 27, 585–92.

Garber, J. L. & Madison, J. B. (1991) Signs of abdominal pain caused by disruption of the small intestine mesentery in three postparturient cows. *Journal of the American Veterinary Medical Association* 198, 864–6.

Gardner, E. (1950) Physiology of movable joints. *Physiological Reviews* 30, 127–76.

Gaskill, H. V., Sirinek, K. R. & Levine, B. A. (1984) Prostacyclin selectively enhances blood flow in areas of GI tract prone to stress ulceration. *Journal of Trauma* 24, 397–402.

Gelberman, R. H., Eaton, R. & Urbaniak, J. R. (1993) Peripheral nerve compression. *Journal of Bone and Joint Surgery* 75A, 1854–78.

Gennarelli, T. A. & Thibault, L. E. (1982) Biomechanics of acute subdural hematoma. *Journal of Trauma* 22, 680–86.

Gentilello, L. M. (1995) Advances in the management of hypothermia. *Surgical Clinics of North America* 75, 243–56.

Gentle, M. J., Hughes, B. O., Fox, A. & Waddington, D. (1997) Behavioural and anatomical consequences of two beak trimming methods in 1- and 10-day old domestic chicks. *British Poultry Science* 38, 453–63.

Geverink, N. A., Engel, B., Lambooij, E. & Wiegant, V. M. (1996) Observations on behaviour and skin damage of slaughter pigs and treatment during lairage. *Applied Animal Behaviour Science* 50, 1–13.

Gilbert, F. F. & Gofton, N. (1982) Terminal dives in mink, muskrat and beaver. *Physiology & Behavior* 28, 835–40.

Gillin, J. C., Seifritz, E., Zoltoski, R. K. & Salin-Pascaul, R. J. (2000) Basic science of sleep. In: *Comprehensive Textbook of Psychiatry*, Vol. 1 (eds B. J. Sadock & V. A. Sadock), pp. 199–209. Lippincott Williams & Wilkins, Philadelphia.

Glen, J. B. & Scott, W. N. (1973) Carbon dioxide euthanasia of cats. *British Veterinary Journal* 129, 471–9.

Gooden, B. A. (1992) Why some people do not drown. Hypothermia versus the diving response. *Medical Journal of Australia* 157, 629–32.

Goodwin, R. F. W. (1957) The concentration of blood sugar during starvation in the newborn calf and foal. *Journal of Comparative Pathology* 67, 289–96.

Gordon, R. G. (1918) A study of epileptiform convulsions in soldiers. *Seale Hayne Neurological Studies* 1, 159–66.

Grafe, T. U., Döbler, S. & Linsenmair, K. E. (2002) Frogs flee from the sound of fire. *Proceedings of the Royal Society B* 269, 999–1003.

Grant, R. (1950) Emotional hypothermia. *American Journal of Physiology* 160, 285–90.

Graven-Nielsen, T. & Meuse, S. (2001) The peripheral apparatus of muscle pain: evidence from animal and human studies. *Clinical Journal of Pain* 17, 2–10.

Gray, P. (1994) *Lameness*. J. A. Allen & Co, London.

Greenwald, A. J., Allen, T. H. & Bancroft, R. W. (1969) Abdominal gas volume at altitude and at ground level. *Journal of Applied Physiology* 26, 177–81.

Gregory, N. G. (1998a) *Animal Welfare and Meat Science*. CABI Publishing, Wallingford.

Gregory, N. G. (1998b) Physiological mechanisms causing sickness behaviour and suffering in diseased animals. *Animal Welfare* 7, 293–305.

Gregory, N. G. (2001) Profiles of currents during electrical stunning. *Australian Veterinary Journal* 79, 844–5.

Gregory, N. G. & Constantine, E. (1996) Hyperthermia in dogs left in cars. *Veterinary Record* 139, 349–50.

Gregory, N. G. & Lister, D. (1981) Autonomic responsiveness in stress sensitive and stress resistant pigs. *Journal of Veterinary Pharmacology and Therapeutics* 4, 67–75.

Gregory, N. G. & Shaw, F. D. (2000) Penetrating captive bolt stunning and exsanguination of cattle in abattoirs. *Journal of Applied Animal Welfare Science* 3, 215–30.

Gregory, N. G. & Wilkins, L. J. (1991) Broken bones in the common pigeon. *Veterinary Record* 128, 154.

Gregory, N. G. & Wilkins, L. J. (1995) Effects of age on bone strength and the prevalence of broken bones in perchery laying hens. *New Zealand Veterinary Journal* **44**, 31–2.

Gregory, N. G. & Wotton, S. B. (1981) Studies on the sympathetic nervous system: T wave vectorcardiogram in cattle. *Research in Veterinary Science* **30**, 75–8.

Gregory, N. G. & Wotton, S. B. (1990) Comparison of neck dislocation and percussion of the head on visual evoked responses in the chicken's brain. *Veterinary Record* **126**, 570–72.

Gregory, N. G., Robins, J. K., Thomas, D. G. & Purchas, R. W. (1998) Relationship between body condition score and body composition in dairy cows. *New Zealand Journal of Agricultural Research* **41**, 527–32.

Groenestein, C. M., Hol, J. M. G., Vermeer, H. M., Den Hartog, L. A. & Metz, J. H. M. (2001) Ammonia emission from individual- and group-housing systems for sows. *Netherlands Journal of Agricultural Science* **49**, 313–22.

Grøndahl, A. M. & Engeland, A. (1995) Influence of radiographically detectable orthopedic changes on racing performance in Standardbred trotters. *Journal of the American Veterinary Medical Association* **206**, 1013–17.

Gross, D. (1982) Contralateral local anaesthesia in the treatment of phantom limb and stump pain. *Pain* **13**, 313–20.

Gross, T. L. & Carr, S. H. (1990) Amputation neuroma of docked tails in dogs. *Veterinary Pathology* **27**, 62–92.

Guth, L. (1956) Regeneration in the mammalian peripheral nervous system. *Physiological Reviews* **36**, 441–78.

Guthery, F. S. & Beasom, S. L. (1978) Effectiveness and selectivity of neck snares in predator control. *Journal of Wildlife Management* **42**, 457–9.

Guy, A. W. & Chou, C.-K. (1982) Effects of high-intensity microwave exposure of rat brain. *Radio Science* **17**, 169S–78S.

Hall, W. M. & Corey, E. L. (1950) Anoxia in explosive decompression injury. *American Journal of Physiology* **160**, 361–5.

Hammer, J. & Phillips, S. F. (1993) Fluid loading of the human colon: effects on segmental transit and stool composition. *Gastroenterology* **105**, 988–98.

Handley, S. L. & McBlane, J. W. (1993) An assessment of the elevated X-maze for studying anxiety and anxiety-modulating drugs. *Journal of Pharmacolgical and Toxicological Methods* **29**, 129–38.

Hardaway, R. M. (1967) Disseminated intravascular coagulation in experimental and clinical shock. *American Journal of Cardiology* **20**, 161–73.

Hardaway, R. M., Dumke, R., Gee, T. *et al.* (1980) Influence of fibrinogen levels in dogs on mortality from haemorrhagic and traumatic shock. *Journal of Trauma* **20**, 417–19.

Hardy, J. D. & Stolwijk, J. A. J. (1966) Tissue temperature and thermal pain. In: *Touch, Heat and Pain* (eds A. V. S. de Reuck & J. Knight), pp. 27–56. J. & A. Churchill Ltd, London.

Harlow, H. F. (1965) Total social isolation effects on Macaque monkey behavior. *Science* **148**, 666.

Harris, J. C. (1989) Experimental animal modelling of depression and anxiety. *Psychiatric Clinics of North America* 12, 815–36.

Harrison, D. G., Beaver, D. E., Thomson, D. J. & Osbourn, D. F. (1975) Manipulation of rumen fermentation in sheep by increasing the rate of flow of water from the rumen. *Journal of Agricultural Science* 85, 93–101.

Harvey, E. N., McMillen, J. H., Butler, E. G. & Puckett, W. O. (1962) Mechanism of wounding. In: *Wound Ballistics* (eds J. B. Coates & J. C. Beyer), pp. 144–235. Office of the Surgeon General, Medical Department of the US Army, Washington, D.C.

Hattingh, J. & van Pletzen, A. J. J. (1974) The influence of capture and transportation on some blood parameters of fresh water fish. *Comparative Biochemistry and Physiology* 49A, 607–609.

Haug, T. T., Svebak, S., Hausken, T., Wilhelmsen, I., Berstad, A. & Ursin, H. (1994) Low vagal activity mediating mechanism for the relationship between personality factors and gastric symptoms in functional dyspepsia. *Psychosomatic Medicine* 56, 181–6.

Heller, K. E., Houbak, B. & Jeppesen, L. L. (1988) Stress during mother–infant separation in ranch mink. *Behavioural Process* 17, 217–27.

Hepper, P. G. (1991) Transient hypoxic episodes: a mechanism to support associative fetal learning. *Animal Behaviour* 41, 477–80.

Hesterman, H., Gregory, N. G. & Boardman, W. S. J. (2001) Deflighting procedures and their welfare implications in captive birds. *Animal Welfare* 10, 405–19

Hocking, P. M., Maxwell, M. H. & Mitchell, M. A. (1996) Relationships between the degrees of food restriction and welfare indices in broiler breeder females. *British Poultry Science* 37, 263–78.

Hofer, M. A. (1975) Studies on how early maternal separation produces behavioral change in young rats. *Psychosomatic Medicine* 37, 245–64.

Holland, G. R. & Robinson, P. P. (1990) The number and size of axons central and peripheral to inferior alveolar nerve injuries in the cat. *Journal of Anatomy* 173, 129–37.

Holland, M. & Jennings, D. (1997) Use of electromyography in seven injured wild birds. *Journal of the American Veterinary Medical Association* 211, 607–609.

Holmstad, P. R. (1998) Do bag records of willow ptarmigan underestimate hunting mortality? *Fauna-Oslo* 51, 94–6.

Hong, C. C. & Ediger, R. D. (1978) Self-mutilation of the penis in C57BL/6N mice. *Laboratory Animals* 12, 55–7.

Horch, K. W. & Lisney, S. J. W. (1981) On the number and nature of regenerating myelinated axons after lesions of cutaneous nerves in the cat. *Journal of Physiology* 108, 1137–42.

Hori, T., Oka, T., Hosoi, M., Abe, M. & Oka, M. (2000) Hypothalamic mechanisms of pain modulatory actions of cytokines and prostaglandin E_2. *Annals of the New York Academy of Sciences* 917, 106–20.

Hornberger, W. (1950) Decompression sickness. In: *German Aviation Medicine, World War II*, Vol. 1, pp. 354–94. Department of the Air Force, Washington.

Horowitz, S. H. (2001) Venipuncture-induced neuropathic pain: the clinical syndrome, with comparisons to experimental nerve injury models. *Pain* 94, 225–9.

Houghton, K. J., Rech, R. H., Sawyer, D. C. *et al.* (1991) Dose-response of intravenous butorphanol to increase in visceral nociceptive threshold in dogs. *Proceedings of the Society of Experimental Biology and Medicine* **197**, 290–96.

Hubbs, C. L. & Rechnitzer, A. B. (1952) Report on experiments designed to determine effects of underwater explosions on fish life. *California Fish and Game* **38**, 333–66.

Humphreys, D. J. (1978) A review of recent trends in animal poisoning. *British Veterinary Journal* **134**, 128–45.

Husseini, R. H., Sweet, C., Collie, M. H. & Smith, H. (1982) Elevation of nasal viral levels by suppression of fever in ferrets infected with influenza viruses of differing virulence. *Journal of Infectious Diseases* **145**, 520–24.

Hutchins, D. R. & Rawlinson, R. J. (1972) Eventration as a sequel to castration of the horse. *Australian Veterinary Journal* **48**, 288–91.

Hutchinson, R. R., Ulrich, R. E. & Azrin, N. H. (1965) Effects of age and related factors on the pain–aggression reaction. *Journal of Comparative and Physiological Psychology* **59**, 365–9.

Iinuma, M., Yoshida, S. & Funakoshi, S. (1994) A role of periodontal sensation in development of rhythmical chewing in dogs. *Comparative Biochemistry and Physiology* **107A**, 389–95.

Indo, Y., Tsurata, M., Hayashida, Y. *et al.* (1996) Mutations in the TRKA/NGA receptor gene in patients with congenital insensitivity to pain with anhidrosis. *Nature Genetics* **13**, 485–8.

Ingvar, M. & Hsieh, J.-C. (1999) The image of pain. In: *Textbook of Pain* (eds P. D. Wall & R. Melzack), 4th edn, pp. 215–33. Churchill Livingstone, Edinburgh.

Irwin, M., Mascovich, A., Gillin, C. *et al.* (1994) Partial sleep deprivation reduces natural killer cell activity in humans. *Psychosomatic Medicine* **56**, 493–8.

Irwin, M., McClintick, J., Costlow, C., Fortner, M., White, J. & Gillin, J. C. (1996) Partial night sleep deprivation reduces natural killer and cellular immune responses in humans. *Federation of American Societies for Experimental Biology Journal* **10**, 643–53.

Irwin, R. J., Lerner, M. R., Bealer, J. F., Mantor, P. C., Brackett, D. J. & Tuggle, D. W. (1999) Shock after blast wave injury is caused by a vagally mediated reflex. *Journal of Trauma* **47**, 105–10.

Ivy, A. C. (1943) The treatment of shock in the dog. *Veterinary Journal* **99**, 81–6.

Jackson, D. L. (2000) Living without oxygen: lessons from the freshwater turtle. *Comparative Biochemistry and Physiology* **125A**, 299–315.

Jacobs, B. L., Wilkinson, L. O. & Cornal, C. A. (1990) The role of brain serotonin: a neurophysiologic perspective. *Neuropsychopharmacology* **3**, 473–9.

Jacobson, A. & Schrader, S. C. (1987) Peripheral nerve injury associated with fracture or fracture-dislocation of the pelvis in dogs and cats: 34 cases (1978–1982). *Journal of the American Veterinary Medical Association* **190**, 569–72.

Jarcho, S. (1967) Marshall Hall on crush injury and traumatic shock. *American Journal of Cardiology* **20**, 853–6.

Järvi, T. (1989) The effect of osmotic stress on the anti-predatory behaviour of Atlantic salmon smolts: a test of the maladaptive anti-predator behaviour hypothesis. *Nordic Journal of Freshwater Research* **65**, 71–9.

Jarvis, A. M., Messer, C. D. A. & Cockram, M. S. (1996) Handling, bruising and dehydration of cattle at the time of slaughter. *Animal Welfare* **5**, 259–70.

Jarvis, S., McLean, K. A., Chirnside, J. *et al.* (1997) Opioid-mediated changes in nociceptive threshold during pregnancy and parturition in the sow. *Pain* **72**, 153–9.

Jeffery, N. D. & Blakemore, W. F. (1999) Spinal cord injury in small animals. 1. Mechanisms of spontaneous recovery. *Veterinary Record* **144**, 407–13.

Jennings, P. B. (1982) Hypovolaemic shock in the military working dog. *Military Medicine* **147**, 372–6.

Jensen, D. D. (1964) Paramecia, Planaria, and pseudo-learning. *Animal Behaviour Supplement* **1**, 9–20.

Jensen, T. S., Krebs, B., Nielsen, J. & Rasmussen, P. (1983) Phantom limb, phantom pain and stump pain in amputees during the first six months following limb amputation. *Pain* **17**, 243–56.

Johansson, G., Jönsson, L., Thorén-Tolling, K. & Häggendal, J. (1981) Porcine stress syndrome – a general response to restraint stress. In: *Porcine Stress and Meat Quality*, pp. 32–41. Agricultural Food Research Society, Ås, Norway.

Jones, I. H., Stoddart, D. M. & Mallick, J. (1995) Towards a sociobiological model of depression. A marsupial model (*Petaurus breviceps*). *British Journal of Psychiatry* **106**, 475–9.

Jones, J. B., Burgess, L. R., Webster, A. J. F. & Wathes, C. M. (1996) Behavioural responses of pigs to atmospheric ammonia in a chronic choice test. *Animal Science* **63**, 437–45.

Juanes, F. & Smith, L. D. (1995) The ecological consequences of limb damage and loss in decapod crustaceans: a review and prospectus. *Journal of Experimental Marine Biology and Ecology* **193**, 197–223.

Juhler, M. (1993) Medical diagnosis and treatment of torture survivors. In: *International Handbook of Traumatic Stress Syndromes* (eds J. P. Wilson & B. Raphael), pp. 321–32. Plenum Press, New York.

Kabat, H. (1940) The greater resistance of very young animals to arrest of the brain circulation. *American Journal of Physiology* **130**, 588–99.

Kalin, N. H. (1989) The HPA system and neuroendocrine models of depression. In: *Animal Models of Depression* (eds G. F. Koob, C. L. Ehlers & D. J. Kupfer), pp. 57–73. Birchaüser, Boston.

Kamada, R. O. & Smith, J. R. (1972) The phenomenon of respiratory failure in shock: the genesis of 'shock lung'. *American Heart Journal* **83**, 1–4.

Kaplan, J. M. & Horvitz, H. R. (1993) A dual mechanosensory and chemosensory neuron in *Caenorhabditis elegans*. *Proceedings of the National Academy of Science* **90**, 2227–31.

Kavaliers, M., Hirst, M. & Teskey, G. C. (1983) A functional role for an opiate system in snail thermal behavior. *Science* **220**, 99–101.

Keele, C. A. & Armstrong, D. (1964) *Substances Producing Pain and Itch*. Edward Arnold (Publishers) Ltd, London.

Keep, J. M. (1970) Gunshot injuries to urban dogs and cats. *Australian Veterinary Journal* **46**, 330–4.

Keep, J. M. & Fox, A. M. (1971) The capture, restraint and translocation of kangaroos in the wild. *Australian Veterinary Journal* **47**, 141–5.

Kestin, S. C. (2001) Review of welfare concerns relating to commercial and special permit (scientific) whaling. *Veterinary Record* **148**, 304–307.

Kiernan, J. A. (1979) Hypotheses concerned with axonal regeneration in the mammalian nervous system. *Biological Reviews* **54**, 155–97.

Killgore, K. J., Maynord, S. T., Chan, M. D. & Morgan, R. P. (2001) Evaluation of propeller-induced mortality on early life stages of selected fish species. *North American Journal of Fisheries Management* **21**, 947–55.

King, W. S. & Moller, A. W. (1943) Experiences of air bombardment in an urban area. *Veterinary Journal* **99**, 258–68.

Kirkbride, C. A. & Frey, R. A. (1967) Experimental water intoxication in calves. *Journal of the Veterinary Medical Association* **151**, 742–6.

Klenerman, L. (1962) The tourniquet in surgery. *Journal of Bone and Joint Surgery* **44B**, 937–43.

Kluger, M. J. & Vaughn, L. K. (1978) Fever and survival in rabbits infected with *Pasteurella multocida*. *Journal of Physiology* **282**, 243–51.

Knight, P. K. & Evans, D. L. (2000) Clinical abnormalities detected in post-race examinations of poorly performing Standardbreds. *Australian Veterinary Journal* **78**, 344–6.

Kolata, R. J., Kraut, N. H. & Johnston, D. E. (1974) Patterns of trauma in urban dogs and cats: a study of 1000 cases. *Journal of the American Veterinary Medical Association* **164**, 499–502.

Koltzenburg, M. (2000) Neural mechanisms of cutaneous nociceptive pain. *Clinical Journal of Pain* **16**, S131–8.

Koob, G. F. (1989) Anhedonia as an animal model of depression. In: *Animal Models of Depression* (eds G. F. Koob, C. L. Ehlers & D. J. Kupfer), pp. 162–83. Birhaüser, Boston.

Kreeger, T. J., White, P. J., Seal, U. S. & Tester, J. R. (1990) Pathological responses of red foxes to foothold traps. *Journal of Wildlife Management* **54**, 147–60.

Kumer, R., Berger, R. J., Dunsker, S. B. & Keller, J. T. (1996) Innervation of the spinal dura: myth or reality? *Spine* **21**, 18–25.

Landrum, L. M., Thompson, G. M. & Blair, R. W. (1998) Does postsynaptic α_1-adrenergic receptor supersensitivity contribute to autonomic dysreflexia? *American Journal of Physiology* **274**, H1090–98.

Lang, D. R. (1964) Ovulations in Merino ewes moved by road or rail in Queensland. *Proceedings of the Australian Society of Animal Production* **5**, 53–7.

Latner, A. L. (1942) The low-pressure phase of blast. *Lancet* ii, 303–304.

Lau, V.-K. & Viano, D. C. (1981) Influence of impact velocity on the severity of nonpenetrating hepatic injury. *Journal of Trauma* **21**, 115–23.

Lay, D. C., Friend, T. H., Bowers, C. L., Grissom, K. K. & Jenkins, O. C. (1992) A comparative physiological and behavioral study of freeze and hot-iron branding using dairy cows. *Journal of Animal Science* **70**, 1121–5.

Leach, M. C., Bowell, V. A., Allan, T. F. & Morton, D. B. (2002) Degrees of aversion shown by rats and mice to different concentrations of inhalational anaesthetics. *Veterinary Record* **150**, 808–15.

Le Couter, R. A. & Child, G. (1995) Diseases of the spinal cord. In: *Textbook of Veterinary Internal Medicine*, Vol. 1 (eds S. J. Ettinger & E. C. Feldman), pp. 629–96. W. B. Saunders Co, Philadelphia.

Levine, M. & Wolff, H. C. (1932) Cerebral circulation. Afferent impulses from the blood vessels of the pia. *Archives of Neurology and Psychiatry* **28**, 140–50.

Levine, S. (1957) Infantile experience and resistance to physiological stress. *Science* **126**, 405.

Lewis, A. R., Pinchin, A. M. & Kestin, S. C. (1997) Welfare implications of the night shooting of wild impala (*Aepyceros melampus*). *Animal Welfare* **6**, 123–31.

Lewis, A. R. & Wilson, V. J. (1977) An evaluation of a fence in the control of wild ungulates under extensive conditions in Africa. *British Veterinary Journal* **133**, 379–87.

Lewis, T. & Hess, W. (1933) Pain derived from the skin and the mechanism of its production. *Clinical Science* **1**, 39–61.

Lewis, T. & Love, W. S. (1926) Vascular reactions of the skin to injury. Part III. Some effects of freezing, of cooling and of warming. *Heart* **13**, 27–60.

Littin, K. E., O'Connor, C. E., Gregory, N. G., Mellor, D. J. & Eason, C. T. (2002) Behavior, coagulopathy and pathology of brushtail possums (*Trichosurus vulpecula*) poisoned with brodifacoum. *Wildlife Research* **29**, 259–367.

Lorrain-Smith, J., Ritchie, J. & Dawson, J. (1915) Clinical experimental observations on the pathology of trench frostbite. *Journal of Pathology and Bacteriology* **20**, 159–89.

Lowe, T. E., Gregory, N. G., Fisher, A. D. & Payne, S. R. (2002) The effects of temperature elevation and water deprivation on lamb physiology, welfare and meat quality. *Australian Journal of Agricultural Research* **53**, 707–14.

Lown, B., Verrier, R. & Corbalan, R. (1973) Psychologic stress and threshold for repetitive ventricular response. *Science* **182**, 834–6.

Luescher, U. A., McKeown, D. B. & Halip, J. (1991) Stereotypic or obsessive–compulsive disorders in dogs and cats. *Veterinary Clinics of North America* **21**, 401–13.

Luikkonen-Anttila, T., Saartoala, R. & Hissa, R. (2000) Impact of hand-rearing on morphology and physiology of the capercaillie (*Tetrao urogallus*). *Comparative Biochemistry and Physiology* **125A**, 211–21.

Luisada, A. A. (1967) Mechanism of neurogenic pulmonary edema. *American Journal of Cardiology* **20**, 66–8.

McBride, B. & Whitelaw, W. A. (1981) A physiological stimulus to upper airway receptors in humans. *Journal of Applied Physiology* **51**, 1189–97.

McCarroll, J. R., Braunstein, P. W., Cooper, W. *et al.* (1962) Fatal pedestrian automative accidents. *Journal of the American Medical Association* **180**, 127–33.

Macdonald, A. J. R. (1980) Abnormally tender muscle regions and associated painful movements. *Pain* **8**, 197–205.

McCreath, C. F. P. (1993) Docking of dogs. *Veterinary Record* **133**, 303.

McEwen, B. S. & Magarinos, M. (1997) Stress effects on morphology and function of the hippocampus. *Annals of the New York Academy of Sciences* **821**, 271–84.

McGeown, D., Danbury, T. C., Materman-Pearson, A. E. & Kestin, S. C. (1999) Effect of carprofen on lameness in broiler chickens. *Veterinary Record* **144**, 668–71.

McKinney, W. T. (1992) Animal models. In: *Handbook of Affective Disorders* (ed. E. S. Paykel), pp. 209–17. Churchill Livingstone, Edinburgh.

McMeekan, C. M., Mellor, D. J., Stafford, K. J., Bruce, R. A., Ward, R. N. & Gregory, N. G. (1998) Effects of local anaesthesia of 4 to 8 hours' duration on the acute cortisol response to scoop dehorning in calves. *Australian Veterinary Journal* **76**, 281–5.

McQueen, C. (1972) Hyperthermia in cattle in Northern Australia. *Australian Veterinary Journal* **48**, 128.

Madding, G. F. & Kennedy, P. A. (1971) *Trauma to the Liver*, 2nd edn. W. B. Saunders Co, Philadelphia.

Maes, M., Song, C., Lin, A.-H. *et al.* (1999) Negative immunoregulatory effects of antidepressants: inhibition of interferon-γ and stimulation of interleukin-10 secretion. *Neuropsychopharmacology* **20**, 370–79.

Magerl, W. & Treede, R.-D. (1996) Heat-evoked vasodilatation in human hairy skin: axon reflexes due to low-level activity of nociceptive afferents. *Journal of Physiology* **497**, 837–48.

Malechek, J. C. & Smith, B. M. (1976) Behavior of range cows in response to winter weather. *Journal of Range Management* **29**, 9–12.

Manefield, G. W. & Tinson, A. H. (1996) *Camels – a Compendium.* University of Sydney Post Graduate Foundation in Veterinary Science, Australia.

Marchant, B. (1986) Improving wether production and reducing stains through pizzle dropping and testosterone implants. *Wool Technology and Sheep Breeding* **34**, 67–71.

Marcus, P. & Belyavin, A. (1978) Thermal sensation during experimental hypothermia. *Physiology and Behavior* **21**, 909–14.

Marcus, P. & Redman, P. (1979) Effect of exercise on thermal comfort during hypothermia. *Physiology and Behavior* **22**, 831–5.

Marshall, B. L. (1977) Bruising in cattle presented for slaughter. *New Zealand Veterinary Journal* **25**, 83–6.

Mason, G. J. (1993) Forms of stereotypic behaviour. In: *Stereotypic Animal Behaviour: Fundamentals and Applications to Welfare* (eds A. B. Lawrence & J. Rushen), pp. 7–40. CAB International, Wallingford.

Mason, G. & Littin, K. E. (2003) The humaneness of rodent pest control. *Animal Welfare* **12**, 1–37.

Mathews, C. A. & Freimer, N. B. (2000) Genetic linkage analysis of the psychiatric disorders. In: *Comprehensive Textbook of Psychiatry*, Vol. 2 (eds B. J. Sadock & V. A. Sadock), pp. 184–98. Lippincott Williams & Wilkins, Philadelphia.

Meddings, J. B. & Swain, M. G. (2000) Environmental stress-induced gastrointestinal per-meability is mediated by endogenous glucocorticoids in the rat. *Gastroenterology* **119**, 1019–28.

Mee, J. F. (1993) Bovine perinatal trauma. *Veterinary Record* **133**, 555.

Meek, P. D., Jenkins, D. J., Morris, B., Ardler, A. J. & Hawksby, R. J. (1995) Use of two humane leg-hold traps for catching pest species. *Wildlife Research* **22**, 733–9.

Meier, G. W. (1965) Maternal behaviour of feral- and laboratory-reared monkeys follow-ing the surgical delivery of their infants. *Nature* **206**, 492–3.

Meischke, H. R. C., Ramsay, W. R. & Shaw, F. D. (1974) The effect of horns on bruising in cattle. *Australian Veterinary Journal* **50**, 432–4.

Meisel, S. R., Kutz, I., Dayan, K. I. *et al.* (1991) Effect of Iraqi missile war on the inci-dence of acute myocardial infarction and sudden death in Israeli civilians. *Lancet* **338**, 660–61.

Mellor, D. J. & Gregory, N. G. (2003) Responsiveness, behavioural arousal and awareness in fetal and newborn lambs: experimental, practical and therapeutic implications. *New Zealand Veterinary Journal* **51**, 2–13.

Melzack, R., Wall, P. D. & Ty, T. C. (1982) Acute pain in an emergency clinic: latency of onset and descriptor patterns related to different injuries. *Pain* **14**, 33–43.

Mench, J. A. (1993) Problems associated with broiler breeder management. In: *Fourth Euro-pean Symposium on Poultry Welfare* (eds C. J. Savory & B. O. Hughes), pp. 195–207. UFAW, Potters Bar.

Mercadente, S. (1997) Malignant bone pain pathophysiology and treatment. *Pain* **69**, 1–18.

Mercer, P. (1992) Docking of dogs. *Veterinary Record* **131**, 374–5.

Miller, N. E. & Di Cara, L. (1967) Instrumental learning of heart rate changes in curarized rats. *Journal of Comparative and Physiological Psychology* **63**, 12–19.

Mitler, M. M., Boysen, B. G., Campbell, L. & Dement, W. C. (1974) Narcolepsy–cataplexy in a female dog. *Experimental Neurology* **45**, 332–40.

Mock, H. E. (1943) Refrigeration anesthesia in amputations. *Journal of the American Medical Association* **123**, 13–17.

Molloy, R. G., Holzheimer, R., Nestor, M., Collins, K., Mannick, J. A. & Rodrick, M. L. (1995) Granulocyte-macrophage colony-stimulating factor modulates immune function and improves survival after experimental thermal injury. *British Journal of Surgery* **82**, 770–76.

Monaghan, E. P. & Glickman, S. E. (1992) Hormones and aggressive behavior. In: *Behav-ioral Endocrinology* (eds J. B. Becker, S. M. Breedlove & D. Crews), pp. 261–85. MIT Press, Massachusetts.

Morag, M. (1967) Influence of diet on the behaviour pattern of sheep. *Nature* **213**, 110.

Morag, M., Yirmiya, R., Lerer, B. & Morag, B. (1998) Influence of socio-economic status on behavioural, emotional and cognitive effects of Rubella vaccination: a prospective, double blind study. *Psychoneuroendocrinology* **23**, 337–51.

Morley, F. H. W. (1949) Comparison of Manchester operation with Mules operation modifications in prevention of flystrike in sheep. *Agricultural Gazette of New South Wales* **60**, 543–8, 571–5, 655–7.

Moss, B. W. & Trimble, D. (1988) A study of the incidence of blemishes on bacon carcases in relation to carcase classification, sex and lairage conditions. *Record of Agricultural Research* **36**, 101–107.

Mouttotou, N. & Green, L. E. (1999) Incidence of foot and skin lesions in nursing piglets and their association with behavioural activities. *Veterinary Record* **145**, 160–65.

Mouttotou, N., Hatchell, F. M. & Green, L. E. (1999) Foot lesions in finishing pigs and their associations with the type of floor. *Veterinary Record* **144**, 629–32.

Muir, I. F. K., Barclay, T. L. & Settle, J. A. D. (1987) *Burns and their Treatment*, pp. 14–18, 103, 139. Butterworths, London.

Murison, R., Ursin, R., Coover, G. D., Lien, W. & Ursin, H. (1982) Sleep deprivation procedure produces stomach lesions in rats. *Physiology and Behavior* **29**, 693–4.

Murphy, M. J. (1994) Toxin exposures in dogs and cats: pesticides and biotoxins. *Journal of the American Veterinary Medical Association* **205**, 414–21.

Murray, E. A. (1991) Contributions of the amygdalar complex to behavior in macaque monkeys. *Progress in Brain Research* **87**, 167–80.

Murray, M. G., Lewis, A. R. & Coetzee, A. M. (1981) An evaluation of capture techniques for research on impala populations. *South African Journal of Wildlife Research* **11**, 105–109.

Murray, S. A. (1971) Shock effects on *Euglena gracilis*: the effect of the pressure duration. *Experientia* **27**, 757.

Nass, R. D. (1977) Mortality associated with sheep operations in Idaho. *Journal of Range Management* **30**, 253–8.

Nelson, K. L. (1998) Catch-and-release mortality of striped bass in the Roanoke river, North Carolina. *North American Journal of Fisheries Management* **18**, 25–30.

Newton, S. A., Knottenbelt, D. C. & Eldridge, P. R. (2000) Headshaking in horses: possible aetiopathogenesis suggested by the results of diagnostic tests and several treatment regimes used in 20 cases. *Equine Veterinary Journal* **32**, 208–16.

Noble, R. L. (1945) Observations on various types of motion causing vomiting in animals. *Canadian Journal of Research* **E23**, 212–25.

Norman, F. I. (1976) The incidence of lead shotgun pellets in waterfowl (*Anatidae* and *Rallidae*) examined in south-eastern Australia between 1957 and 1973. *Australian Wildlife Research* **3**, 61–71.

Nose, H., Yawata, T. & Morimoto, T. (1985) Osmotic factors in restitution from thermal dehydration in rats. *American Journal of Physiology* **249**, R166–71.

Noss, A. J. (1998) The impacts of cable snare hunting on wildlife populations in the forests of the Central African Republic. *Conservation Biology* **12**, 390–98.

O'Brien, P. H. (1988) The toxicity of sodium monofluoroacetate (Compound 1080) to captive feral pigs, *Sus scrofa*. *Australian Wildlife Research* **15**, 163–70.

O'Brodovich, H. M., Stalcup, S. A., Pang, L. M., Lipset, J. S. & Mellins, R. B. (1981) Bradykinin production and increased pulmonary endothelial permeability during acute respiratory failure in unanaesthetized sheep. *Journal of Clinical Investigation* **67**, 514–22.

Øen, E. O. (1995a) Description and analysis of the use of cold harpoons in the Norwegian Minke whale hunt in the 1981, 1982 and 1983 hunting seasons. *Acta Veterinaria Scandinavica* **36**, 103–10.

Øen, E. O. (1995b) A Norwegian penthrite grenade for minke whales: hunting trials with prototypes and results from the hunt in 1984, 1985 and 1986. *Acta Veterinaria Scandinavica* **36**, 111–21.

Ohkuda, K., Nakahara, K., Binder, A. & Staub, N. C. (1981) Venous air emboli in sheep: reversible increase in lung microvascular permeability. *Journal of Applied Physiology* **51**, 887–94.

Øverli, O., Pottinger, T. G., Carrick, T. R., Øverli, E. & Winberg, S. (2002) Differences in behaviour between rainbow trout selected for high- and low-stress responsiveness. *Journal of Experimental Biology* **205**, 391–5.

Paech, M. J. (1991) The King Edward Memorial Hospital 1000 mother survey of methods of pain relief in labour. *Anaesthesia in Intensive Care* **19**, 393–9.

Pallis, C. (1982) Diagnosis of brain stem death. *British Medical Journal* **285**, 1641–4.

Pavlov, P. M. & Hone, J. (1982) The behaviour of feral pigs, *Sus scrofa*, in flocks of lambing ewes. *Australian Wildlife Research* **9**, 101–109.

Pearlman, M. D., Tintinalli, J. E. & Lorenz, R. P. (1990) Blunt trauma during pregnancy. *New England Journal of Medicine* **323**, 1609–1613.

Pearson, W. H., Skalski, J. R. & Malme, C. I. (1992) Effects of sounds from a geophysical survey device on behavior of captive rockfish (*Sebastes* spp). *Canadian Journal of Fisheries and Aquatic Sciences* **49**, 1343–56.

Peek, I. S. (1995) Docking of puppies' tails. *Veterinary Record* **136**, 302–303.

Penny, R. H. C., Edwards, M. J. & Mulley, R. (1972) Gastric ulcer in the pig: a New South Wales abattoir survey of the incidence of lesions of the pars oesophagea. *British Veterinary Journal* **128**, 43–9.

Petrie, N. J. (1994) *Assessment of tail docking and disbudding distress and its alleviation in calves*. MSc thesis, Massey University.

Petrie, N. J., Mellor, D. J., Stafford, K. J., Bruce, R. A. & Ward, R. N. (1996) Cortisol responses of calves to two methods of disbudding used with or without local anaesthetic. *New Zealand Veterinary Journal* **44**, 9–14.

Phillips, Y. Y. & Zajtchuk, J. T. (1989) Blast injuries of the ear in military operations. *Annals of Otology, Rhinology and Laryngology. Supplement* **140**, 3–4.

Pietras, R. J., Stavrakos, C., Gunnar, R. M. & Tobin, J. R. (1968) Phosphorus poisoning simulating acute myocardial infarction. *Archives of Internal Medicine* **122**, 430–34.

Plaut, S. M., Thal, A., Haynes, E. E. & Wagner, J. E. (1974) Maternal deprivation in the rat: prevention of mortality by nonlactating adults. *Psychosomatic Medicine* **36**, 311–20.

Pluske, J. R. & Williams, I. H. (1996) Reducing stress in piglets as a means of increasing production after weaning: administration of amperozide or comingling of piglets during lactation? *Animal Science* **62**, 121–30.

Poole, G. V., Ward, E. F., Muakkassa, F. F., Hsu, H. S. H., Griswold, J. A. & Rhodes, R. S. (1991) Pelvic fracture from major blunt trauma. *Annals of Surgery* **213**, 532–9.

Procacci, P., Zoppi, M. & Maresca, M. (1999) Heart, vascular and haemopathic pain. In: *Textbook of Pain* (eds P. D. Wall & R. Melzack), 4th edn, pp. 621–39. Churchill Livingstone, Edinburgh.

Proulx, G., Onderka, D. K., Kolenosky, A. J., Cole, P. J., Drescher, R. K. & Badry, M. J. (1993) Injuries and behavior of racoons (*Procyon lotor*) captured in the Soft Catch™ and Egg™ traps in simulated natural environments. *Journal of Wildlife Diseases* 29, 447–52.

Pynoos, R. S., Steinberg, A. M., Ornitz, E. M. & Goenjian, A. K. (1997) Issues in the developmental neurobiology of traumatic stress. *Annals of the New York Academy of Sciences* 821, 176–93.

Quinn, R. H., Danneman, P. J. & Dysko, R. C. (1994) Sedative efficacy of droperidol and diazepam in the rat. *Laboratory Animal Science* 44, 166–71.

Racine, C. H., Walsh, M. E., Roebuck, B. D. *et al.* (1992) White phosphorus poisoning of waterfowl in an Alaskan salt marsh. *Journal of Wildlife Diseases* 28, 669–73.

Racotta, I. S. & Hernández-Herrera, R. (2000) Metabolic responses of the white shrimp, *Penaeus vannamei*, to ambient ammonia. *Comparative Biochemistry and Physiology* 125A, 437–43.

Radeleff, R. D. (1970) *Veterinary Toxicology*, 2nd edn. Lea & Febiger, Philadelphia.

Rainey, J. W. (1933) Shooting as a means of painless despatch. *Veterinary Journal* 89, 307–12.

Raj, A. B. M. & Gregory, N. G. (1996) Welfare implications of the gas stunning of pigs. 2. Stress of induction of anaesthesia. *Animal Welfare* 5, 71–8.

Ratcliffe, H. L., Luginbühl, H., Schnarr, W. R. & Chacko, K. (1969) Coronary arteriosclerosis in swine: evidence of a relation to behavior. *Journal of Comparative and Physiological Psychology* 68, 385–92.

Ray, B. S. & Wolff, H. G. (1940) Experimental studies on headache: pain-sensitive structures of the head and their significance in headache. *Archives of Surgery* 41, 813–56.

Recher, H. F., Gowing, G. & Armstrong, T. (1985) Causes and frequency of deaths among birds mist-netted for banding studies at two localities. *Australian Wildlife Research* 12, 321–6.

Reece, R. L., Beddome, V. D., Barr, D. A. & Scott, P. C. (1992) Common necropsy findings in captive birds in Victoria, Australia (1978–1987). *Journal of Zoo and Wildlife Medicine* 23, 301–12.

Rees, W. D. (1972) The distress of dying. *British Medical Journal* 3, 105–107.

Reinert, H.-K. (1990) A profile and impact assessment of organized rattlesnake hunts in Pennsylvania (USA). *Journal of the Pennsylvania Academy of Science* 64, 136–44.

Richards, M. P. M. (1966) Maternal behaviour in virgin female golden hamsters (*Mesocricetus auratus* Waterhouse): the role of the age of the test pup. *Animal Behaviour* 14, 303–309.

Riddell, C., Helmboldt, C. F., Singsen, E. P. & Matterson, L. D. (1968) Bone pathology of birds affected with cage layer fatigue. *Avian Diseases* 12, 285–97.

Riesen, A. H. & Zilbert, D. E. (1975) Behavioral consequences of variations in early sensory environments. In: *The Developmental Neuropsychology of Sensory Deprivation.* Academic Press, New York.

Riley, V. (1975) Mouse mammary tumors: alteration of incidence as apparent function of stress. *Science* **189**, 465–7.

Rivers, J. F., Orr, G. & Lee, H. A. (1970) Drowning: its clinical sequelae and management. *British Medical Journal* **ii**, 157–61.

Rogers, T. J., Steele, A. D., Howard, O. M. Z. & Oppenheim, J. J. (2000) Bidirectional heterologous desensitisation of opioid and chemokine receptors. *Annals of the New York Academy of Sciences* **917**, 19–28.

Roine, R. O., Hillbom, M., Valle, M. *et al.* (1988) Fatal encephalitits caused by a bat-borne rabies-related virus. *Brain* **111**, 1505–16.

Rose, J. D. (2002) The neurobehavioral nature of fishes and the question of awareness and pain. *Reviews in Fisheries Science* **10**, 1–38.

Ross, D. D. & Alexander, C. S. (2001) Management of common symptoms in terminally ill patients: Part 1. Fatique, anorexia, cachexia, nausea and vomiting. *American Family Physician* **64**, 807–14.

Ross, J. (1972) Zoological and wildlife review. Myxomatosis and the rabbit. *British Veterinary Journal* **128**, 172–6.

Rossen, R., Kabat, H. & Anderson, J. P. (1943) Acute arrest of cerebral circulation in man. *Archives of Neurology and Psychiatry* **50**, 510–28.

Rowland, N. E. & Antelman, S. M. (1976) Stress-induced hyperphagia and obesity in rats: a possible model for understanding human obesity. *Science* **191**, 310–12.

Rushen, J. (1987) How can we tell if a sheep is in pain? *Applied Animal Behaviour Science* **17**, 374.

Sackett, G., Griffin, G. A., Pratt, C., Joslyn, W. D. & Ruppenthal, G. (1967) Mother–infant and adult female choice behavior in rhesus monkeys after various rearing experiences. *Journal of Comparative and Physiological Psychology* **63**, 376–81.

Salminen, A. & Vihko, V. (1983) Endurance training reduces the susceptibility of mouse skeletal muscle to lipid peroxidation in vitro. *Acta Physiologica Scandinavica* **117**, 109–13.

Saunders, C. & Platt, M. (1999) Pain and impending death. In: *Textbook of Pain* (eds P. D. Wall & R. Melzack), 4th edn, pp. 1113–22. Churchill Livingstone, Edinburgh.

Schill, D. J. & Scarpella, R. L. (1997) Barbed hook restrictions in catch-and-release trout fisheries: a social issue. *North American Journal of Fisheries Management* **17**, 873–81.

Schmidt, J. P. (1968) Psychosomatics in veterinary medicine. In: *Abnormal Behavior in Animals* (ed. M. W. Fox), pp. 365–97. W. B. Saunders Company, Philadelphia.

Schoenen, J. & Sándor, P. S. (1999) Headache. In: *Textbook of Pain* (eds P. D. Wall & R. Melzack), 4th edn, pp. 761–98. Churchill Livingstone, Edinburgh.

Schwei, M. J., Honore, P., Rogers, S. D. *et al.* (1999) Neurochemical and cellular reorganization of the spinal cord in a murine model of bone cancer pain. *Journal of Neuroscience* **19**, 10886–97.

Schwilch, R., Grattarola, A., Spina, F. & Jenni, L. (2002) Protein loss during long-distance migratory flight in passerine birds: adaptation and constraint. *Journal of Experimental Biology* 205, 687–95.

Seddon, H. R. (1935) Blowfly attack in sheep: its prevention by fold removal (Mules' Operation). *Journal of the Council for Scientific and Industrial Research* 8, 25–6.

Seksel, K. & Lindeman, M. J. (2001) Use of clomipramine in treatment of obsessive-compulsive disorder, separation anxiety and noise phobia in dogs: a preliminary, clinical study. *Australian Veterinary Journal* 79, 252–6.

Seltzer, Z. (1995) The relevance of animal neuropathy models for chronic pain in humans. *Seminars in the Neurosciences* 7, 211–19.

Seltzer, Z., Beilin, B., Ginzburg, R., Paran, Y. & Shimko, T. (1991) The role of injury discharge in the induction of neuropathic pain behavior in rats. *Pain* 46, 327–36.

Shasteen, S. P. & Sheehan, R. J. (1997) Laboratory evaluation of artificial swim bladder deflation in largemouth bass: potential benefits for catch-and-release fisheries. *North American Journal of Fisheries Management* 17, 32–7.

Sheridan, J. F., Stark, J. L., Avitsur, R. & Padgett, D. A. (2000) Social disruption, immunity, and susceptibility to viral infection. *Annals of the New York Academy of Sciences* 917, 894–905.

Sherman, R. A., Sherman, C. J. & Parker, L. (1984) Chronic phantom and stump pain among American Veterans: results of a survey. *Pain* 18, 83–95.

Shields, B. A., Engelman, R. W., Fukaura, Y., Good, R. A. & Day, N. K. (1991) Caloric restriction suppresses subgenomic mink cytopathic focus-forming murine leukemia virus transcription and frequency of genomic expression while impairing lymphoma formation. *Proceedings of the National Academy of Sciences* 88, 11 138–42.

Shutt, D. A., Fell, L. R., Connell, R., Bell, A. K., Wallace, C. A. & Smith, A. I. (1987) Stress-induced changes in plasma concentrations of immunoreactive β-endorphin and cortisol in response to routine surgical procedures in lambs. *Australian Journal of Biological Sciences* 40, 97–103.

Simonsen, H. B., Klinken, L. & Bindseil, E. (1991) Histopathology of intact and docked pig tails. *British Veterinary Journal* 147, 407–12.

Simpson, J. A. (1963) Current neurophysiological concepts of spinal cord injuries. In: *Spinal Injuries. Proceedings of a Symposium held in the Royal College of Surgeons of Edinburgh*, pp. 10–15. Morrison and Gibb Ltd, London.

Skolnick, P., Ninan, P., Insel, T., Crawley, J. & Paul, S. (1984) A novel chemically-induced animal model of human anxiety. *Psychopathology* 17 suppl. 1, 25–36.

Skuse, D. H. (2000) Behavioural neuroscience and child psychopathology: insights from model systems. *Journal of Child Psychology and Psychiatry* 41, 3–31.

Smith, A. U. (1958) The resistance of animals to cooling and freezing. *Biological Reviews* 33, 197–253.

Smith, A. U. (1959) Viability of supercooled and frozen mammals. *Annals of the New York Academy of Sciences* 80, 291–300.

Smith, E. N., Johnson, C. & Martin, K. J. (1981) Fear bradycardia in captive eastern chipmunk, *Tamias striatus. Comparative Biochemistry and Physiology* 70A, 529–32.

Spatz, H. (1950) Brain injuries in aviation. In: *German Aviation Medicine, World War 2*, pp. 616–40. Department of the Air Force, Washington.

Stafford, K. J. & Mellor, D. J. (1993) Castration, tail docking and dehorning – what are the constraints? *Proceedings of the New Zealand Society of Animal Production* 53, 189–94.

Standfast, H. A. & Dyce, A. L. (1968) Attacks on cattle by mosquitoes and biting midges. *Australian Veterinary Journal* 44, 585–6.

Starec, M., Mráz, M., Zídek, Z. *et al.* (1994) Genetic differences in immunomodulation, behavior, and stress-induced organ lesions. *Annals of the New York Academy of Sciences* 741, 252–62.

Steckler, T. & Holsboer, F. (1999) Corticotropin-releasing hormone receptor subtypes and emotion. *Biological Psychiatry* 46, 1480–508.

Steel, J. D. (1969) Abnormalities of gait in the racehorse, referred to as tying-up syndromes. *Australian Veterinary Journal* 45, 162–5.

Stephens, T. (1975) Nutrition of orphan marsupials. *Australian Veterinary Journal* 51, 453–8.

Stermer, R. A., Brasington, C. F., Coppock, C. E., Lanham, J. K. & Milam, K. Z. (1986) Effect of drinking water temperature on heat stress of dairy cows. *Journal of Dairy Science* 69, 546–51.

Sternbach, R. A. (1968) *Pain. A Psychophysiological Analysis.* Academic Press, New York.

Stevenson, J., Batten, N. & Cherner, M. (1992) Fears and fearfulness in children and adolescents: a genetic analysis of twin data. *Journal of Child Psychology and Psychiatry* 33, 977–85.

Stewart, O. W., Russel, C. K. & Cone, W. V. (1941) Injury to the central nervous system by blast. *Lancet* **1941** i, 172–4.

Strejffert, G. (1992) Report on tail injuries in Shorthaired German Pointer dogs born in Sweden 1989. *MS penes me.*

Sulman, F. G., Pfeifer, Y. & Superstine, E. (1977) The adrenal exhaustion syndrome: an adrenal deficiency. *Annals of the New York Academy of Sciences* 301, 918–30.

Sutherland, M. A., Mellor, D. J., Stafford, K. J. *et al.* (1999) Acute cortisol responses of lambs to ring castration and docking after the injection of lignocaine into the scrotal neck or testes at the time of ring placement. *Australian Veterinary Journal* 77, 738–41.

Sutherland, M. A., Mellor, D. J., Stafford, K. J. *et al.* (2002) Effect of local anaesthetic combined with wound cauterisation on the cortisol response to dehorning in calves. *Australian Veterinary Journal* 80, 36–8.

Sutherland, S. P., Cook, S. P. & McClesky, E. W. (2000) Chemical mediators of pain due to tissue damage and ischemia. *Progress in Brain Research* 129, 21–38.

Taddio, A., Katz, J., Ilerisch, A. L. & Koren, G. (1997) Effect of neonatal circumcision on pain response during subsequent routine vaccination. *Lancet* ii, 599–603.

Takahashi, S., Fang, J., Kapás, L., Wang, Y. & Kreuger, J. M. (1997) Inhibition of brain interleukin-1 attenuates sleep rebound after sleep deprivation in rabbits. *American Journal of Physiology* 273, R677–R682.

Tavin, G. & Prata, R. G. (1980) Lumbrosacral stenosis in dogs. *Journal of the American Veterinary Medical Association* **177**, 154–9.

Taylor, M. J. & White, K. R. (1997) Response: trout mortality from baited barbed and barbless hooks. *North American Journal of Fisheries Management* **17**, 808–809.

Thornton, P. D. & Waterman-Pearson, A. E. (1999) Quantification of the pain and distress responses to castration in young lambs. *Research in Veterinary Science* **66**, 107–18.

Tigner, J. R. & Larson, G. E. (1977) Sheep losses on selected ranches in southern Wyoming. *Journal of Range Management* **30**, 244–52.

Toth, L. A. & Kreuger, J. M. (1988) Alteration of sleep in rabbits by *Staphylococcus aureus* infection. *Infection and Immunity* **56**, 1785–91.

Turner, S. W. & Hough, A. (1993) Hyperventilation as a reaction to torture. In: *International Handbook of Traumatic Stress Syndromes* (eds J. P. Wilson & B. Raphael), pp. 725–32. Plenum Press, New York.

Tyler, D. B. & Bard, P. (1949) Motion sickness. *Physiological Reviews* **29**, 311–69.

Ungley, C. C. & Blackwood, W. (1942) Peripheral vasoneuropathy after chilling. 'Immersion foot and immersion hand'. *Lancet* **ii**, 447–51.

Valentino, R. J., Curtis, A. L., Page, M. E. *et al.* (1998) The locus coeruleus – noradrenergic system as an integrator of stress responses. *Progress in Psychobiology and Physiological Psychology* **17**, 91–126.

Vallée, M., Mayo, W., Dellu, F., Le Moal, M., Simon, H. & Maccari, S. (1997) Prenatal stress induces high anxiety and postnatal handling induces low anxiety in adult offspring: correlation with stress-induced corticosterone secretion. *Journal of Neuroscience* **17**, 2626–36.

Van Ballenberghe, V. (1984) Injuries to wolves sustained during live-capture. *Journal of Wildlife Management* **48**, 1425–9.

Vandegraaff, R. (1976) Squamous-cell carcinoma of the vulva in Merino sheep. *Australian Veterinary Journal* **52**, 21–3.

Vaughan, L. C. (1969) Locomotory disturbance in pigs. *British Veterinary Journal* **125**, 354–65.

Vecchiotti, G. G. & Galanti, R. (1986) Evidence of heredity of cribbing, weaving and stall-walking in thoroughbred horses. *Livestock Production Sciences* **14**, 91–5.

Verstraete, F. J. M., van Aarde, R. J., Nieuwoudt, B. A., Mauer, E. & Kass, P. H. (1996) The dental pathology of feral cats on Marion Island, Part II: periodontitis, external odontoclastic resorption lesions and mandibular thickening. *Journal of Comparative Pathology* **115**, 283–97.

Vestweber, J. G. E. & Al-Ani, F. K. (1985) Venous blood pressure relative to the development of bovine udder edema. *American Journal of Veterinary Research* **46**, 157–9.

Vos, J. G., Dybing, E., Grein, H. A. *et al.* (2000) Health effects of endocrine-disrupting chemicals on wildlife, with special reference to the European situation. *Critical Reviews in Toxicology* **30**, 71–133.

Wall, P. D., Devor, M., Inbal, R. *et al.* (1979) Autotomy following peripheral nerve lesions: experimental anaesthesia dolorosa. *Pain* **7**, 103–13.

Wall, P. D., Waxman, S. & Basbaum, A. I. (1974) Ongoing activity in peripheral nerve injury discharge. *Experimental Neurology* **45**, 576–89.

Warburton, B. (1992) Victor foot-hold traps for catching Australian brushtail possums in New Zealand: capture efficiency and injuries. *Wildlife Society Bulletin* **20**, 67–73.

Warburton, B., Gregory, N. & Bunce, M. (1999) Stress response of Australian brushtail possums captured in foothold and cage traps. In: *Mammal Trapping* (ed. G. Proulx), pp. 53–66. Alpha Wildlife Research & Management Ltd, Alberta, Canada.

Warburton, B., Gregory, N. G. & Morriss, G. (2000) Effect of jaw shape in kill-traps on time to loss of palpebral reflexes in brushtail possums. *Journal of Wildlife Diseases* **36**, 92–6.

Watts, J. E. & Marchant, R. S. (1977) The effects of diarrhoea, tail length and sex on the incidence of breech strike in modified mulesed Merino sheep. *Australian Veterinary Journal* **53**, 118–23.

Weis, E. B., Pritz, H. B. & Hassler, C. R. (1983) Experimental automobile–pedestrian injuries. *Journal of Trauma* **17**, 823–8.

White, P. J., Kreeger, T. J., Seal, U. S. & Tester, J. R. (1991) Pathological responses of red foxes to capture in box traps. *Journal of Wildlife Management* **55**, 75–80.

White, R. G., DeShazer, J. A., Tressler, C. J. *et al.* (1995) Vocalization and physiological response of pigs during castration with or without a local anesthetic. *Journal of Animal Science* **73**, 381–6.

Wiepkema, P. R., van Hellemond, K. K., Roessingh, P. & Romberg, H. (1987) Behaviour and abomasal damage in individual veal calves. *Applied Animal Behaviour Science* **18**, 257–68.

Wiggers, C. J. (1918) The initial and progressive stages of circulatory failure in abdominal shock. *American Journal of Physiology* **45**, 485–99.

Willner, P. (1984) The validity of animal models of depression. *Psychopharmacology* **83**, 1–16.

Willson, R. L. (1966) Assessment of bush fire damage to stock. *Australian Veterinary Journal* **42**, 101–103, 328–9.

Wilmore, D. W., Mason, A. D., Johnson, D. W. & Pruitt, B. A. (1975) Effect of ambient temperature on heat production and heat loss in burn patients. *Journal of Applied Physiology* **38**, 593–7.

Wittenburg, N. & Baumeister, R. (1999) Thermal avoidance in *Caenorhabditis elegans*: an approach to the study of nociception. *Proceedings of the National Academy of Science* **96**, 10477–82.

Witting, N., Svensson, P., Arendt-Nielsen, L. & Jensen, T. S. (1998) Differential effect of painful heterotropic stimulation on capsaicin-induced pain and allodynia. *Brain Research* **801**, 206–10.

Wolff, H. G. & Forbes, H. S. (1928) The cerebral circulation. V. Observations of the pial circulation during changes in intracranial pressure. *Archives of Neurology and Psychiatry* **20**, 1035–47.

Wood-Gush, D. G. M. (1973) Animal welfare in modern agriculture. *British Veterinary Journal* **129**, 167–74.

Woods, A., Smith, C., Szewczak, M., Dunn, R. W., Cornfeldt, M. & Corbett, R. (1993) Selective serotonin re-uptake inhibitors decrease schedule-induced polydipsia in rats: a potential model for obsessive compulsive disorder. *Psychopharmacology* **112**, 195–8.

Woolf, C. J. & Walters, E. T. (1991) Common patterns of plasticity contributing to nociceptive sensitisation in mammals and *Aplysia. Trends in Neuroscience* **14**, 74–8.

Wythes, J. R., Horder, J. C., Lapworth, J. W. & Cheffins, R. C. (1979) Effect of tipped horns on cattle bruising. *Veterinary Record* **104**, 390–92.

Yagil, R., Etzion, Z. & Oren, A. (1983) The physiology of drowning. *Comparative Biochemistry and Physiology* **74A**, 189–93.

Yellowlees, P. M., Alpers, J. H., Bowden, J. J., Bryant, G. D. & Ruffin, R. E. (1987) Psychiatric morbidity in patients with chronic airflow obstruction. *Medical Journal of Australia* **146**, 305–307.

Young, M. D. & Delforce, R. J. (1986) Licensed kangaroo shooting in New South Wales: the people, the money they make and the animals they shoot. *Australian Rangeland Journal* **8**, 36–45.

Zouboulis, C. C. (1998) Cryosurgery in dermatology. *European Journal of Dermatology* **8**, 466–74.

Zuckerman, S. (1940) Experimental study of blast injuries to the lungs. *Lancet* **ii**, 219–24.

Abbreviations

ACE   angiotensin converting enzyme
ACTH   adrenocorticotropic hormone
ATP   adenosine triphosphate
AVMA   American Veterinary Medical Association
CD4$^+$ cluster designation 4$^+$
CGRP   calcitonin gene-related peptide
CNS   central nervous system
CREB   cyclic AMP-responsive element-binding protein
CRH   corticotrophin releasing hormone
CSF   cerebrospinal fluid
CTR   competitive trial ride
dB   decibels
DDT   dichloro-diphenyl-trichloroethane
DIC   disseminated intravascular coagulation
DNIC   diffuse nociceptive inhibitory control
ECG   electrocardiogram
EEG   electroencephalogram
EMG   electromyogram
ER   endurance ride
FFA   free fatty acid
FSH   follicle stimulating hormone
GC-CSF   granulocyte colony stimulating factor
GM-CSF   granulocyte-macrophage colony stimulating factor
H$_1$ histamine$_1$
h^2 heritability coefficient
5-HIAA   5-hydroxyindoleacetic acid
HPA   hypothalamic–pituitary–adrenal axis
5-HT   5-hydroxytryptamine
IAP   intra-abdominal pressure
IFN   interferon
IL   interleukin

kcal   kilocalories
LC   locus coeruleus
LCT   lower critical temperature
LH   luteinizing hormone
LPS   lipopolysaccharide
LTP   long-term potentiation
MAO$_A$ monoamine oxidase type A
MSH   melanocyte stimulating hormone
NGF   nerve growth factor
NIC   nociceptive inhibitory control
NK   natural killer
NMDA   N-methyl-D-aspartate
NREM   non-rapid eye movement
OCD   obsessive compulsive disorder
PAG   periaqueductal grey
p$_a$CO$_2$ arterial carbon dioxide tension
PGE$_2$ prostaglandin E$_2$
p$_a$O$_2$ arterial oxygen tension
POA   pre-optic area
PTSD   post-traumatic stress disorder
REM   rapid eye movement
RVM   rostral ventromedial medulla
SEW   segregated early weaning
sGGT   serum gamma glutamyl transferase
SIA   stress-induced analgesia
SNS   sympathetic nervous system
TGF   transforming growth factor
Th   T-helper
TNF   tumour necrosis factor
VIP   vasoactive intestinal peptide

Index

Page numbers in *italics* refer to figures, those in **bold** to tables.

Printed and bound by CPI Group (UK) Ltd, Croydon, CR0 4YY

18/03/2025

14642005-0001